Godiva Books

The Moon over Matsushima

Insights into Moxa and Mugwort

"This is a unique book. It brings together kn‹ focus on the practice of moxa.

"It takes us through a breathtaking vista of i keeps down-to-earth practice front and cente expand our knowledge of this traditional therapy readable way and stuffs the book with practical information.

"The treatment list at the end is the most comprehensive I have yet come across."

Professor Stephen Birch PhD
Associate Professor, University College of Health Sciences
– Campus Kristiania, Oslo, Norway
Acupuncturist, Author and Researcher

"No one has spent as much time thinking about moxa in so many different contexts as Merlin Young.

"If you are interested in the history, and in the clinical potential of Moxibustion, you will find the "the Moon over Matsushima" a fascinating read, and you will understand moxa in a new light."

Charles ("Chip") Chace
Acupuncturist and Author, Boulder, Colorado
– published extensively on
the application of pre-modern Chinese medical ideas
in modern clinical practice in the West

"Meticulously researched, timely and thought-provoking.

"Part historical epic in the spirit of Simon Winchester, part scientific inquiry, part call to action, this book is both a salient work and a must-read for any acupuncturist and moxibustion practitioner."

Todd Howard DTCM
President and Founder of the Pacific Rim College
Victoria, British Columbia, Canada
and Director of its Global Outreach Program

The Moon over Matsushima

Insights into Moxa and Mugwort

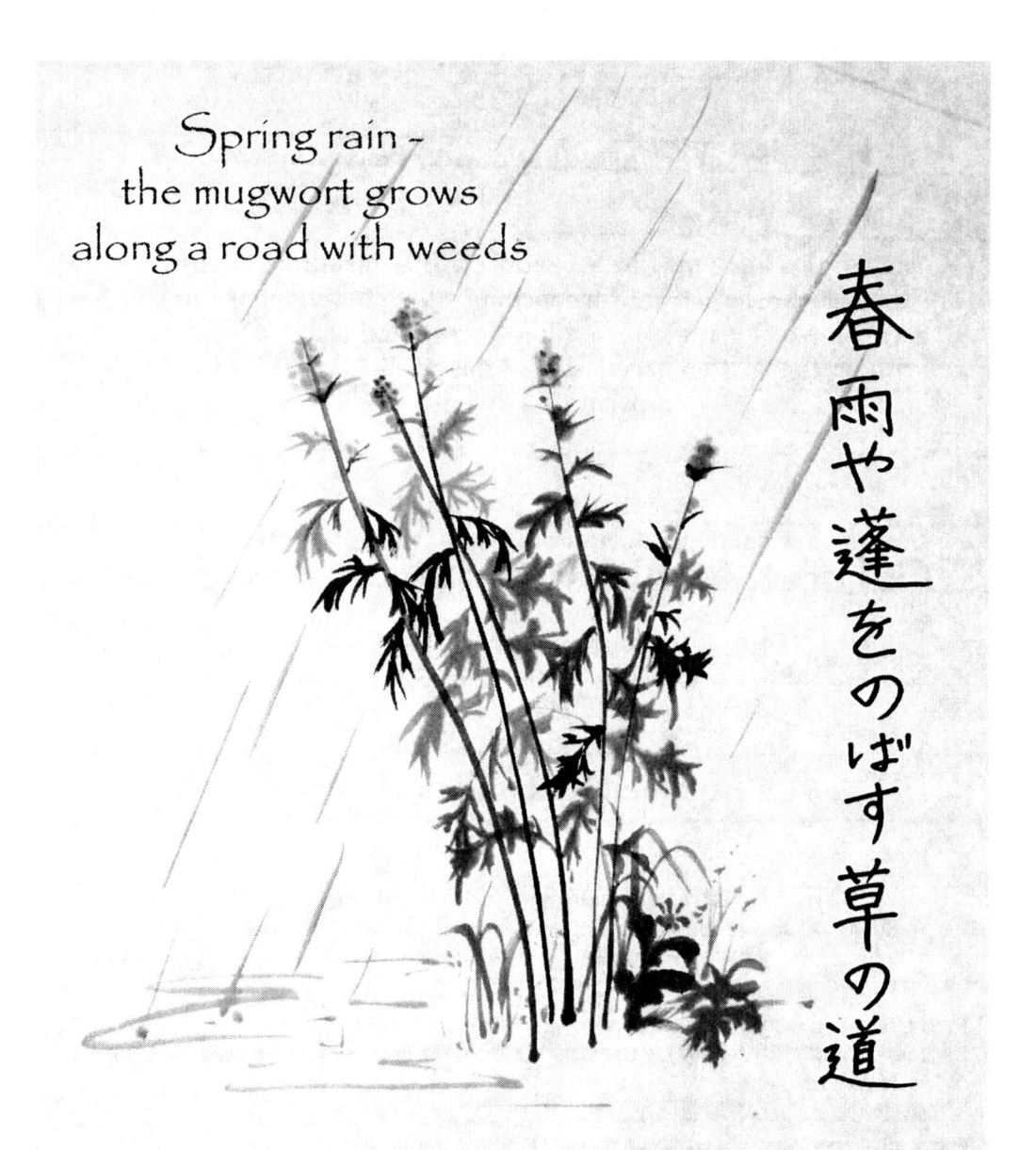

Spring rain –
the mugwort grows
along a road with weeds

春雨や蓬をのばす草の道

a poem by Matsuo Bashō
1694

All rights reserved

Copyright © 2012 Merlin Young

No part of this book may be reproduced or transmitted in any form or by any means, electronic or mechanical, including photocopying, recording or by any information storage and retrieval system, without the written permission of the publisher, except where permitted by law.

For further information e-mail the author at:
godivabooks@gmail.com or visit: http://godivabooks.com/

ISBN: 978 - 0 - 956633262

Published by Godiva Books

Printed in the United Kingdom
(using FSC accredited paper originally sourced from sustainable forests)

Front Cover: woodblock "Moonrise at Futago Island", Matsushima, 1933 by Kawase Hasui (1883-1957) – used with kind permission of the Tokyo Museum of Modern Art.

Back cover: Copy of Li Tang's Song Dynasty painting of moxa being burnt on a patient's back. Copy painting by Yoshio Manaka and used with the kind permission of Morinomiya College of Medical Arts and Sciences' Museum of Traditional Medicine (*Hari Kyu* Museum).

Frontispiece: watercolour painting of mugwort in the rain by Jenny Craig with calligraphy of Bashō's haiku about mugwort by Yuki Itaya.

Cover design: Olaf Waltmann.

In memory of Frank at Lyantonde…

and in hope for Kenneth

..and dedicated to Allen, Magdalene and Achiro in Uganda;

and to Thoko, Margaret, Zandile, Nyameka and the rest of the team in South Africa

Table of Contents

Foreword (by Lorraine Wilcox) i
Preface – the Smoke and the Glow iii
Acknowledgements xi
Time Chart xii

Part 1 – the Roots

Moxibustion's Relationship with Acupuncture 1
Tomb Findings 2
Early Channel/Vessel Theory 6
Evolving Medical Knowledge at the Time of the Han 11
The Origins of the Chinese Character *jiu* 灸 19
The Word "Moxa" and the Dutch East India Company 21
Moxa arrives in Europe 30
The earlier Portuguese Reports 33
A Diversion into the "Greek" Connections 35
The Importance of the Silk Trade 36
Early Trading across Central Asia and the Persian Empire 37
Ancient China and its Furthermost Western Reaches 41
The Nomadic Peoples of Central Asia 45
The Tinder Fungus 46
The Trade of Jade 48
The *Yuezhi* 49
The Mummies of Central Asia 54
 "Mister White" 55
Further Thoughts on the Origin of the Word "moxa" 57
The Ultimate Origins of Moxibustion 60

The Development of *jingluo* Channel Theory 62

Mugwort and Moxibustion – the Very Earliest References 63

The History of Moxibustion through the Centuries 66

The Role of Technology 70

Moxibustion in other Early Texts 72

Acumoxa in Japan 77

Later Chinese Texts 79

More Current Use of Moxa 80

Part 2 – the Stalk

The Nature of Mugwort 85

Mugwort Processing for Moxa 90

The Arcana of Mugwort 93

Mugwort's Chemistry 101

Part 3 – the Branches

Tonification and Dispersion in the Classical Texts 105

The Business of Tubes 115

Heat Perception Moxa (*chinetsukyu*) Technique 118

Direct and Indirect Techniques 123

Indirect Moxa with the Moxa Pole and Tonification and Dispersion 123

Indirect moxa on Intermediary Materials 124

Indirect Moxa-on-the-Needle-Head Technique 127

One other Indirect Method 128

"Stick-on" Proprietary Moxa 129

Undifferentiated Moxa Treatment 130

Moxa-only Treatment Protocols from China 132

Longevity and Moxibustion 135
Moxa and Home Treatment 138
Stomach 36, Bladder 43, Ren 8, the Four Flowers, Suffering Gate, Sp17 and Ren4 140
The Possible Nature of these "Moxa" Points 151
Warming Moxibustion 153
Moxa and the Divergent Channels 154
Moxa and the Muscle/Sinew Channels 158
Moxa and the Akabane Balancing Protocol 164
Moxa and Koryo Sooji Chim Hand Microsystem 167
Moxa and Needling Combined 174

Part 4 – the Stems

The Actions of Moxibustion 179
Moxibustion and White Blood Cell Count 183
Wei Qi and the Immune System 188
Moxibustion and Tuberculosis 196
Auto-immune Disorder 199
Moxibustion and the Immune Response – the Research Evidence 201
Professor Abo's Theories of Immune Response and its Implications 206
Animal Research 210
Immune Response and Specific Acupoints 211
Moxa and Temperature 214
Moxa on Skin 222
Body Temperature and Immune Function 223
What happens in the skin when it heats up and burns? 225
The Additional Impact of Chemical Components on Immune Response 227
Smokey versus Smokeless 232

The Possible Mechanisms with Indirect Techniques 235

Moxa and the Channel Pathways (or Photonic Release) 242

Direct Moxibustion – Dosage and the Issue of Scars and Blisters 243

Alternative Views on the Necessity of Blistering 246

Moxafrica's Very First Patient 248

Contra-indications around Heat and Hypertension 252

Moxa in Needle-Shock 256

Moxa and Warts 256

Moxa with Breech Presentation – and also in Pregnancy 257

Some Conclusions 261

Part 5 – the Leaves

So Finally 263

Moxa and the Problems of Modern Research 266

Final Conclusions 278

Postcript (the Seed): – page 1 of the Story of Moxafrica 283

Appendix 1   – Preparing and applying small moxa cones 285

                      – Clinical Treatments 289

                      – Locations for the Extra Points 323

Appendix 2   – A selective list of research papers particularly relating to immune response 327

Appendix 3   – Resources 331

Further Reading 332

Index 335

A few things about the author 342

A List of Maps

Map showing the full extent of the Han Empire………………………………………..6

Map showing VOC sailing routes to Batavia …………………………………..25

Map of trading routes between Batavia, Vietnam, and Japan……………..……..…..21

Map showing the proximity of Kos to the mainland of Asia Minor…….…..……..39

Map of the Persian Empire c. 500BC……………………………………………40

Map of the Tarim Basin…………………………………………………...………43

Map of the Kushan Empire………………………………………………..…52

Map of China showing favoured locations for mugwort for moxa…………..………87

Map of Japan showing favoured locations for mugwort for moxa……………..……..88

Foreword (by Lorraine Wilcox PhD)

You are a lucky reader; you are about to embark on a marvellous quest! What are the secrets of mugwort and moxibustion? This book will be your guide.

Reading the first two parts of *The Moon over Matsushima*, I feel as if I am sitting in a teashop sipping tea with an old friend who has just returned from a journey through time and space. I listen with wonder to the customs and habits of people throughout the world in regard to the miraculous herb, mugwort, and its many uses. The images are described so vividly that they fill my mind. I am grateful to undertake this journey by listening or reading; there is no need to pad my own shoes with mugwort to dispel the fatigue of the road, there is no need to carry talismans of mugwort in my clothes to ward off the dangers of the journey.

In the next section, I sit at the feet of my teacher and listen to his instruction on the mechanisms of moxibustion according to the theories of East Asian medicine, especially the medicine of Japan. I am the apprentice, trying to absorb a deeper understanding of this marvellous healing technique. I know this deepening will enable me to practice this medical art in a more profound way.

Finally, in the last two parts, I enter the world of modern medicine, clinical trials, and the laboratory. Here I see Western medicine attempting to understand the complexity of moxibustion and how it may heal patients. Is it the heat? The smoke? The tar? Which part of the immune system does moxibustion boost? Which diseases can it remedy? These questions are not yet resolved, but I am presented with intriguing clues and sharp analysis. I can also now see clearly how difficult it is to analyze holistic medicine through reductionist thought. Yet this is the challenge we face in the 21st century if we want to bring traditional medicine into the mainstream.

Throughout all of this, Merlin Young acts as our tour guide. He is a gracious host, friendly and eloquent. Beyond this, he knows the power of moxibustion as his life has led him to treat serious diseases with this ancient form of medicine. Many modern practitioners are only comfortable treating pain, gynaecological disorders, digestive problems and so forth in a modern relatively urban environment. While this is also good work, Merlin Young (along with Jenny Craig) has had the audacity and vision to use ancient methods to treat tuberculosis in underdeveloped countries, just as people did in ancient times. Preliminary reports suggest that moxibustion may have a powerful effect. If so, this is a great boon for the sufferer and a dramatic indication of the power of the humble mugwort plant.

Lorraine Wilcox Los Angeles, California. March 5th, 2012.
The 13th day of the second lunar month of the Ren Chen year
On the day of the Awakening of Insects (驚蟄 Jing Zhe)

The Moon over Matsushima

Preface

Asama yori
Hiroki kiburu wa
Ibuki-yama

MORE WIDELY SMOKING
THAN ASAMA VOLCANO
IS MOUNT IBUKI[1]

What I learnt about moxibustion when first studying acupuncture, frankly, wasn't all that much. It was very positively identified as a powerful and even essential part of our therapeutic toolbox, but no particular focus was directed towards it and the information provided lacked any real authority. We were told that moxa was "tonifying"; that it counteracts cold and damp; that it nourishes *yang*; that it's good for chronic disease and could and should be used prolifically during the winter. We were also told that its use was "10,000 years old" (which I assume now to mean of some indeterminate vintage), and that it is made from mugwort (*Artemisiavulgaris latiflora*), a plant which somehow becomes suffused with the pure *yang* power of the sun. We were proscribed from using it with hot or inflamed conditions, told never to use it with patients with high blood pressure, and also told not to use it in pregnancy. There was also some confusion in what was presented regarding what are referred to as direct and indirect techniques. I suspect that these were the sorts of things that many of us trainee acupuncturists heard wherever we may have trained, or maybe I just wasn't paying such good attention that day – or maybe two days...

So what is moxa or moxibustion? Basically it is the burning, or smouldering, of a herb over the skin. It's a traditional treatment, used in China, Japan, Korea, Vietnam, Tibet, Nepal and Mongolia, though actually not always with the same material, and certainly not in identical ways. This "smouldering" can be roughly broken down into two simple categories, and they can be reasonably described as follows: "**indirect moxa**" – on the handles of inserted acupuncture needles, or by waving a cigar-shaped stick of the stuff over the skin, or by using intermediary materials between the "nap" (the refined processed herb) and the skin, or by burning it in special "boxes" or even in bowls; and "**direct moxa**" – by careful smouldering on the skin itself to heat points or even deliberately blister the

---

[1] This poem in its original Japanese is an ironic *senryu* poem in *haiku* format. I have taken the liberty of translating it literally into a *haiku* format in English. Mount Asama is Japan's Central Island's largest currently active volcano. Mount Ibuki, as we will see, is a traditional locational source of prime mugwort for moxibustion.

skin[2]. Most often the herb used is mugwort, although, as we shall see, this is not actually always the case.

Perhaps this smokey/smouldering therapy all comes over as a little too bizarre and primitive for the evidence-based brigade, something which might help explain how its use has pretty much escaped their scientific investigations to date, at least in the West. It might also explain why it has hardly been highlighted by those who write the majority of the books on acumoxa which appear in the English language. By the standards of high-tech medicine it does most certainly appear both primitive and strangely foreign compared to a modern medical technique, but then so does the use of maggots on suppurative wounds, a practice which has recently been re-introduced within a specific niche of modern medicine. I am hoping that the contents of this book might promote the value of re-examining this curious practice in the light of some of the challenges which not only face the modern acumoxa practitioner, but which also face the whole of medicine and mankind.

Something which is pretty indisputable is that currently, with some notable exceptions, moxibustion plays a secondary supportive role to acupuncture, if or when it plays any role at all. This is not just true now, but it has generally been true throughout the larger part of the story of traditional East Asian medicine. Part of what follows is an attempt to find out whether it really deserves this "poor relative" status, as well as to review how and why it came to play this subordinate role.

More than a cursory investigation into moxibustion reveals that its use today is fraught with misunderstandings. Some of the dogma as taught to trainee acupuncturists (at least in my case) is very clearly challengeable, if not actually flawed. As a result what follows is also an attempt to tease out these conceptions or misconceptions, and to investigate just how much better use this therapy might be put to in the modern acupuncture clinic.

Few specialist books have been written in English to date on the subject of moxa, so this work is most definitely also an attempt to fill a gap. Generally, moxibustion claims space in the form of no more than a few references in most books on acumoxa. Two earlier publications, both of them creditworthy and still of interest to the general acumoxa practitioner, are now unfortunately out of print (which hopefully does not bode ill for this current work). These were Royston Low and Roger Newman Turner's "Moxibustion, its Principles and Practice" and Sung Baek's "Classical Moxibustion Skills in Contemporary Clinical Practice". So, unless the modern student has access to a good second-hand book shop or a library at their acupuncture school which manages to retain its books, he or she will find little around on the subject.

---

[2] This distinction is not quite as simple as it initially appears, as will be discussed in Part 3 the Branches.

Whilst in the process of preparing this current work, however, a landmark publication appeared in the form of Lorraine Wilcox's "Moxibustion, the Power of Mugwort Fire". This book stands head and shoulders above anything previously published on the subject, and truly provides a treasure trove of scholarly research for the student of the history of East Asian medicine, let alone of acumoxa. Its focus, however, is (relatively speaking) confined to one period in one country (Ming Dynasty China) which Lorraine quite rightly views as a golden age of moxibustion practice. Moxa techniques from this era, however, are generally impossible to replicate today for reasons of modern standards of practice relating to patient safety, so, whilst the writings of these Ming masters undeniably ring out loud and clear across the centuries and call for a proper re-examination of this therapy, they unfortunately also present real difficulties for us to meaningfully replicate in our treatment rooms. So I felt happy to continue to pursue my labours believing that I might helpfully still fill this gap.

But Lorraine did it again, well before this book was finished, publishing a second book entitled "Moxibustion: a Modern Clinical Handbook" – and with this she has given us a classic modern English-language moxibustion textbook. Meticulously researched and clearly presented, she offers us practical interpretations of the therapy, with many applications skillfully extrapolated directly from the pages of her first book.

As a result I began to wonder whether it was worth completing what I had started! I realised over time, however, that I might still have further perspectives to offer which might enrich the subject for anyone interested enough to examine them – perspectives which come from picking up alternative clues as to how best we might try and put this all together today. I think that some of these clues may not have been of such immediate interest to Lorraine with her skills and focus directed on the historical Chinese perspectives – and I am hoping that developing them within the pages of this book might help make even more compelling sense of this beguiling therapy. I suspect that some of them have particularly revealed themselves to me because of my own exposure to moxibustion from the perspective of Japanese traditions rather than from Chinese ones. If, however, it feels that at times in the following pages I have crossed too far into the territory that has been so well staked out by Lorraine herself, it was far from my intention; in order to offer something that can stand alone in its own right, however, I have simply had to accept this risk.

The book is split into five main parts, exploring firstly moxibustion's origins and history ("the Roots"), secondly the properties of mugwort ("the Stalk"), thirdly some clinical applications ("the Branches"), and the next its possible mechanisms and potentials ("the Stems"). A fifth part attempts to tie a few of the various themes together ("the Leaves") and offers one or two further provocative ideas. By approaching the subject in this way, I hope to provide a comprehensive source of study for any serious student of acumoxa, and as importantly to provoke argument, ideas and possible inspiration in the minds of creative practitioners. I have also taken the occasional liberty of challenging some of the assumptions which may be burdening or bedevilling contemporary understandings of this treatment.

My intention has been to collate as much information as might be of relevance to a modern practitioner as possible, particularly since so much of it is not that widely available. This inevitably results in inconsistencies and contradictions, something which is typical of any honest examination of traditional East Asian medicine. In such instances, and indeed in many others, I have attempted to weigh up some of the possibilities inherent in each viewpoint, and have also tried to make some kind of general sense of these by subsequent "discussion" in light of my own personal experiences and also more generally in the light of simple clinical reality. In some instances, I have even been rash enough to invent some contradictions of my own and attempt to evaluate them as well.

Lorraine, in "Mugwort Fire" helpfully quotes Wang Zhizhong (who in 1220 wrote the "Classic of Nourishing Life with Acupuncture and Moxibustion"). Wang enigmatically summed up such contradictions as follows: "You cannot be tied down with one theory without also knowing that surely there is another theory". This insight lies at the heart of any general appreciation of East Asian medicine particularly when reviewed across the centuries, and absorbing the spirit of Wang's idea should serve to enrich our appreciation of the subject we study as much as it might simultaneously trouble our Western mind sets. Whilst I must take full responsibility for any errors in this text, I can at least hide behind Wang's wisdom in excusing myself for making some of them. In fact it is omissions that I am much more conscious of, and I'm sure that there are many.

The early history of East Asian medicine really offers us today something of a paint-by-numbers picture, with large areas still remaining white, incomplete and unnumbered. It is also quite fair to suggest that some of the colours that have been added to this canvas by scholars across the centuries may not have been done with much more than very well-educated guesswork, and it is even possible that some of these may even have been applied mistakenly. As a result, the true image of the traditions which present themselves to us today is far less coherent or complete than many of us may wish or believe it to be – in fact it may even in certain instances be not at all what the original artists in the distant past were intent on presenting to their contemporaries. We are sometimes inclined to look back at the history of acumoxa through rosier spectacles than are appropriate.

As the reader will quickly realise, I have taken the liberty of painting in a few paint-by-numbers colours of my own, sometimes even having the temerity to do so over existing ones, and I am well aware that I have sometimes done so based on my own set of prejudices. Some of these areas I have even deliberately and quite consciously painted over in white for reasons which will become clearer towards the end of Part 1 the Roots. I am also well aware that I have used both brush and palette at times a little too liberally for more scholarly tastes, but I have done so quite deliberately in order to attempt to transport the reader's imagination in consideration of this ever-evolving therapy whose true story has unquestionably been lost in the mists of time and place. Such colourful diversions include personal and tentative speculation, but they also contain ideas which are deliberately intended to bring the subject more alive, even if the reader sometimes might find him or herself at odds with some of them. These flights of imagination (which on occasion they unapologetically are) touch down in unexpected places, and amongst unlikely people and things – luminaries from ancient Greece, Jesuit monks, the steppes of Central Asia, Dutch venture capitalists, mummies separated by thousands of miles and thousands of years in Egypt, China and Austria, an erotic novel and even in apocalyptic events of the nuclear age. Most of these connections are highly tentative. My intention is to provide food for thought and to offer up a territory of possibility; to add, not just colour, but also taste and smell to parts of the study which might otherwise prove difficult to digest. Too many times, in my opinion, important discourses on the history of our medicine are presented too drily to be digested by the average reader and the profession is rendered poorer in its understanding of itself as a result.

In one sense this study is inspired by Stephen Birch's and Robert Felt's "Understanding Acupuncture". This work did an extraordinary job in terms of gathering together many different therapeutic perspectives on acupuncture whilst still relating them to its philosophical, contextual and historical roots. As a text on acupuncture practice, it stands tall in its field, perhaps taller than any other text in the English language. It was tempting to consider using "Understanding Moxibustion" as my working title as a result, but I am increasingly convinced that there is too little about moxibustion that we actually *do* yet comprehensively understand, so it would have been a dishonest title. "An Attempt at Understanding Moxibustion" might perhaps have been more honest, but as a title it plainly has little going for it. I have ultimately resorted to a more enigmatic one, "The Moon over Matsushima". It is one which metaphorically reflects a moment in a master poet's journey of life when he was preparing to set out on a long and dangerous journey to an iconic destination with a vision of what he might encounter on his arrival. Better sense of this will be found in Part 3 and at the end of Part 5. The title reflects the idea that we may be only at the very beginning of a decent understanding of this therapy, whilst offering an enigmatic glimpse of what such an understanding ultimately might imply.

The title also hints at the fact that there has been a personal journey unravelling behind this study, and that it too has yet to reach its destination. Working on this book unexpectedly gave spontaneous birth to a compellingly bothersome idea or vision of its own. It was something which materialised of its own will into something truly daunting - the MoxafricaProject – co-delivered into some measure of reality with the help of my valued and trusted friend and colleague Jenny Craig, and through the efforts of our new-found friends in Uganda and South Africa. Jenny, it should be well noted, also deserves more than a little credit for some important parts of this work, as well as for providing some of the beautiful artwork.

In truth, the book that you hold in your hand actually started life as a modest essay on moxibustion, prepared for some friends in a private study group. From there it developed incrementally into what now comprises this larger work, something which is genuinely intended to be of interest to both serious students and practitioners of East Asian medicine. Issues which relate to my own perspectives on the subject, however, also leave me hoping that this work might also offer a little something to the sum of the wider history of medical anthropology – but much more importantly might sow fresh seeds in the financially barren and unfurrowed soil at the fringes of the fields of potentiality in modern medical care.

The book you are about to read, therefore, is most definitely a study of moxa, but each and every part is also unapologetically touched by the darker shadow of a secondary story which is very much still unravelling at the time of publication, the story of a desperate battle to protect the most vulnerable millions of humanity from a modern plague of drug-resistant disease. It is a story of appalling neglect. The agenda of the Moxafrica Project is to ascertain whether moxa may be able to contribute to this battle. The project's final outcome remains uncertain, as does the fate of many, many lives. It's just possible that Moxafrica might yet offer a novel chapter in the history of acumoxa, and if so it will be one with something of a twist. Our therapy does not normally inconveniently encroach upon some of the most fundamentally troubling topics of our times – those of poverty, of inequality and powerlessness, and of the widespread abuse of the human right to access decent health care. Such subjects lie normally well outside the confines of a conventional academic study or clinical textbook of traditional East Asian medicine, but the Moxafrica project has irresistibly shuffled this humble therapy of moxibustion towards such unfamiliar academic specialities, ones which include sociology, anthropology, medical ethics, medical economics and even geo-politics.

Notwithstanding this, I am hoping that this study will also offer some other unexpected and unanticipated food for thought for the modern acumoxa practitioner plying his or her therapeutic business in the world of modern allopathic medicine. It is a world which has become increasingly dominated by what appear superficially to be quite reasonable demands for evidence of efficacy, but such demands are almost invariably made on awkward terms for body therapies generally and are also predicated by the necessity of having access to substantial financial resource accompanied by an expectation of a rich marketplace with potential for return and subsequent profit. None of these form much of the day to day life of the average acumoxa therapist (nor have they ever been part of the story of moxa practice, as evidence in the following pages should prove). This makes the world of acumoxa practice and the world of modern medical research something of a clumsy encounter, though one that deserves to be much better attempted.

Preface

I trust that some of these latter issues and tensions, some of which already lie semi-concealed between the lines of even the earliest history of moxibustion, might prove of interest to any reader, but particularly to any who are interested in the current state of modern medicine. In Japan in the 1930s, Shimetaro Hara, a doctor who used direct moxa to treat just about anything patients brought through his clinic door, called moxa a "proletarian" medicine. Such a term sounds anachronistic and even a little pejorative today. In some sense moxa has suffered from such an image for two millennia, something which has been both its underbelly and its intrinsic strength. From the perspective of so many millions of our fellow human beings who struggle to survive with such limited access to the sorts of standards of heath care which most of us would consider a basic right, any form of medicine which is cheap, patent-free and fundamentally low-tech surely deserves better investigation. If moxa is as effective as it apparently has been (and as Moxafrica's studies are so far revealing it to be in Uganda and South Africa today), the possibility definitely exists that it might yet prove able to throw a telling slingshot or two at one of the true Goliath-like plagues of our times.

Merlin Young
Birmingham, United Kingdom
WHO International TB Day
March 24, 2012.

The Moon over Matsushima

ACKNOWLEDGEMENTS

This book would never have been possible without the help of many people most of whom I simply cannot name because of space.

First of all a huge thank you to my wonderful wife Jo, who has had to endure so much as this book has developed – often as the first sounding board for many of the ideas contained within its pages (more often than not at the most inopportune moments), but also as the proof-reader for my clumsy typing and endlessly long sentences. Her life has (in the truest sense of "for better or for worse") been hijacked by moxa and Moxafrica – and she has been generous enough not just to embrace this intrusion but, particularly as far as Moxafrica itself is concerned, to give the project her unqualified and constant support.

Jenny Craig has contributed hugely, and has done so with extraordinary but characteristic generosity. In 2007 we somehow both found ourselves entrusted with an unexpected task, revealed (I'm ashamed to say) in my case through the fog of a terrible hangover. The task was to develop the Moxafrica Project from scratch as best we could, and to guide its initial ideas towards some sort of reality. I'm still unclear exactly why or how this happened (when there are so many better qualified and equipped), but somehow it felt like we never really had much choice in the matter. Jenny's skills, good sense and compassion have been and continue to be vital for Moxafrica's systematic development. As if this weren't enough, her own words, her artistic talents, her editorial skills, her research-mindedness and some excellent photos all grace the pages of this book, particularly in Parts 3 and 4.

I must also add my heartfelt gratitude to Lorraine Wilcox for her generosity in writing the foreword, and also in identifying some embarrassing errors in my final drafts, some of which would have particularly exposed my ignorance of the subtleties of translating from Chinese. She deserves a second special round of thanks, however, for the world of moxa is lucky to have someone, not only as generous, but also as knowledgeable and inquisitive, as its principle advocate in the West.

Steve Birch and Junko Ida helped gave birth to so much of this. I thank both of them for introducing me to the wonders of Japanese moxibustion, but I also thank them for giving me the confidence to explore the subject critically on my own, and for some very important corrections in the final draft.

Olaf Waltmann designed the cover, and has worked tirelessly on the maps. This was a challenge for both of us, and we've both learnt a little about English ales in the process. He has also generously helped by taking most of the photographs. *Danku Weil!*

Atsuko Cowley translated sections of Doctor Hara's book. Given that it was written in old Japanese, this was no simple task but it has been so invaluable. Hara's words have spoken loudly to me for several years now through her translation. Without them this book would be much poorer, as would my perception of some of moxa's potentials.

I must also thank the extraordinary generosity of both Junji Mizutani and Stephen Brown – both moxa experts in their own right. Also so very many thanks to Todd Howard for so much, and finally I want to thank my publisher and editor, Phil Biggerton of Godiva Books, who had immediate and instinctive faith in the idea behind the book and has constantly encouraged me to complete it.

Dynastic period	Moxa events	General and acupuncture events	Philosophical Influences	Events in Central Asia	Events in Asia Minor or the "West"
Pre-Shang, Shang, and Zhou		Bronze arrives in China c. 1300BC. Fu Hao interred in Yellow River basin with Tarim jade in tomb, c. 1200 BC.	Divination by burning (*jiu*) on tortoise shells and ox scapulae.	The Indo-European *Yuezhi* migrate East over the Pamirs (unknown date). Blonde-haired Eurasian mummies interred in East Asian Tarim Basin c. 1800BC	Ötzi is killed in Alps, c. 5300 BC. Mediterranean Bronze Age 2000-1200 BC. Silk buried in tomb in Egypt 1070BC.
Spring and Autumn BC 770-475	The *Shi Jing* (Book of Odes) mentions collecting mugwort.	Stable feudal society in China.	Confucius 551-479. Laozi (dates unkown).	The Persian empire stretches westwards to Anatolia, and eastwards to the Pamirs.	Death of Cyrus the Great of Persia 530 BC. Fall of Kos to the Greeks from the Persians 479.
Warring States 475-221	Zhuangzi & Mengzi separately allude to moxa or moxibustion. c.300-200 Mawangdui texts originally written	Feudal system breaks down. Great Wall begun. Canals, roads and palaces built. *Guo Yu* "Discourse of the States" refers to *mai* and *qi*.	Mozi 480-390 (Mohism). Yin-Yang philosophy. Mengzi 372-299 (Confucian). Han Feizi d.233 (Legalism). Zuangzi 379-301. Zou Yan (350-270)(*Wu Xing* five phase theory).	The "Yingpan Man" buried in Tarim Basin 5th-4th century.	5th century BC first reference to the *Seres* by Ctesias. 4th century BC – Hippocratic Corpus developed on Kos including cauterization with *mykes* (vegetable matter).

Dynastic period	Moxa events	General and acupuncture events	Philosophical Influences	Events in Central Asia	Events in Asia Minor or the "West"
Qin 221-207		The Burning of the Books 213 BC.	Legalism triumphs. Repression.		
Western Han BC 207-9 AD	Mawangdui tomb closed 168 BC. Shuangbaoshan figurine 150BC.	*Shiji* refers to acupuncture. Earliest gold and silver metal needles 113BC. Earliest blast furnace in China c.100BC. Probable earliest collation of the *Neijing Suwen* & *Lingshu* (*Zhenjing*). The *Lingshu* refers to *Hao Zhen* (hair needles)	Confucianism predominates as official philosophy. Han library collections 26C.	The *Xiongnu* migrate southwards to harass China's borders, and the *Yuezhi* migrate westwards over the Pamirs to Bactria. Official "opening" of Silk Roads by Zhang Qian 139BC.	
Hsin 9-23		Yellow River changes course. Capital city moves. Civil war			

The Moon over Matsushima

Dynastic period	Moxa events	General and acupuncture events	Philosophical Influences	Events in Central Asia	Events in Asia Minor or the "West"
Eastern Han 23-220	Master Cao's Classic (lost).	Recovery of civilization 25-74. *Nanjing* (no moxa mentioned). Invention of paper. First Chinese dictionary. *Shang Han Lun* herbal text c.200	Buddhist texts appear in China from Kushan India.	Kanishka the Great, the Kushan king officially adopts and promotes Buddhism. Kushan Empire flourishes.	Stability and peace in Roman Empire 96-192.
Six Dynasties 220-589	Moxa used on intermediary substances by Ge Hong.	Huang Fumi's Systematic Classic 282. Wang Shu-he's Pulse Classic.	Development of organised Daoism. Golden age of Buddhism. Cha'an (Zen) Buddhism begins.		
Sui 589-618					
Tang 618-906	Sun Simiao writes extensively on moxa - 652. Wang Tao advocated moxa over acupuncture 752. Moxa practice develops.	Oldest extant copy of *Neijing* edited by Wang Bing 762. Acumoxa arrives in Japan (562) First printed books in China.	Cultural health. Searchings for alchemical immortality.		

xiv

Dynastic period	Moxa events	General and acupuncture events	Philosophical Influences	Events in Central Asia	Events in Asia Minor or the "West"
Ten Kingdoms/ Five Dynasties 906-960	Debate begins on moxa with heat conditions.		Buddhism begins to relatively decline.		
Sung & Southern Song 960-1270	Zhuang Chuo writes "Moxibustion on Gaohuangshu" 1127. Dou Cai writes the "Book of Bian Que's Heart" 1146. Shen Zhen tradition begins, mixing moxa with herbs in poles.	"Classic of the Bronze Man" 1027. Golden age for acupuncture.			
Yuan 1270-1368	Zhu Danxi on treating Heat conditions with moxa.		Neo-Confucianism. Daoist books Burnt.		

xv

Dynastic period	Moxa events	General and acupuncture events	Events in Asia	Events in Japan	Events in Europe
Ming 1368-1660	Zang Jiebin, Li Shi Zhen & Yang Zizhou Each write on moxa in China. Goto Konzan writes on moxa in Japan.	Waichi Sugiyama develops the guide tube and begins tradition of blind "hari" acupuncturists in Japan.	War between China and Japan fought in Korea. Trade between China and Japan stopped but taken through Vietnam, then taken over by the Dutch.	Early Portuguese connections. Dutch trading post founded 1636. Japan formally closed 1637.	Papal Donation 1493. Japanese "Herbal fire buttons" reported back in Europe by Fransiscans in Japan 1601. VOC Founded 1602. Founding of Batavia 1618. *Het Podagra* published 1674.

The Moon over Matsushima

Part 1 – the Roots

"harusame ya
yomogi o nobasu
kusa no michi"

SPRING RAIN –
THE MUGWORT GROWS
ALONG A ROAD WITH WEEDS[3]

Moxibustion's Relationship with Acupuncture

From the earliest records of both therapies it would appear most likely that "moxa" is actually something best described as acupuncture's slightly older half-breed orphaned sibling.

You can find plenty of fanciful references to acupuncture's supposed antiquity, some of which suggest it to be is as much as five thousand years old, with "needles" (*bian*) of stone, or ones of bamboo, all offered as explanation of how it may have been used prior to China's uncharacteristically late development in metallurgy in comparison with that of the Mediterranean basin. However, we have to wonder how a stone *bian* might have been used, given its shape, as anything other than a tool for incision and bloodletting.

In fact it is more generally accepted by scholars that the "art" of acupuncture as we understand it today is at best celebrating its two thousandth-and-a-bit birthday (still a pretty respectable age, of course). But old China was pretty good at serially destroying much of its literature and written cultural history during unsettled times as well as having it destroyed by natural disaster, so it's difficult to be in any way certain about the subject.

But what about the age of moxibustion as a therapeutic practice?

Some context is needed to better understand the period during which the early history of acumoxa emerged. The earliest genuine authentic evidence of acupuncture emerges hazily from the early Han dynasty which began in 206 BC. China had been languishing for centuries in what is now known as the "Warring States Period", during which it had become divided into separate competing nation states. Despite these being such turbulent times, this was also a period of cultural, philosophical and technological growth. In the fields of philosophy it saw the development of Daoism, the refining of Confucianism, as well as the birth of Mohism, and Legalism. This era has become known as that of the "hundred schools" of philosophy, but it was one which also saw the beginning of the

---

[3] A *haiku* by Matsuo Bashō (from 1694) as previously shown in the frontispiece.

tradition of serious canal building and wall construction, as well as the start of China's Iron Age. All of these impacted in different ways on the development of Chinese medicine. It ended abruptly in 221 BC, when the Qin from the West unexpectedly united the country, brutally founding the first imperial dynasty, the Qin dynasty, albeit it lasted a mere fourteen years.

Right in the middle of this brief dynastic tsunami a particularly dramatic event occurred – the "Burning of the Books" in 213BC. It was an event which witnessed the short-lived triumph of Legalism over the other competing philosophical doctrines of the time and provides testimony to a concerted attempt by the Qin to totally suppress and eradicate all alternative philosophies. It is in the context of this event and its aftermath, together with the fact that it involved the loss of a mass of Chinese cultural history, that we need to begin to consider and review how both of these therapies, acupuncture and moxibustion, emerged during the Han.

The Qin were ruthless warriors of a despotic bent who were exceptional even by Chinese standards. As despots are wont to do, they assumed that eradicating any alternative philosophies to the one which supported their right to rule would effectively preserve their dynasty for ever. Doing so included, not just burning books, but summarily burying some of those philosophers connected with such literature whilst still alive. The brevity of their dynasty (just fourteen years) amply demonstrates the folly of their assumption, but the damage they wreaked on Chinese culture in so short a period is still shocking to this day.

Tomb Findings

Certain hard evidence in the form of archaeological findings suggests a sequence of developments directly after the demise of the Qin which fleshes out this dearth of reliable surviving written testimony. The most significant of these for our story was the discovery in 1973 of two particular previously unknown medical texts which devoted themselves specifically to moxa and its therapeutic use. They were discovered in a prince's tomb at Mawangdui in China, part of a larger hoard which was one of the major archaeological finds of the twentieth century. The significance of these particular texts lies in the fact that, not only do they predate any other previously authenticated medical texts from China, but also that they contain no reference at all to acupuncture. In fact there is no mention of needle therapy anywhere else in the silks or bamboo slips which were found in the cache alongside them. This tomb was known to have been sealed in 168 BC, in early Han times in other words. These two particular moxa silks (silk cloths on which these texts were written) were certainly written some time earlier, quite probably prior to the Qin in the heart of the times of the Warring States between 300 and 200 BC based on the calligraphic style and the formations of the characters.

In the context of the early history of East Asian medicine, however, these texts hold particular significance because they also provide us with the very earliest topological or anatomical descriptions of what have come to be known in English as the meridians or channels, the energetic pathways which have subsequently formed the foundation for traditional acupuncture treatment.

Both texts explicitly described eleven bilateral vessels/meridians – the details of which we will discuss later in this section. The word "meridian", incidentally, as is regularly used to describe these lines on the body, is a mildly contentious one. Coined in the early twentieth century by George Soulie de Mourant, the French diplomat and scholar, to describe the Chinese word *jingluo*, 經络, the word has comfortably passed into the acumoxa vernacular. The compound word *jingluo* actually suggests the idea of a warp and weft, terms used to define the vertical and horizontal threads used in weaving. All of the regular meridians are vertical, which could have suggested using the word warp as a more accurate translation, but de Mourant would appear to have preferred the word meridian not just to reflect their vertical axes – but also their topographical insubstantiality.

These meridians were not described at all by using the term *jingluo* in these early texts, however, but rather by the term *"mai"*. This is not a word that is used to describe the regular meridians at all today, and as such suggests that they may have been initially understood slightly differently to the vertical *jing* channels as we now understand them. In slightly later times to these Mawangdui texts, the word *mai* was also used to describe ideas that have been widely translated by scholars as "vessels" (as in the Eight Extraordinary Vessels, the *Qi Jing Ba Mai*) and also as the pulse (as in the *Mai Jing* or Pulse Classic).

This earlier phenomenon of meridians or channels being defined by using the word *mai* recurs in some other medical texts of similar age excavated at Zhangjiashan, although these other channel texts are frustratingly unidentifiable as relating specifically to either moxa or acupuncture. There were other medical texts discovered at Mawangdui, along with arcane, esoteric and even magical ones, but what remains of such particular interest to the early history of Chinese medicine is that there was not a single allusion to acupuncture[4].

We are left with the very plausible idea, therefore, that the theories of acupuncture developed directly from these seminal understandings of some sort of "vessels" (if that is the best terms we can use today) which traverse the topography of the human body, and also that the use of moxa probably predates acupuncture, at

---

[4] It is of course possible that the word *mai*, as used in these early texts to describe what has subsequently been described by the composite character *jing luo*, suggests not simply a prototypical foundation for what later developed into the theory of the circulatory theory of *qi* (on which the more mature edifice of acumoxa is built) but even something conceptually fundamentally different from it.

least in the sense of any needle therapy which is based on any sort of *jingluo* channel theory.

A further archaeological find, excavated in 1993 from a tomb in Shuangbaoshan in Szechuan, deepens this idea. It is a fascinating 30cm high lacquered wooden representation of a human body. This figurine is dated at between 179 and 141 BC. It has lines drawn down its body, but no points – in similar vein, in one sense, to the Mawangdui texts (as we shall soon see) because it implies lines, but has no identifiable sign of treatment points along them.

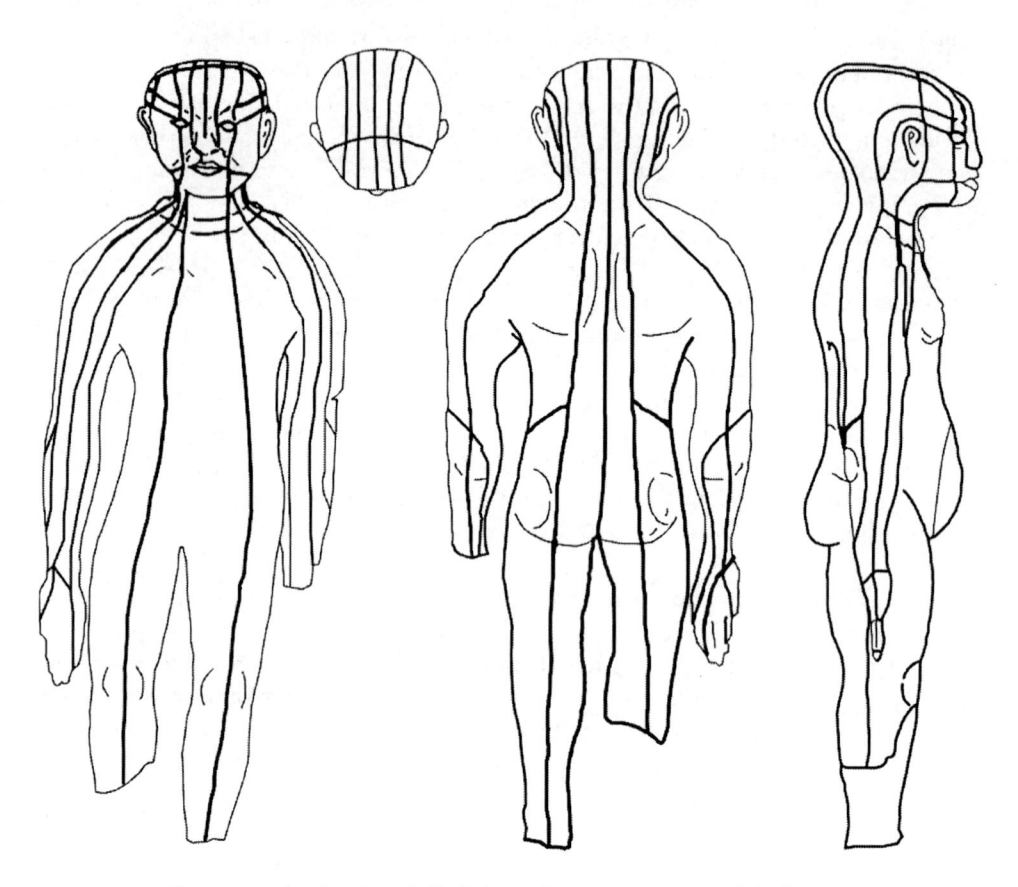

Representative drawing of the figurine showing trajectories of the lines.
This drawing is derived directly from the drawing in Vivienne Lo's "Imaging Practice: Sense and Sensuality in Early Chinese Medical Thought"

The Shuangbaoshan figure, however, is suggested as showing a total of only nine converging lines as opposed to an anticipated bilateral twenty-two (if such a figure were to have accurately reflected the Mawangdui texts). This in turn suggests that it might have been a model for use with some form of therapy similar to the Mawangdui or Zhangjiashan texts but not quite the same one. One of the reasons that we can propose this possibility arises is because of the fact that the figurine is nude, something which marks it out from other examples of contemporary grave figures all of which to date have been found fully robed. Self-evidently, of course, a robed figure would serve no purpose at all as a model for lines drawn on the skin; it just may be, therefore, that this figure represents an alternative or even a more seminal school of moxibustion – or at least some other vessel theory than that suggested by the Mawangdui scrolls. It might even offer us a variant representation of earlier vessel/channel theory. The figurine almost certainly post-dates the moxa texts, however, although this does not necessarily mean that any therapy associated with it might also postdate the therapy associated with them.

It might seem puzzling that soemthing which might be reflective of acumoxa as we understand it today could be associable with this figurine given that only lines (not points) are identifiable on it. The same, however, can be said of the Mawangdui texts which describe lines but no points, and these were **definitely** moxa texts.

Unfortunately no further information is associated with the figurine apart from the fact that the resident of the tomb was probably someone of some military significance, a conclusion based on the other contents found within it.

This military link may provide a clue to one possible early use for moxibustion. Vivienne Lo, an English scholar, translates for us from a bamboo slip originating from the archives of the Jiaqu Defence Company Headquarters recording how "a commanding officer of a beacon unit along the line of defences in the remote North-West of China treated a soldier with moxa-cautery in two places on his back[5]". This slip dates from the Eastern Han Dynasty 24 AD to 220 AD, rendering it later than the texts quoted above, but it suggests that moxa might have, at the very least, been used as a kind of emergency front-line remedy available to the Han soldier in one of the most remote fortresses of the Great Wall in the farthest reaches of the empire. It was being used perhaps in the absence of a more sophisticated medical intervention such as herbs, or even of acupuncture, and it was apparently performed by a senior soldier, presumably with rudimentary medical training. This association of moxibustion with lay or bare-foot medicine will be encountered repetitively in our investigations, in fact right up to the twenty-first century.

So we must continue to ponder on exactly what the word *mai* may have meant to those using it in these early times. Lo particularly suggests that the *mai*, these seminal channels (if that is what they are) which are described in the early texts and quite possibly are shown on the figurine, might reflect perceived routes of

---

[5] Vivienne Lo 2007. "Imaging Practice: Sense and Sensuality in Early Chinese Medical Thought" (in "The Warp and the Weft: Graphics and Text in the Production of Technical Knowledge in China". Metailie and Dorofeeva eds. Leiden: Brill) p 397

pain as much (or more) than their being a reflection of blood vessels or anything similar. Other ideas about this create a richer perspective, however.

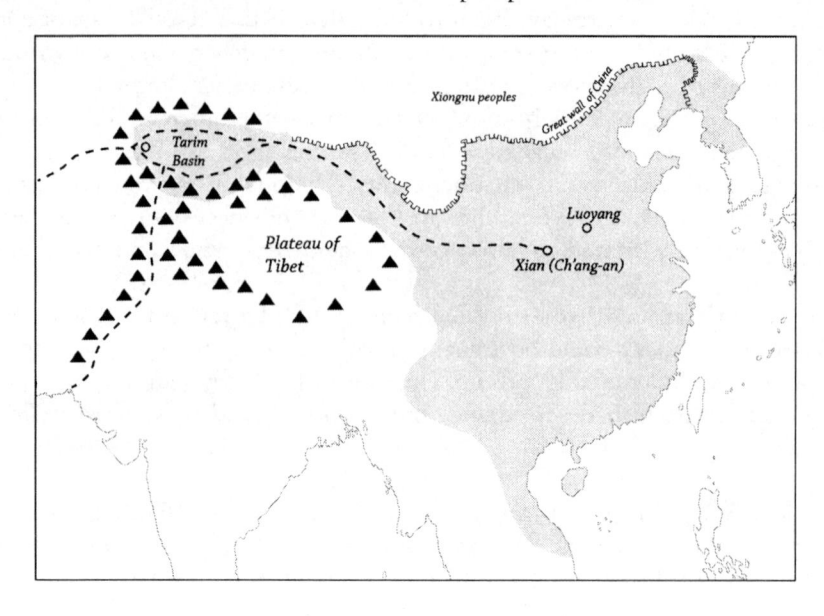

Map showing the full extent of the Han Empire, and the two ancient capitals at Luoyang and Xian. The dotted lines show the trading routes in and out of China

Early Channel/Vessel Theory

Keiji Yamada, a modern Japanese scholar and authority on these early texts, fascinatingly considers that channel theory originated from an earlier conception that a network of similar vessels existed in the earth itself, the manipulation or modification of which might create beneficial effects in agriculture or even in the wider world. He identifies the earliest extant example of the characters of both *qi* and *mai* together (in other words of *qi*-filled vessels or channels similar in any sense to those types described in the Mawangdui texts) as being found in the *Guo Yu* (a "Discourse on the States"), a text from the Warring States period[6]. This was most definitely not talking about medicine: it concerned the nature of the earth itself. "If the earth is not shaken (moved) and overturned" he translates "the *qi* will overflow in the earth's vessels (*mai*) and disaster will strike. When the *yang* is thick and plentiful, the *qi* of the earth begins to move."[7]

---

[6] The *Guo Yu* was reportedly written by Zuoqui Ming to record the sayings of nobles in different states during the last years of the Western Zhou Dynasty (c. 11th century B.C. to 770 B.C.)

[7] Keiji Yamada 1998 "The Origins of Acupuncture, Moxibustion, and Decoction" – (Kyoto: Nichibunken, International Research Centre for JapaneseStudies)

The ideas expressed in this particular text thus link early vessel theory with equally early agricultural theory, but they also tellingly associate seismological portents with the health of the state. Elsewhere, the text reads: "*Yang* was stuck and could not get out, *yin* was suppressed and could not evaporate, so an earthquake was inevitable. Now the earthquakes around the three rivers are due to *yang* losing its place and *yin* being pressed down. *Yang* is forsaken under *yin* so the source of rivers has been blocked. If the foundation of rivers is blocked the country will definitely collapse. This is because of the fact that the flowing water and flourishing land are necessities for the people's lives. If the water and land cannot sustain the people's living conditions, the country will inevitably fall".

Actually, the idea of "*yang* losing its place and *yin* being pressed down" could serve as a rather poetic explanation of what is termed today as a subduction zone at which one continental plate moves inexorably beneath another, potentially creating both earthquake and eruption. Notwithstanding this, in a country like China that has been regularly afflicted with catastrophic earthquakes, such seismological ideas may have taken instant intuitive hold on the collective imagination, and the translation of these ideas into ones concerning human health, therefore, might not be considered as that surprising. In early Chinese thought, for instance, the idea persisted that the source of the Yellow River lay far to the west in the distant mountains of the Kunlun and Tian ranges, but that the run-offs from these ranges went underground for hundreds of miles only to resurface far to the East, nearer to the agricultural centre of China itself. Such an idea in fact finds clear reflection in the later emergent understandings of the channels, and also with their interior pathways.

There is also an interesting echo of these seismological ideas in the *Yin Yang Shuyi Mai Jiu Jing* (one of the two Mawangdui moxa texts). This text describes each channel formulaically, starting with a description of its pathway, followed by the repeated clause "When this vessel *is moved* ..." followed by a list of symptoms associated with the specific channel being described. The idea of pathogical "movement" in these vessels reflecting ill health in the human is not dissimilar to the idea of abnormal "movements" in the earth spelling out catastrophe for the state as described in the *Guo Yu*. No actual idea of causation of these movements is suggested or discussed. The broad principle underlying this emerging idea, however, reveals itself to be an intellectual association between particular "movements" within these vessels and specific sets of symptoms: and a rectification of these movements through the application of moxibustion would logically result in a more normal state and a resultant resolution of these very symptoms.

It is at least arguable that this particular Mawangdui text (the *Yin Yang Shuyi Mai Jiu Jing*) is in fact the earlier of the two texts, simply because it seems, at least from our perspective, to be less cohesive and coherent in terms of the later *Nei Jing* texts which, as we will see, may well directly derive from them.

It is also possibly more than co-incidental that the character subsequently used for *xue*, the acupoint (more literally a "hole"), etymologically depicts a hole beneath the ground or a cave, suggesting a further subsequent link with this geomantic connection.

穴 *xue* the acupoint

It has been widely observed that the language in the earlier acumoxa texts time and again relates to water regulation and irrigational practices which clearly represented the dominant technology of the time (and much evidence can be found for this connection[8]), but the true sources of channel theory might reside as much or more in seismological and geomantic theory (and its consequent secondary effects on the major waterways) rather than in water management *per se*.

It can also be readily observed that much of the language in these early texts describes topographical landscape and geography, as do, of course, many of the names of the subsequent acupoints themselves. In a country in which huge earthquakes are not uncommon, and are at times so devastating that they have actually changed the course of the massive Yellow River by hundreds of miles with undoubted catastrophic consequences[9], this seminal linkage between the contours of the world at large and the contours of the human body, of the unpredictable *qi* of the earth (and its associated movements), the *qi* of the waterways, and the uncertainties of the movements of the *qi* in the human body seems quite a striking but also understandable one.

Interestingly Lo suggests that the nine lines on the figurine bear no particular resemblance to the later fully fledged channel system which may or may not have evolved from it. In support of this, she identifies that the *yin* meridians of the leg are ignored, and that the focus of the lines on the sensory organs of the face point to alternative understandings than those that have subsequently evolved and survived. She may be being a little unfair since at least one interpretation of the lines of the figure suggest otherwise. There is a central dorsal line which can very clearly be interpreted as the *Du* vessel; there are two parallel channels down the back and the back of the legs which are identifiable as the Leg *Taiyang* Bladder channels; there are also two subsidiary lines (generally not counted within the nine) which bifurcate from these back channels just above the waist and which from this point run down the sides of the legs following a pathway very similar to the Leg *Shaoyang* Gall Bladder channels. In fact, the description of the pathway of

---

[8] Donald Harper indicates an essay on water from the 3rd century BC in the *Guangzi* in this connection, linking *qi* with *mai*, a passage which he believes predates both *yinyang* and five phase theories. It seems probable that the *Guo Yu* was written even earlier.

[9] The Yellow River changed course right across Shandong as recently as 1852 causing death and devastation. Two thousand years earlier a similar shift in river course had precipitated the demise of the Western Han.

the Leg *Shaoyang* channel in one of the *Mawangdui* texts almost exactly reflects the line on the figurine. There are also four bilateral channels running down the figurine's arms which bear some strong resemblances to the pathways of the five vessels of the arm as described in the *Mawangdui* texts. The Leg *Yangming* Stomach channel is also quite clearly identifiable on the frontal aspect of the figure. All the *yin* channels of the leg, however, as well as two channels of the arm including the *jueyin* channel (which is not identified for us by the writers of the *Mawangdui* scrolls either) are missing, as is the *Ren* vessel.

Certain fascinating resonances with the *phlebes* of Greek medicine exist with this small figure. The "salient common supposition" about these tubes, ducts or channels as conceived and described in Hippocratic medicine was that they originated in the head[10]. In similar fashion, all of the lines on the figurine originate or end (we have no idea which) at the head. There may or may not be connections here which we will explore in more depth shortly.

The fact that these lines do clearly converge on the sensory organs of the head actually does seem to reinforce this exclusive *yang* channel interpretation. All the conventional *yang* channels to this day are also understood to connect to the very same organs of sensory perception, either converging on them (the *yang* channels of the arm) or originating from them (those of the leg). They might arguably even be defined by this association. We will also see later that, when described in one of the Mawangdui texts, what we have since come to understand as the Arm *Yangming* Large Intestine and Arm *Shaoyang* Triple Burner channels were referred to as the "Mouth vessel" and the "Ear vessel" respectively, so this sensory association may have been more than theoretical. The arm *Taiyang* channel incidentally was referred to as the "Shoulder vessel" in one of these texts[11].

The idea that these *mai* vessels converge on the sensory organs of the head, which is implicit in the lines on the figurine, also accords with the etymological interpretation of the Chinese character for *mai* itself, an interpretation of which intriguingly lends itself to neither of the conventional later translations of the term – as vessel or pulse.

Nigel Wiseman describes the character as representing a confluence of waterways, particularly that of a tributary into a main waterway[12].

脈 – *mai* (the full character)

---

[10] E M Craik 2004 "Knife and fire: medical practice of east and west" in *Proceedings of COE* meeting held at Kyoto November, 2003 (published as *Globalization*, Kyoto, Iwanami Shoten) pp 227–43

[11] See chart on page 60

[12] Nigel Wiseman 2003 "Chinese Medical Characters vol 1" (Paradigm Publications)

The image of this ancient figurine, with one line converging into another, reflects this same idea as clearly as anywhere, much more clearly in fact than the channel descriptions in the later texts. In a similar sense, so do those early Chinese ideas of the origins of their waterways, beginning as the run-off water from the western ranges flowing into deep underwater streams to emerge many miles away to turn into a single mighty river. The idea is both pervasive and persuasive, suggesting that, certainly in terms of the early texts, the word *mai* might quite acceptably be translated as "channel", just as accurately as "vessel".

The association of moxibustion with that which is *yang*, an unavoidable observation based on any study of the moxibustion literature across the centuries, serves to further suggest that this figurine might be linked with moxibustion practice. For instance, it might reflect a school which associated the application of moxa almost exclusively with the *yang* surfaces of the body and with *yang* in general, particularly since most of the indications for treatment in the early records seem to be predicated by findings of excess. Another Mawangdui text (the "Death Signs of the *Yin Yang* Vessels" or *Yin Yang Mai Sihou*) actually suggested that the *yin* vessels are more associable with death and the *yang* vessels more with life. So perhaps the inclusion only of *yang* lines on the figurine renders it no more than a symbolic type of talisman of life for the dead in the afterlife.

To create a clearer picture for ourselves, however, we need to review the turbulent history that was taking place at the time of these early texts in a little more detail. Part of the possible historical significance of these earliest texts lies in the fact that, although they did not survive further, they must at least have escaped the destructive hands of those "burners of books" by dint of their being interred in the posterity of sealed tombs after the event itself.

We know that Chinese civilisation, philosophy and medical theory, as well as society itself, were all in a phase of rapid and turbulent transition during this same period. It is generally accepted today that medical texts (as opposed, for instance, to philosophical ones) were generally preserved by decree from the Burning of the Bookssimply because this is what historians have since recorded. It is also accepted that the Han scholars were exhaustive in their subsequent efforts to build up libraries in order to preserve what was left or what could be recreated from what had survived. Neither supposition may be quite as true as is generally accepted to be the case, however, particularly since so little of the earlier medical literature would actually seem to have survived. We need to consider, for instance, whether some or indeed most of these earlier texts might have represented approaches which were considered simply too unorthodox for the dominant emergent philosophical authorities to see them as being medical. If so, they might still have found themselves on a shortlist for destruction by fire.

Additionally, in an era which predates the invention of printing, this confiscation of written material, whether for burning or indeed for recopying into the more modern Han script, must have involved the requisitioning of scrolls which may have been rare if not unique. Just how protective might their owners have felt about them?

Evolving Medical Knowledge at the Time of the Han

Nathan Sivin, a modern scholar and sinologist, has thoroughly explored the likely methods of transmission of medical knowledge in the Han[13]. From evidence available from the *Shi Ji* of the great historian Sima Qian, and the *Nei Jing Suwen* and *Lingshu*, all emanating from 100BC onwards, it seems most likely that medical knowledge, at least among more elite and literate physicians, was passed on through transmission of texts from teacher to student, the process of which included both the intellectual absorption of specific texts and some form of ritual ceremony which (according to some passages in the *Lingshu*) may have included fasting, purification and the smearing of blood. Such transmission certainly included the reading, rote learning and copying of medical texts which appear to have been regarded as almost sacred. As such these were precious and exclusive documents, implicitly the preserve of a relatively select and chosen few. Would such physicians willingly have allowed them to be handed over either to the Legalist thought police of the Qin, or even to the Han Confucian scribes? Might they have seen it as a preferable gift for eternity or even as a duty to their ancestors that they be securely entombed rather than entrusted to the vicissitudes of more volatile political whim?

Moreover, might these Confucian "guardian" librarians or scribes who were entrusted with preserving China's literate past in the characters of the new age simply have transliterated those scrolls of more unorthodox or even heretical provenance into the new script and then sent them straight to the secure confines of politically secure storage – or, worse still, might they even have just sent them straight to oblivion by not copying them at all? If either of these were the case, the chance of their survival into later ages would have been decidedly reduced.

The curious fact that no moxa texts survived into the Han period suggests at the very least that not everything may have been quite as it has been subsequently presented. It strongly suggests that the history of the period may not be quite as it has since been recorded, and even hints that the preservation order protecting medical texts may not necessarily have been interpreted in exactly the way that it has since been understood to have been.

Four questions arise. How confidently can we truly accept the supposition that **all** medical texts (as we might define them today) really were exempt from destruction in the fires of the *Qin*? In addition, how certain can we be that such surviving texts would have been readily given up subsequently to the Han scholar scribes who were entrusted with collating and recording China's dismembered

---

[13]Nathan Sivin 1995 "Text and Experience in Classical Chinese Medicine" in "Knowledge and the Scholarly Medical Tradition" (Cambridge University Press)

cultural past? And just what was the real definition of the word "medical" at the time, given that paradigms were in a state of flux? Finally, how confidently can we assume that these Han librarians were as assiduously impartial in their copying as we might hope they were?

Such questions seem quite reasonable based simply on the telling fact that, only shortly after this period, in the third century AD, Huangfu Mi found himself obliged to compile the "Systematic Classic" (the *Jiu Jia Yi Jing*) from **only three** texts because so little was available to him, and he was quite frank that a decent understanding even of these was already both limited and confusing. Huangfu was a Han scholar who contracted a serious illness during middle age as a result of which he focused most of his attentions for the rest of his life to the study of existing medical texts since he was so concerned that their authentic messages were already being lost.

Suppose, for instance, that the earlier moxa literature and even some less orthodox early acupuncture literature were not seen as "acceptable" to either the officials of the Qin or the Han. What might this have implied? Perhaps they were seen to have been grounded in a quasi-medicine of a more magical or demonic orientation in contrast to the emerging more orthodox medical theories which were more dependent on newly emerging ideas of the forces of Nature and the related perceptions of Natural Order and Natural Law. If this were the case, then this very "medical" literature might not have been seen to be so medical after all, and would simply have found itself being peremptorily condemned to the flames of the Qin rather than being preserved as we believe today should have been the case. Or indeed a little later they may have been simply overwritten by the Han scribes. It seems quite possible that either could have been the case, whatever the Han historians may have wanted us to believe on the subject.

So just how might these moxa texts have been viewed in the Han?

It may not be a coincidence that they were interred in a tomb with other texts which frequently also invoked spells and magic to dispel disease, and that these texts were neither preserved nor copied in the imperial libraries either. If burning mugwort, for instance, had evolved directly from demonological medicine and was conceived largely as a way to ward off evil or inauspicious influences, this of itself may have rendered it a style of medicine of less respectability and repute amongst an emerging scholastic class of physician in the Han dynasty. Today, both the lines on the figurine and the channels described in the tomb texts might seem to us intrinsically complementary and compatible with our own understandings of the developing channel system, but during the Han might they have been seen as being embarrassingly and inconveniently at odds with the newer theories that were still undergoing development in the light of new understandings of the world?

It remains a confusing picture. Based on the archaeological evidence, we surely cannot ignore the idea that these slightly inconvenient early moxa texts may have played an important part in the development of *jingluo* channel theory, but it is curious that, apart from these isolated tomb findings, no others have survived or been discovered and any further trace of them from the time seems quite simply to have disappeared. The next definitive textual signpost that is available to us today is in the library records of the Han. These identify the *Huang Di Nei Jing* (which included the *Suwen* and *Lingshu*) among seven other medical classics. The moxa texts do not, however, appear to be amongst them at all.

If the extant *Suwen* and *Lingshu* **are** indeed two parts of this apparent compilation of earlier medical texts as is widely accepted, then they hold the only possible torch available for us today with which to review the possible seminal sources for acupuncture and *jingluo* channel theory. We might logically expect to find within them some vestigial traces of these earlier lost texts. In fact, the *Suwen* does refer to earlier texts, mentioning a substantial total of twenty-seven earlier texts by reference. Not one of them unfortunately is identifiable as a moxa text, nor does a single one of them appear by name in the Han librarian records (although they may of course have been contained within them as single chapters in a larger volume).

Some of them are, however, identifiable in the testimony of Chunyu Yi in the *Shiji*, as recorded by Sima Qian the Han historian. Chunyu helpfully identifies the names of a series of texts that were formally transmitted to him at around 180 BC. None of these named texts are identifiable as being acupuncture texts, but they do hint at being associated with anatomical measurements, diagnosis by pulse and colour, drug treatment, stone needling and some channel/vessel theory which may possibly be associated with moxibustion. The stone needling should not be assumed to be that closely related to acupuncture as we know it today since it does not appear to involve any form of channel theory although it does involve the movement of *qi*.

"I discussed the locations of the loci and how the *qi* should travel up and down, exit and enter, and its proper pathological, abnormal and normal behaviour, in connection with indications for the use of the stone needle and for determining the location for its use and for moxibustion[14]."

Chunyu is quite explicit about the importance of guarding these texts, and the importance of their being passed on appropriately to successive generations of physicians. This theme is picked up in the *Lingshu* itself, when the Thunder Duke laments that: "I fear that [the teachings] will be scattered and become extinct in

---

[14] Nathan Sivin 1995 "Text and Experience in Classical Chinese Medicine" In "Knowledge and the Scholarly Medical Tradition" (Cambridge University Press) pp181-2

later generations, inaccessible to our descendants[15]." How right the Thunder Duke appears to have been.

By Huangfu Mi's time, at around 260AD, as mentioned above, scholarly access appears to have been limited to only three texts, two of which were part of the *Huang di Nei Jing*, with the other one (the *Ming Tang*) remaining relatively unidentifiable both in terms of its origin, and its actual content since it was subsequently lost. The modern scholar Paul Unschuld very tellingly observes: "The absence of all the unearthed texts from the official bibliographies of the time is a clear sign that the latter should be considered selective[16]."

Such confusions to some degree challenge the received mythologies of these venerable medical classics, particularly because the Qin period is generally regarded as such a stain on the tapestry of Chinese history and the Han as such a triumph, as in so many ways of course was the case. A fuller appreciation of the times in which these therapies were emerging reveals perhaps a cloudier context, however, with which paradoxically we might attempt to clarify this confusion.

As previously stated, the Warring States period was a time of massive upheaval in China, a time which served to totally destroy the stable feudal structure of the previous centuries. The figure of Confucius casts long and powerful shadows over both the period before and during the Warring States and also over the one after it, but these shadows are texturally and textually different from each other, a difference may well have proved to have been important to the story of moxibustion.

Confucius (551-479 BC), of course, lived before the Warring States period began. His original teachings, however, even then referred back to a prior "golden age". He specifically advocated layers of hierarchical respect within his philosophy, starting with respect for parents, then to clan, prince or duke, each layer dependent one upon the other. After his death, these teachings were continued during the period of the Warring States itself, particularly by Meng Zi (Mencius). Confucian teachings were far from the dominant philosophical school of the time, however, competing for attention with many others, Daoism being only one.

With the final supremacy of the Qin, however, Confucian thought along with all of the others apart from the triumphant Legalism of Han Fei Zi was quite literally consigned to the fires. Confucians, Daoists, Mohists and others were equally considered by these extremists as "vermin". What separated Confucianism from some of these others, however, was the fact that it survived from these

---

[15] A passage from the *Lingshu* as identified by David J Keegan 1988 in his unpublished doctoral dissertation "Huang -ti Nei-Ching: the Structure and Compilation; the Significance and the Structure" (University of California at Berkeley).

[16] Paul Unschuld 2003 "Huang Di Nei Jing Su Wen – Nature, Knowledge, Imagery in an Ancient Chinese Medical Text"- (University of California Press) p76

iconoclastic times relatively intact, evidenced by its surviving texts. In contrast, Mohism was eradicated completely.

There may be several reasons for its survival, not least of which would have been the bravery of those who risked certain death by hiding their venerated texts from the book-burners. An important reason, however, was the subsequent supremacy of the Han.

Liu Bang, the first Han emperor, is considered today above all to have been a pragmatist. He came to power by exploiting a wave of anti-Qin sentiment, fuelled by the dynasty's cruel repression. Having gained power, however, he had no intention of giving it away, and was far from averse from using a little repression himself, extending to the murder and assassination of both foes and former friends when deemed necessary. Part of this pragmatic process of accumulating and centralising power included a somewhat selective adoption of the codes of Confucianism which thus became the "official" philosophy of the Han in ways that were to some extent reflective of the strategy of the Qin with their adoption of Legalism. It was in some important respects, however, a slightly different form of Confucianism from what had been taught by the Master himself, or indeed from what had been taught by his followers, since it included telling variations. The principle distinction was in the glossing over of the individual layers of hierarchy of respect. Han Confucianism amalgamated these largely into a single layer of respect directed towards the state and the Emperor himself in order to effectively consolidate imperial power. This simple change of emphasis made it critically distinct from the teachings that had gone before.

Thus it can be argued that Liu Bang essentially softened the stringencies of the Qin by cleverly adapting some of the more useful facets of their Legalist codes into Confucian ones. In so doing he appears to have consciously introduced codes which were much more popularly acceptable, whilst still creating a useful prop to his imperial dynasty.

Evidence of Confucian influence can clearly be seen in the medical texts. One of the key Confucian ideas was of a former "golden age" and the very first chapter of the *Suwen* clearly resonates with this same idea. In it Huang Di, the Yellow Emperor, asks his chief physician Qibo how and why, in just such a prior golden age, people had lived to over a hundred years of age, whilst "today" they could barely live to half that age. This question clearly comes from a Confucian worldview, and the response (that their life-style had been based on moderation and living within the laws of Nature) is even more so. Confucius himself had presented his philosophy in exactly such terms – and furthermore suggested that the few surviving texts that were available at his own time, surviving from the earlier Zhou dynasty (from around 1000 BC), contained all of the wisdom necessary for a good life in a benevolent society.

The important eighth chapter of the *Suwen*, which describes the roles of the "twelve officials", also clearly concurs with this Confucian world view. And the Confucian idea that there are "Laws", living contrary to which results in illness and catastrophe, has continued to permeate Chinese medical thought throughout the centuries. They are clearly first seen in these Han era texts and are indisputably Confucian ideas.

It can therefore be suggested that, in contrast to the seminal moxa tomb texts which preceded them, these *Nei Jing* "classics" which now form the foundation for Chinese traditional medical theory and which incorporate and promote needle therapy, do so by reflecting this slightly bowdlerised Han/Confucian thinking reflective of the age in which they were written. Some of the theories of health in the human body as seen by the Han physician can thus be seen to have evolved to resonate, not so much with the earlier seismological ideas which we previously discussed as being seminally influential on the development of channel theory, but rather with the notions contained in the political and philosophical theories enshrined in the emergent Han imperial state.

This new state was tied together by roads and canals, dependent upon granaries for storage, and critically dependent upon hierarchical bureaucratically structured laws for its stability. Such ideas symbolised how Han thinkers considered that the state might best withstand the threats, both internal and external, that had been experienced in the previous centuries – a type of disorder which surely represented as much anathema for the Confucians of the Han as it had for the Legalists of the Qin[17].

This idea may be important because it also logically suggests an opposite – it suggests the possibility that medical theories of health and disease which incorporated an alternative and less orthodox world view to the one which was emerging might not have been promoted as positively as those which more clearly resonated with the political correctness of the time. They might, in fact, not even have been thought worthy of preservation.

Given the political ruthlessness that persisted during the Han, the actions of not preserving or promoting such ideas might well have included both proscription and censorship, and could equally have resulted in the persecution or even execution of their proponents. These were still dangerous times in which to be seen to be challenging the all-powerful *status quo*. Such proscriptions may not even have been seen worthy of being recorded by the historians of the time, who may have been understandably driven by simple good intentions, quite simply in order

---

[17] More detailed consideration of these ideas are discussed in Paul Unschuld 2003 "Huang Di Nei Jing Su Wen – Nature, Knowledge, Imagery in an Ancient Chinese Medical Text" - (University of California Press) pp 338-348.

to impose a fantasy of "completeness and perfection"[18] on ancient works which were self-evidently far from perfect in the forms in which they were being received at the time.

At this time a new class was emerging as well. The feudal elite, which had effectively destroyed itself during the Warring States, was being succeeded by a scholar elite which is accepted today as being altogether more meritocratic. As a further reflection of these sociological shifts, within the field of medicine there also emerged the phenomenon of the "scholar physician", a prototype that came to control the very heart of the emerging acumoxa traditions.

A further relevant archaeological find was revealed in 1968 (five years before the Mawangdui tomb was excavated) in Mancheng County, Hebei Province, in the tomb of Prince Liu Sheng, the son of Emperor Jing Di, who died during the Western Han Dynasty. The tomb had been sealed in 113 BC (fifty-five years after the Mawangdui tomb had been sealed). When excavated it was found to contain four gold and five silver "needles", so far the earliest evidence of metal acupuncture needles.

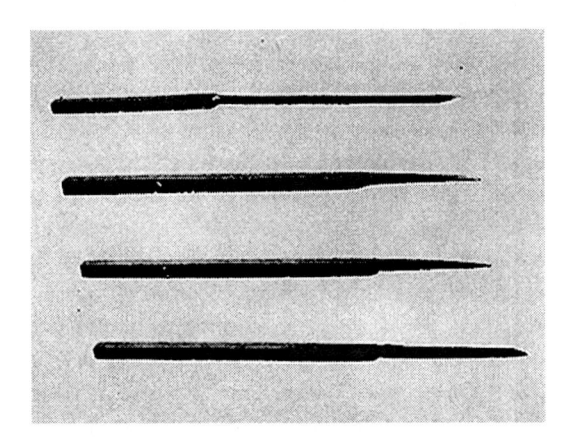

Some of the needles found in the tomb – their shafts being 2-3mm diameter.

No matter how they may be referred to as "acupuncture" needles, however, these quite clearly are not examples of the *hao zhen* or filiform needles as we recognise them today, having a diameter of about two millimetres. Any suggestion that the technology to manufacture finer needles did not then exist is belied by the use of the word *hao* which was used to define this thinner type of needle in the *Lingshu*. "*Hao*" (which is today often simply translated as "filiform") actually is the same character as the one used for "hair". But these gold and silver needles found in the

---

[18] John B Henderson 1991 "Scripture, Canon and Commentary. A Comparison of Confucian and Western Exegesis" (Princeton) p105

tomb in Hebei have little in common with any type of hair, even that of an elephant.

毫針 – *hao zhen*

The requisite technology to manufacture such fine needles is another important component of the emerging picture and will be something we will return to soon. For now we can surmise that, somewhere between 168 and 113 BC, both medical and technological developments were taking place which may have fed each other. These included the formulation of the theoretical foundations of acupuncture and the production of the first real acupuncture needles. The prince at Mawangdui, we can recall, was interred for eternity along with fourteen medically associated scrolls among many others not one of which contained one single reference to acupuncture. It seems safe to assume therefore that, unless he had a personal aversion to needles, it is most likely that moxibustion channel therapy was in widespread use since at least the fourth century BC or even earlier, whilst acupuncture in some simple form was added as the more modern technique some time during the mid to late second century BC[19].

As might be expected, there are plenty of references in the *Suwen* to earlier texts which imply that some form of proto-acupuncture may well have existed, although we will shortly speculate as to whether this was actually possible for technical reasons. There is also evidence of distinct "schools" of medicine already being in existence in the early Han. Working from the bibliological records of the Han librarians, David Keegan, an American scholar, hypothesises that there may have been at least three separate schools in existence. All of them, by definition, must have either survived the pyromantics of the *Qin* or have been invented afterwards – but whichever was the case it would appear that two of them fell into disuse within a couple of centuries. Keegan lists these three schools as the "*Huang Di* school", the "*Bian Que* school" and the "*Bai Shi* (Mister White)" school. Unfortunately, it appears either that almost all of the texts associated with them were subsequently lost, or that they were literally and metaphorically overwritten by the dominant surviving doctrines of the "*Huang Di* school" exemplified in the *Nei Jing* texts. Unfortunately, unless a serendipitous archaeological discovery reveals otherwise, we may never know more, although these references to other texts provide fertile ground for speculation, something which we will shortly attempt ourselves.

What seems fairly incontrovertible is that, from the time of the earliest evidence of needle therapy, the relationship between moxibustion and acupuncture had been a close one. The original and current etymology suggests this. There is no real

---

[19] The information on the Mawangdui texts is sourced from Birch & Felt 1999 "Understanding Acupuncture"- (Churchill Livingstone), and Bai Xinghua 2001 "Acupuncture, a Visible Holism" - (Butterworth Heinemann)

commonly used literal equivalent word for "acupuncture" in Chinese; what we in the West call "acupuncture" is invariably written using two characters 針灸. This is spoken as *zhen jiu* in pinyin Mandarin, *jung gal* in Cantonese, or *shin kyu* in Japanese. The first character represents the metal needle, and the second something which is matured or enduring and is burnt by fire, therefore a much more representative translation of this compound vernacular term *zhen jiu* is often suggested as simply "acumoxa"[20]. A similar composite exists in Korean, *chimgu* and the Korean characters for them are 침구.

In earlier texts alternative compound characters had been used – *ci jiu* (or puncturing-moxa), for instance, and *zhen ai* (needle-mugwort). Intriguingly, according to Yamada[21], in one Eastern Han text (the *Wuwei Han Dai Yi Jian*) excavated in 1972, the use of both *jiu ci* and *zhen jiu* actually refer mainly to moxibustion practice, whilst in another Eastern Han text, the *Jiu Ci Jue*, the two therapies were treated pretty equally. This last text was part of a Daoist Canon, the *Tai Ping Jing*. From this it seems likely that none of these composite terms need be taken completely literally.

The Origins of the Chinese Character *jiu* 灸

This character for *jiu* (moxibustion or cauterisation) deserves some elaboration. The lower part of the character 灸 is the radical ideogram for fire, while the upper part represents something which is "old and twisted" or "bent" (like an old man's back) and is sometimes interpreted as being "matured" or "enduring". This upper part invites speculation, particularly because in those earliest Mawangdui texts the character *jiu* was written simply using this upper part without the fire radical beneath. It may therefore tell us something more about the earliest use of moxa. Wilcox, however, persuasively suggests that it is also quite possible that the upper part 久 was just an abbreviation for the whole character 灸 at a time when the radicals were often optional.

So is this "old and twisted" or "bent" stuff an indicator purely of age, an implicit reference to the ageing process in moxa's production, something which is evidenced by the literature right back to the fourth century BC? Or is it simply an indicator of the "twisting" of the nap to make small cones? Alternatively, is it a reference to the common practice of burning moxa on a patient's bent back, as we

---

[20] Whilst this term "*zhenjiu*" does not seem to have been in as wide a use as it has become subsequently when looked for in the *Suwen*, *Lingshu*, or *Jia Yi Jing*, it was in use nevertheless at the time, including in Sima Qian's *Shiji* of 90BC (although this text significantly fails to mention either the *Suwen* or *Nei Jing* by name).

[21] Keiji Yamada 1998 "The origins of acupuncture, moxibustion, and decoction" - (Kyoto Nichibunken: International Research Centre for Japanese Studies).

shall encounter quite graphically when we look at the practice of moxibustion on Bl43 *Gaohuang shu*, for instance, or on the Four Flowers[22]? Or could it be a hint from the ancients as to the apparent long-term cumulative effects from its repeated use in treating chronic disease, or of its suitability as a treatment for the more senior citizen (although this is certainly not evident from the surviving literature until Tang times)? Or is it merely a reference to the mugwort plant itself from which moxa is processed? At maturation this plant, stands awkwardly crooked and has been associated with the bent stature of a human. There is a wonderful slightly archaic idiom in Japanese – *asa-no-naka-no-yomogi*, which literally translates as "the mugwort amongst the field of hemp", a saying which perfectly exploits in metaphor the plant's normal lopsided stature after flowering, suggesting that even the most crooked person, if surrounded by good people, might struggle to straighten up as mugwort can be found to straighten when found growing in a field of hemp, or stand crooked forever.

We may never know exactly what was truly intended in this character – and we can quite reasonably conclude that it has meant different meaningful things to different users of the treatment across the centuries. It is posited in the *Shuo Wen Jie Zi*, an important Han dynasty dictionary of etymology, that the verb *jiu* 灸 originally referred to the application of heat to the shell of a tortoise or to an ox-bone for the purpose of oracular divination, a practice that was carried out for the guidance of the dynastic rulers of the Shang dynasty prior to 1000 BC. Like much of early Chinese history, this practice has only been fully revealed and interpreted by archaeological findings in the twentieth century[23], quite possibly allowing us a deeper perspective on the subject today than was ever available to the Han etymologists two thousand years ago.

Typically, part of the scapula of an ox or the belly shell of a tortoise was used for such divination. A hole or a deep hollow would be drilled into a selected piece of either material and then intense heat would be applied into the hole. It has occasionally been suggested that this was done by inserting twists of mugwort but this is by no means generally accepted as being the method used, more likely it being done by inserting a burning rod into the shell. However the heatmay haveactuallybeen applied, it was intended that it should crack the bone or shell and that the resulting pattern would then be interpreted. The result of each divination was then carved on to the bone or shell, allowing it to be studied by sinologists three millennia later. These earliest examples of writing in China are known today as "Oracle Bone Inscriptions". Given the high temperature that we know mugwort burns at (see Part 4 the Stems), it has to be said that the idea of

---

[22] Neither practice is recorded in extant literature until at least the Tang, but this does not necessarily rule out the possibility that moxibustion on the back was the most common approach to the therapy in earlier times.

[23] These inscriptions were first identified as writing by an antiquarian scholar in 1899, although farmers had been finding them for many years before this in Henan Province.

mugwort being used in this process would actually make some sense. If this was in fact mugwort, it surely casts extra contrast on the significance of mugwort in the extraordinary story of Chinese civilisation.

And if this was so, it also places the possible origins of moxibustion squarely back many centuries earlier than we have so far suggested, and renders the use of this character at once both more mundane and more mysterious – a contemporary modernisation of a verb which meant applying heat with mugwort for a very specific purpose. All of a sudden, the character is thus enriched by an association with the world of the arcane or semi-occult at the very heart of Shang civilisation. More basically, however, the original etymology of the character 灸 may not be much more than an archaic representation of heat being applied either to the shell of a tortoise or to a shoulder bone of an ox, with the "old man's back" interpretation of *jiu* 久 itself representing no more than a scapula or a tortoise plastron.

The words "moxa" or "moxibustion", as we have them in English, pose their own set of problems, not least of which relate to the fact that they have no relationship to any related word in Chinese. Modern scholars, when presented with this character *jiu* 灸 whilst translating the old texts, tend to favour the word "cautery" or "mini-cautery". There are good reasons for this, but whilst they may linguistically and etymologically serve us as technically preferable translations, this logically leaves us with the optimal literal translations of *zhenjiu* as "needle-cautery" which seems unlikely ever to have much appeal. In what follows we therefore adopt the lower-brow option of using the words "moxa" and "moxibustion" with the intention of reducing confusion.

The Word "Moxa" and the Dutch East India Company

The origin and use of the word itself is a little confusing. In English, "moxa" is often used to mean both the treatment and the material, but in Chinese they are totally separate words. In Chinese, *jiu* 灸 means the treatment, but it does not specify the materials used. A*i* 艾 is the Chinese for mugwort, the most common material for moxibustion, which itself has come to be known as "moxa" in English.

Be that as it may, the origins of the word "moxa" itself give us further indications as to where our deeper investigations will take us. Whilst the word "moxa" (the noun of the processed material used in moxibustion) would raise no immediate recognition in a native speaking Chinese, there may have vague familiarity for a Japanese, since it is popularly understood to have evolved from a corruption of the Japanese word *mogusa* 艾 meaning a "herb which burns" (from the intransitive verb "*mueru*" to burn and the noun "*kusa*" a herb). This is processed from *yomogi*

蓬[24] or mugwort (*Artemisia vulgaris latiflora* or other mugwort types) which provides the therapy's raw material.

It is also proposed, it should be added, that the root of the word may also come from the verb *"momeru"* to knead, suggestive of the way the herb is ground and sieved, and how the cones are rolled into requisite shapes before burning.

This takes us only part of the way, however, since the therapeutic practice of burning the herb is known today in Japan by the word *kyuji* (moxa treatment) – or (with the typically Japanese application of the honorific prefix *"o"* as a mark of rendering something special) *o-kyu* or "honourable moxa"[25]. This word "moxa" (latinised to "moxibustion") was actually first used by Herman Busschof, a Dutch clergyman, who published a report about it (*Het Podagra*), published in Amsterdam in 1674.

His report described the successful treatment of his gout through the application and burning of a "wool-like" substance on his knee whilst he was living in Jakarta, Java[26]. Jakarta was then known as Batavia, the East Indian headquarters of the Dutch colonialists[27]. *"Podagra"* was a word widely used at the time in Europe to describe gout in the foot. Busschof described his treatment as being carried out by a female doctor (he called her an "Indian doctress") who came from Quinam, in what is now Northern Vietnam. Busschof, furthermore, enterprisingly provided a small monopolised supply of this mysterious "moxa" material (which remained unidentified) for sale in Europe via his son, thus stimulating a contemporary interest in its exact nature, although he failed to identify what the material was actually derived from, implying that it was a closely guarded secret.

So exactly why might a Japanese word have been used by a Vietnamese doctor in Java? The story persists that Busschof simply adapted the word from the Japanese *mogusa* – but how and why did he do so when he was a good two and a half thousand miles away from Japan?

---

[24] Actually the same Japanese kanji character 艾 is often used for *yomogi* as well *as mogusa*, as a result of which the phonetic hiragana "spelling" of *mogusa* is popularly used to avoid confusions in modern Japanese.

[25] *Kyu* was (significantly perhaps) the word which Bashō used in 1689 to describe applying moxa to his leg before setting out on his epic journey to Matsushima.

[26] It should be noted that, despite the title of the tract, Busschof did not endorse moxibustion merely for the treatment of gout. He also mentioned it for the treatment of toothache, catalepsy and for "falling sickness", and also catalogued the successful cure of insanity with one of his slaves.

[27] Adding another littke twist to our story, Batavia was actually renamed Jakarta during its occupation by the Japanese in 1942.

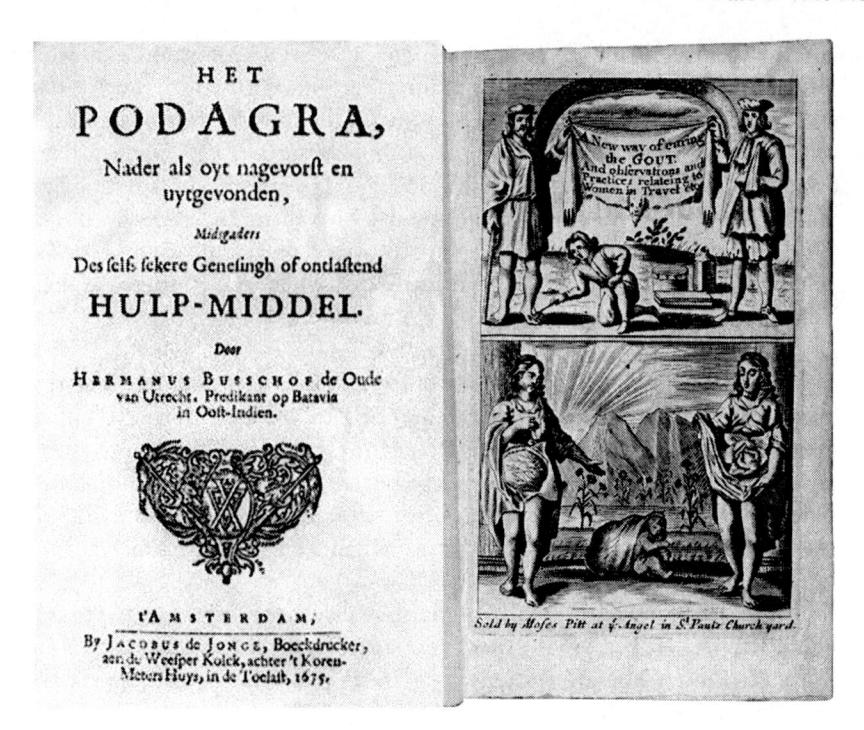

Busschof's text (left – the Dutch frontispiece, and right – a page from the English version)

This seems to be a valid question. Perhaps it was simply that "Japanese moxa", as the German Joseph Cleyer, another adventurer and employee of the Dutch in the East Indies, who was to further describe the material a few years later, was simply the finest quality moxa being traded in East Asia at the time, and was accordingly being widely exported around the shores of the South China Sea. But this does not seem to be the case at least as far as Busschof was concerned, for, although he claimed not to know what the exact material was, he explicitly wrote that the premium moxa was Chinese: "The Chineses do herein far excel the Japoneses; as they also do in preparing and conserving all other sorts of Medicines."

Certainly Java was already the established centre for Dutch trade around East Asia, and the Dutch did have links from there with both Japan and China. But what is curious is that both China and Vietnam are very much nearer than Japan is to Java, so why didn't Busschof pick up a Chinese or even a Vietnamese word?

Perhaps there's a little more to this simple version of events and we will review this small mystery more fully later.

It was an alluring trinity of spices that had drawn the Dutch (and thus also our good Reverend Busschof) to the East Indies – that of pepper, cloves and nutmeg. The spice trade had been initially monopolised by the catholic Portuguese with records of immense profit of as much as 30,000% on a single successful cargo. This trade was initially made available to the Portuguese thanks to the magnanimity of the Papal Donation of 1493 (a year after Columbus's discovery of the West Indies) which had divided the then-known world westwards and eastwards respectively between the kingdoms of Spain and Portugal. This Papal Bull was made by the Spanish Borgia Pope Alexander VI, one of the most controversial pontiffs of his and possibly any age. He favoured his native Spain to the tune of awarding them what he believed to be all of the recently discovered New World in thanks for their support of his own papal military ambitions. The Spanish thus lucked into the gold of the Americas, whilst the Portuguese defaulted into the lucrative spice trade.

It was, incidentally, because of this same Papal Donation and the fact that the most easterly coasts of South America extended to the east of this dividing line that Portuguese is now spoken in Brazil today. The Portuguese took the opportunity to capitalise on this unexpected geographic anomaly and settled this coast since it lay on their side of the line – something which had evidently not been anticipated by Pope Alexander VI, and nor indeed by the Spanish.

Changes in European religious demographics were soon to impinge on the Portuguese East Asian monopoly, however. In 1579, a century after the Donation, the protestant Dutch liberated themselves from the yoke of catholic Spain and formed an independent Netherlands. Their emergent merchant class had no cause to respect the arbitrary whim of a Pope, and looked to snatch a share of the Portuguese spice trade monopoly, losing little time in developing the means to do so. In 1602 the Dutch government formally and historically chartered the Dutch East India Company, the Vereenigde Oost-Indische Compagnie or VOC. The original company directors, the "gentlemen seventeen" as they were famously known, unfortunately found themselves effectively unable to finance this immensely ambitious project on their own, however, nor could they dare to bear the financial risk of failure of a single voyage, and so they innovatively invented the idea of inviting shareholders to help fund the fleets which they planned to send eastwards. The promise of a lucrative 400% profit was tempting enoughfor wealthy investors to share this risk, and the scene was thus set for one of the biggest commercial enterprises in history – the Dutch adventure in East Asia. It also marked the birth of joint stock shareholding and venture capitalism as we know them both today.

The dominance of the Dutch in East Asia at the time of Busschof's residence in Batavia was still quite new – the first tentative Dutch expedition to the east only having taken place in 1596 and the VOC only having been founded in 1602. It had been quickly recognised back in Amsterdam that a regional headquarters was needed, a location for victualling, for making repairs, or for simple rest and recuperation, but also more importantly a port which might act as the hub for further trade and exploration. Batavia was the site that was chosen, initially being founded in 1618.

Its founder was one of the first governor generals of the Company, the legendarily ruthless Jan Pieterszoon Coen whose figure still casts dark shadows over some islands in the Indonesian archipelago to this day. One advantage of its location was that the outpost could be reached by means of the trade winds directly from the Cape of South Africa, thus avoiding possible complications from either Portuguese or British competition in the Arabian Sea and around the coast of India. Seasonal easterly trade winds would take the ships straight across the Indian Ocean towards Australia, hooking northwards towards the end of the voyage towards Batavia.

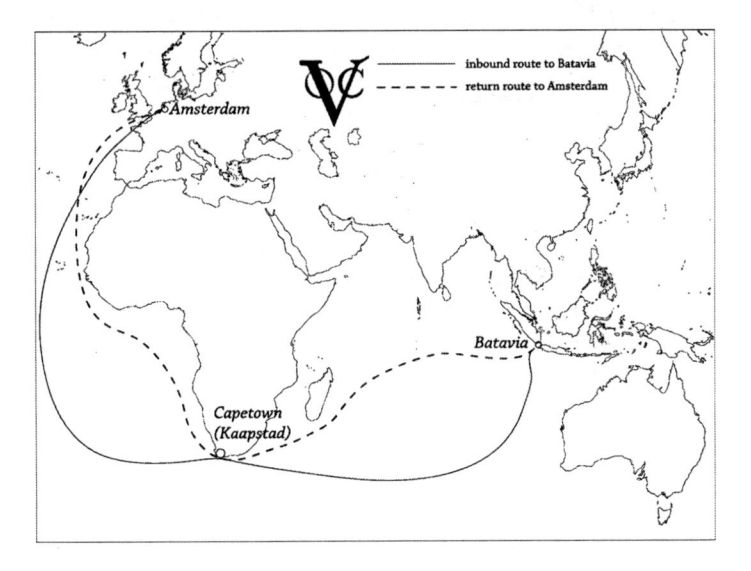

Map showing sailing routes used outbound and inbound to Batavia via Capetown

It was a long three month voyage out of sight of land, however, and one far from devoid of risk. Approaching the Sunda Straits after months at sea with the promise of final landfall, those grateful early colonialists must have thanked their protestant God for their deliverance from the long ocean passage, even as they passed by the island of Krakatoa in the approaches to the Sunda Straits a mere 80 miles from Batavia itself.

This eastern outpost grew quickly, becoming the epicentre of a wider hub-and-spoke trading operation around East Asia with the VOC involving itself not only in importing spices back to Europe but also more widely becoming the carriers in mutual trading between other East Asian countries. The port rapidly developed into what was to become known as the "Queen of the East". In 1673, just a year before Busschof's publication, a census had been taken, and it credited the fortified square mile of Batavia with housing 27,000 inhabitants, only 2,000 of whom were Dutch. Amongst the rest there were Chinese, *Mardijkers* (Portuguese speaking Indians and Malaccans), Macassarese, Balinese, Keralanese, Tamils, and Burmese. Of specific interest to the story of moxa, however, is the fact that the only reference to Japanese in the census was a mention of a few mercenary soldiers brought in to do guard duty. A full sixty percent of the total population, it should be added, were slaves. There can be no question that this is strong evidence of a lack of direct contact with Japan and with the Japanese at the time.

In fact, a tiny outlying VOC trading outpost in Japan itself **had** also been established as early as 1609, a decade or so earlier even than the founding of Batavia. It was, spawned from a disastrous attempt at circumnavigation by a Dutch fleet in 1600. The expedition's last eighteen sorry survivors had washed up on Japanese shores, but had managed to swiftly impress the Shogun nevertheless. Firstly they appeared much less interested in converting Japanese people to Christianity than the eager Portuguese Jesuits had been, but secondly they also had some rather useful weaponry on board their wrecked ship. The cannons were salvaged from the wreck of their ship and then quickly put to productive use in a military campaign with the Dutch as military advisors. The campaign was successful, leaving the Shogun very positively predisposed to befriending any subsequent Dutch traders – although they were still severely restricted in their activities. A tiny outpost was thus established by the VOC to attempt to exploit the existing (and significant) flourishing trading partnership specifically between Japan and Vietnam, something which had only recently developed. Several factors were at work: firstly the banning of Chinese citizens from trading directly with the Japanese by order of the Ming emperor; secondly by the closure of Japan itself to foreigners apart from the Dutch at Deshima; and thirdly the total ban of Japanese from leaving Japan itself.

China, particularly on its south-eastern coast, had been suffering for years from constant raids by Japanese pirates who are recorded as sacking towns and cities on the coast and carrying off citizens for ransom. By the end of the sixteenth century these raids had formalised into a full blown war between the two countries, a war which was fought mainly in Korea, culminating in a consequent Chinese ban on trade with Japan.

This trading ban effectively strangled the voracious Japanese appetite for Chinese silk, but commerce invariably finds its own creative way to satisfy such a demand, and the use of an intermediary neutral trading post in the shape of the Vietnamese port of Hội An had provided just the answer. Hội An was actually the largest port at this time in Vietnam. Thus for a short period in the seventeenth century a vibrant trading route between Japan and Vietnam had been created.

By the early seventeenth century a substantial Japanese quarter (known as a *nihonmachi*) had grown up in Hội An to house the seasonal influx of Japanese traders, and it is recorded that the Japanese and Vietnamese (and Chinese) mixed there quite amicably. The Japanese arrived each spring with their ships' holds full of devalued or banned Japanese coinage, and stayed for several months awaiting the return of the trade wind to take their ships home in late summer, carrying cargoes of Chinese silk, sugar, spices and sandalwood.

Today the port is long since silted up, but a small and picturesque city survives and has now been granted the status of a world heritage site. It contains the so-called "Japanese Bridge", also poetically known as *Lai Vien Kieu* (the "Bridge of Friends from Afar") which might suggest that it marked the entrance to the quarter's main street, but unfortunately it is not built in a style that is definitively Japanese and it is not actually known today which part of the city comprised the *nihonmachi* of four centuries ago.

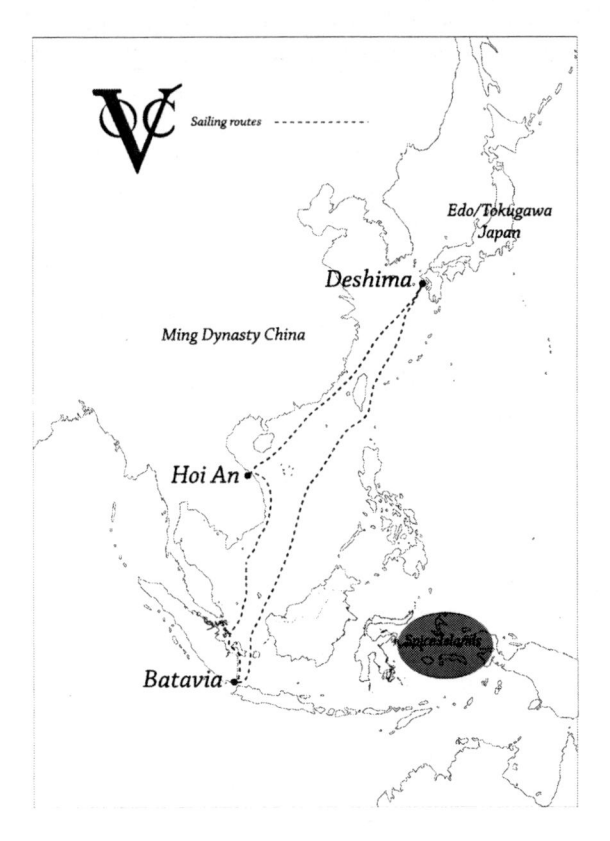

Map of seasonal trading routes between Batavia, Vietnam, and Japan

It was inevitable that from 1619 after the founding of Batavia in Java as the VOC headquarters, direct links would be established between Hội An in Vietnam and Batavia itself as the VOC grew to become as much a trader between countries in East Asia as it was an importer of spices to Europe. The earlier decades of the century had proved problematic in this regard but it briefly became a very profitable port for the Dutch. They set up a post there in 1636, the very year before the Shogun closed down his country for the next two hundred years to everyone except the Dutch, and denied the right of his people to travel outside of Japan. The Japanese community in Hội An dwindled almost immediately, and the Dutch were thus able to capitalise for a few short decades on this trade route themselves, sailing direct between Vietnam and their tiny trading outposts in Japan itself, first at Hirado and later at Deshima, in much the same way that the Japanese fleets had done previously.

At Busschof's time, two much needed Company hospitals existed back in Java but supplies of drugs were expensive and their application risky, particularly because of the understandable unfamiliarity of the Dutch traders with the newly encountered virulent tropical diseases. Utilising or adapting local resources and local physicians must have held some considerable attraction. Busschof's gout, however, was far from tropical. Its cause can be found in a declaration made by the founder of Batavia Jan Pieterszoon Coen himself. "Our nation must drink or die," he famously declaimed.

The average Dutchman in Batavia was said to have taken his (or her) first neat glass of genever gin before breakfast, and would continue throughout the rest of the day with regular glasses of local arack spirit. Poor Busschof had found himself in agony from his gout, and was persuaded by his wife to be administered to by a Vietnamese female physician who had treated some of their slaves as well as his daughter. We can guess that the "doctress" herself had suggested to Mrs Busschof that she might be able to ease the reverend's distress. Initially Busschof had refused the treatment, not liking the idea of the "caustick", but his ongoing agony led him to change his mind. After he had received his treatment from this physician whom he misleadingly described as an "Indian doctress" (and who we can reasonably assume had come to Batavia herself from Hội An on a VOC ship) the alcoholic reverend miraculously found himself relieved of his pain.

"Having demanded a lighted candle," he wrote "and solicitously search'd for that part of the place affected where the greatest pain was: And thereupon she burned with her *Moxa* (of which hereafter) on my feet and knees, (to my best remembrance) about twenty little Escars, which looked like little gray specks, without raising any blisters, or causing any after-pain; whereupon also all the pain of the Gout vanish'd. ... most heartily thanking God Almighty for his goodness to me, and duly acknowledging the operation of this Indian woman, admiring withal the powerfulness of this remedy against so contumacious an evil, as is the Gout[28]."

Unfortunately the mysterious "doctress" is also recorded as having died "not long after" and so she vanishes from the story. Busschof himself, incidentally, only survived the publication of his tract by a couple of years.

---

[28] "To the Reader" in Herman Busschof and Hendrick Roonhuyse's "Two Treatises, the One Medical,of the Gout, and Its Nature More Narrowly Search'd into Than Hitherto; Together with a New Way ofDischarging the Same / by Herman Busschof Senior, of Utrecht, Residing at Batavia in the East-Indies, in the Service of the Dutch East-India Company. The Other Partly Chirurgical, Partly Medical ... By Henry Van Roonhuyse" (1676). Bussschof's contribution was the translated version of the *Het Podagra* tract, anonymously "englished out of the Dutch by a careful hand."

Actually, it may be a gross slander to assume that the reverend was simply afflicted by gout because of his drinking habits, though the likelihood does exist given the habits of the times. What is quiet clear, however, is that he was also a thorough and well-read scholar. His text[29] not only discusses moxa for the treatment of gout, but also discusses the affliction itself with some authority, particularly in terms of its causes and effects. He ascribed its cause primarily to dampness quoting various authorities, and suggested that "this evil [gout] raigns as well in those parts of the world [China and Japan] as in Europe, and even among the Hottentots on the Cape of Good Hope."

He waxed lyrically on moxibustion itself. "This art is by those nations (Chineses and Japoneses) so valued that they will not for any mony communicate it to other Nations, but do keep it for a great secret". Whether this was true is debatable, of course, but further on he elaborated further, claiming that they "carry it in whole bales through those vast empires."

He suggested that it could help not just with gout, but also with "Head-pains, Tooth-ach, Pleurisies, Colick and even the Falling Sickness," although he believed that all of these were caused by a similar dampness as caused *Podagra*. His description of the cure oftheir "mad Female-Slave" Ursula is particularly vivid. She was struck by sudden insanity after encountering a drowned corpse in the harbour whilst out buying fish. The doctress, assisted by other slaves to hold poor Ursula down, applied moxa to her head and neck after which she fell asleep and awoke fully cured.

He described how the wool-like moxa "catches fire sooner than any tinder" but only "causes a little grey speck [escar] at the site of the burn," which he was adamant should be allowed to drop off naturally, often helped by covering it with "vegetable plaisters."

On dosage, he was equally clear: "Ordinarily thrice upon the weak and tender limb; but upon other places, if need be, so often till the pain be removed, although you should (for example in sciatica) on one and the same place kindle 25, yea, 50 pellets."

As far as point location was concerned he referred back to Hippocrates: "And here the rule of Hippocrates must be applied: Burn where the pain is." He developed this idea a little further, however, suggesting that the tender area should be palpated to identify the most painful location.

---

[29] The following excerpts from Busshof's tract are sourced from Kyushu University's Institutional Repository, accessed via https://qir.kyushu-u.ac.jp/dspace/bitstream/2324/2936/4/Buschoff_1676_hi_res.pdf on 30/10/2010.

As for the practitioner, he rather wonderfully described how she should be "a person of good sight, not unwieldy of body, having steady and dry, not trembling nor sweaty hands."

Moxa arrives in Europe

He must have thought that both he and the VOC might be on to something special and hurriedly wrote and sent his paper back to his son in Utrecht along with a good supply of moxa suggesting that it "will be worth the while, since it will prove a gainful commodity in Europe and be of no burthen in the ships."

He favourably compared the efficacy of moxa treatment to the treatment prescribed by Hippocrates himself which could take as long as forty days to take effect: "But this our moxa, by means of burning described, draws this wolf with speed out of his den, and delivers the patient instantly from his pains and anguish." Tellingly, in the Dutch version, at its end there was an advertisement telling the reader how moxa might be obtained (from Busschof's brother). In the English version, the same advertisement said it could be obtained from a bookseller at St Paul's in London[30].

Back in Europe two years later, the English diplomat and essayist, Sir William Temple (1629-1699), picked up on the treatment in The Hague[31]. In 1676, about to depart to help in negotiating a peace treaty at Nijmegen between the Dutch and the French, he found himself incapacitated by the same dreaded gout. He described its cure in detail in "An Essay upon the Cure of the Gout" and actually bought some of the still mysterious moxa moss directly from Busschof's son.

"Monsieur Zulichem came to see me (among the rest of my friends) who, I think, never came into company without saying something that was new, and so he did upon my occasion. For, talking of my illness, and approving of my obstinacy against all the common prescriptions; he asked me, whether I had never heard the Indian way of curing the gout by Moxa? I told him no; and asked him what it was? He said it was a certain kind of moss that grew in the East-Indies; that their way was, whenever any body fell into a fit of the gout, to take a small quantity of it,

---

[30] The bookseller was Moses Pitt, who, subsequent to his own imprisonment following bankruptcy wrote the heartfelt "The Cry of the Oppressed: Being a True and Tragical Account of the Unparallel'd Sufferings of Multitudes of Poor Imprison'd Debtors In Most of the Gaols in England".

[31] For the account of Sir William Temple's experience of moxibustion I am indebted to the thesis of Ruben E. Verwaal2009 entitled "Hippocratesmeetsthe Yellow Emperor **On the Reception of Chinese and Japanese Medicine in EarlyModern Europe"** retrieved from the internet in August 2011http://igitur-archive.library.uu.nl/student-theses/2010-0812-200203/Verwaal

and form it into a figure broad at bottom as a two-pence, and pointed at top; to set the bottom exactly upon the place where the violence of the pain was fixed; then with a small round perfumed match (made likewise in the Indies) to give fire to the top of the moss; which burning down by degrees, came at length to the skin, and burnt it till the moss was consumed to ashes: that many times the first burning would remove the pain; if not, it was to be renewed a second, third, and fourth time, till it went away, and till the person found he could set his foot boldly to the ground and walk….

"Next morning I looked over the book which Monsieur Zulichem[32] had promised me, written by the Minister at Batavia..And the author affirms it happens often there, that upon the last burning, an extreme stench comes out of the skin where the fire had opened it…..

"I was confirmed in this resolution by a German physician, Doctor Theodore Coledy, who was then in my family, a sober and intelligent man, whom I dispatched immediately to Utrecht, to bring me some of the Moxa, and learn the exact method of using it, from the man that sold it, who was son to the Minister of Batavia. He returned with all that belonged to this cure, having performed the whole operation upon his hand by the man's direction. I immediately made the experiment in the manner before related, setting the Moxa just upon the place where the first violence of my pain began, which was the joint of the great toe, and where the greatest anger and soreness still continued, notwithstanding the swelling of my foot, so that I had never yet, in five days, been able to stir it, but as it was lifted….

"Upon the first burning, I found the skin shrink all round the place; and whether the greater pain of the fire had taken away the sense of a smaller one or no, I could not tell; but I thought it less than it was: I burnt it the second time, and upon it observed the skin about it to shrink, and the swelling to flat yet more than at first. I began to move my toe, which I had not done before; but I found some remainders of pain. I burnt it the third time, and observed still the same effects without, but a much greater within; for I stirred the joint several times at ease; and, growing bolder, I set my foot to the ground without any pain at all. After this, I pursued the method prescribed by the book; and the author's son at Utrecht, and had a bruised clove of garlic laid to the place that was burnt, and covered with a large plaister of Diapalma, to keep it fixed there; and when this was done, feeling no more pain, and treading still bolder and firmer upon it, I cut a slipper to let in my foot, swelled as it was, and walked half a dozen turns about the room, without any pain or trouble, and much to the surprise of those that were about me, as well as to my own."

---

[32] Diplomat and poet Sir Constantijn Huygens de Zulichem.

It will be noted that the two treatments (of Busschof and of Temple) differed a little in terms of cone size and overall approach.

A German physician, Andreas Cleyer, was the next to significantly contribute to the subject three years later in 1679. Cleyer is a perplexing character. He appears to have arrived in East Asia as a soldier of the VOC but subsequently rose to the rank of physician and also of rector, altogether a curious combination of professions but suggestive perhaps of the extraordinary opportunities that must have been open to those who dared to take them at the time. It seems reasonable to suggest that he was something of an adventurer. At one stage he was actually in charge of the tiny VOC trading outpost at Deshima in Japan, but was expelled by the Japanese because of problems with smuggling. It is far from difficult to believe that he may have had a personal hand in it.

Cleyer definitively identified for Europe that this curious material was not just "moxa" but was "Japanese moxa". Busschof had not actually identified it as being Japanese at all in his original text, as a result of which it was being referred to back in Europe merely as "ost-indische Wolle" by those parties most interested in it. Cleyer further revealed that it was made from the dried and "hackled" leaves of the mugwort plant, and further stated that a particular preparation and processing of the material seemed to be important for its efficacy. Cleyer had been encouraged in this research by the *"Collegium Naturae Curiosorum"*, an academic German society of which he was a member. This society had picked up on Busschof's earlier report, and had even debated whether the *materia medica* of this as-yet unknown plant material were essential for the reported effects or whether it was simply the heat itself which provided its mechanism of effect. As we will see in later sections, this is something which remains not totally clear to this day.

Up until Cleyer's publication opinion was split about what exactly this "wool" was. The Dutch naturalist Anthoni van Leeuwenhoek had started to investigate the exotic plant "out of curiosity only" in 1677. He wrote: "I have more than once examined this *Moxa* by my Microscope, and do not find it to be such a curious preparation of an excellent dryed herb; but that 'tis only some lanuginose expiration or protrusion of a fruit, such as is the *lanugo* seen upon a Peach, Quince, or the like; and I was of opinion, that I might have gather'd very near the like substance from some herbs; but that I have hitherto failed of." It seems reasonable to assume from this that the moxa which Busschof had sent back to Europe was highly refined with little in the way of extraneous leaf matter visible to Van Leuwenhook's microscope.

Cleyer may have simply reported his findings as part of his responsibilities for supplying the two pharmacies in Java. Clearly, however, there were also commercial possibilities in this newly identified commodity. If the source of a new remedy for a gout-ridden Europe could be secured for the company, it could doubtless further add to company and shareholder profits as well as his own wealth, something which seems to have also already occurred to the Reverend Busschof and his son.

The earlier Portuguese Reports

In fact, if only they had known it, descriptions of this mysterious therapy had actually already come back quite independently to Europe via Jesuit missionaries nearly a century earlier and they had even correctly identified mugwort, but these reports had been ignored – perhaps because of the lack of any motive (commercial or otherwise) to investigate them further. Treatments describing the use of "herbal fire-buttons" were reported in letters sent back to Portugal in 1584, a full decade even before the first Dutch expedition to East Asia and a full ninety years before Busshcof's famous tract. In the following year, 1585, Luis Frois, one of the leading Jesuit missionaries in Japan at the time, described how he had "over three thousand fire buttons" made from leaves into pellets "the size of large pomegranate seeds" burnt on his back and his knees to treat a variety of pains as well as his eye disease.

These Jesuit descriptions, incidentally, reflected a contemporary European practice with which the missionaries would already have been familiar – that of cauterisation. Moxibustion, actually, (as already mentioned) is sometimes described as "mini-cautery" or "moxa cautery", and is quite possibly better translated as such. Cautery itself, however, was a technique well known in Europe, occasionally known by the actual words "button cautery", which defined a treatment when a small iron disk about 6mm thick and 12mm in diameter was heated and applied to the skin. Hence the descriptor naturally chosen by the Jesuits of "herbal fire buttons" was something that would be instantaneously recognisable to a European reader.

In 1601, a Franciscan report from the Japanese archipelago succinctly summed up the use of these herbal fire buttons: "With this procedure they burn the flesh with small balls which look like wool, until a blister develops. They ease many sufferings by this means, because they say that all diseases are caused by coolness[33]."

The constituent material of the "herbal fire buttons" was definitively identified as mugwort as early as in 1604 (a full seventy years before Reverend Busschof's report and the coining of the word "moxa") in the supplement to the Jesuit dictionary *Vocabulario da Lingow de Iapam*. There were several Japanese words quoted in it to describe the treatment (*mogusa, kyuji, yaito, yaihi*), though none of

---

[33] Wolfgang Michel 1993 "Fruehe westliche Beobachtungen zur Moxibustion und Akupunktur" (Sudhofs Archiv Vol 77 No2 - in German)

them at that time had passed into the European vernacular as happened after Busschof's text in 1674.

Listing over thirty-two thousand Japanese words, including some thirteen hundred alone from the field of medicine, this huge dictionary of 1604 was the first instance that the word *mogusa* appeared in a Western reference book. There had in fact been even earlier descriptions of the herbal *botao de fogo* (the herbal fire buttons) in dictionaries, histories and letters from both Jesuits and Franciscans in Japan prior to this, however. It seems curious that none of these had used this particular word *mogusa*. The slightly earlier and more modest Japanese-Latin-Portuguese dictionary of 1595, for instance, included both *yaito* and *kyuji* in relation to moxibustion, but omitted *mogusa* from its inclusion of eight terms from the field of acumoxa. The great poet Bashō, incidentally, used *kyu* rather than *mogusa* to describe burning moxa on his leg in 1694. We might conclude from this that *mogusa* was only one of several contemporary words used to describe moxibustion at the time, and it may well not have been the most widely used or perhaps was used only regionally. Literary references in Japanese prior to this, in *Waka* poems[34] for instance, used the clumsier word "*sashimogusa*" (さし藻草)[35] to describe mugwort for cautery treatment, so it is clear that the word "*mogusa*" was indeed in some sort of use, though not necessarily in its simpler form, nor necessarily was it the most common descriptor.

(A rather wonderful archaic word for mugwort exists in Japanese; this is *tsukuroigusa* which metaphorically translates as the "herb that darns", although it seems the good Doctor Busschof would have found this too difficult to Europeanise if he had encountered it himself in Java.)

So what can we conclude from all of this about the origin of this word? It is probable that Busschof picked up the word *mogusa* from the Vietnamese "Doctress", who in turn had picked up the word from Japanese traders at Hội An in Vietnam when she had lived there possibly three decades earlier. There may be other factors, however, which we will look at shortly.

To complete this excursion into early modern medicine in Europe, meanwhile, it would appear that moxa fell out of favour within a mere thirty years of Busschof's publication. Thomas Sydenham in his work "A Treatise of the Gout and Dropsy"

---

[34] *Waka* poems are a form of Japanese poems, normally short, and often with Buddhist connotations. They date back as far as the 8th century.

[35] "*Sashimogusa*" contains the prefix verb "*sasu*", which either means to "finger" or "point", perhaps indicating the manipulation of the fingers in the rolling of the cone, or (with a different character) to "stab" or "bite", perhaps reflecting the hit of heat from direct application. The literal meaning might then render itself as "the herb which burns and bites." One other archaic meaning of "sasu" is to "light". It has actually been impossible to ascertain which meaning was implied.

all but dismissed "the *Indian* Moss, called *Moxa*, much esteemed of late for the Cure of the Gout." What is interesting, however, is that Sydenham claimed that the practice of moxibustion was not "wholly unknown to the Europeans" before it had been "received from the Oriental *Indians*". He quoted Hippocrates' "Treatise on Diseases" in which it was encouraged that crude flax could be burned when other options were exhausted. "Now," Sydenham concluded, "I suppose, none will think that there is any specifick Difference betwixt the Flame of Flax and of this *Indian* Moss[36]."

This connection with Hippocratic medicine in fact provokes another fascinating diversion which again takes us far away from East Asia.

A Diversion into the "Greek" Connections

Cauterisation in the West goes right back to the Hippocratic medicine of the 5th century BC and quite possibly earlier. Whilst not immediately seemingly relevant to the subject at hand this connection offers us the valuable opportunity for a short excursion back a full two millennia before the Dutch expansion into East Asia, an excursion which tentatively dares to cast a deeper perspective not only on the possible wider roots of the word "moxa" but even, more surprisingly, on the possible roots of moxa therapy itself. Initially, these discussions will take us away from the subject of moxibustion, but they will be found to finally return to it in a way which, it is hoped, is at least a little provocative.

Some recent scholars have attempted to identify links between these ancient Mediterranean medical traditions and the traditions of medicine both in India and China, so it may not be so completely indulgent in taking this diversion, even if the possibilities of connections may seem at first unlikely. Part of the scholastic reasoning behind making such a connection between medicinal developments at either end of Asia relates to similar developments that were taking place at the time. The newly formulated Hippocratic approaches to medicine focused on a recently developed idea of *techne* or skill, and on the beginnings of recognisable science in medical practice. It is in fact widely accepted that something similar appears to have been taking place at either end of the Eurasian landmass at around this same time. In the West, this new approach effectively displaced the previously dominant philosophies which lay behind prior medical practice in the Mediterranean basin, concepts which had been based primarily on ideas of the supernatural. It has been further suggested that this shift constituted the first dawning of the scientific age. At the end of the Warring States period in China, a similarly more scientific and technologically based medicine was also emerging,

---

[36] Busschof himself had quite favourably compared moxibustion with the "Aegyptian manner of burning" using "cotton and stramineous [strawlike] linen".

and it also was superseding the previously dominant attitudes which were more resonant with magic and demonology.

Elizabeth Craik, an eminent scholar of early Greek medicinal writings, has identified an extraordinary co-incidence: at the time of Hippocrates, his native island of Kos was not only developing as the epicentre of Hellenic medicine, but it was also the Mediterranean centre for sericulture, which used wild silk worms for raw silk production (an art that had been originally, of course, mastered and refined by the Chinese). In Kos this art was subsequently lost, and was only re-introduced into the Mediterranean a thousand years later[37].

Since sericulture indisputably originated in China, the potential for some curious if unlikely interconnection between the island of Kos and ancient East Asia implied by the simple fact that raw silk was being produced in Kos does definitely tantalise the imagination.

The Importance of the Silk Trade

Silk was adored and coveted by both Greeks and Romans, and there had existed various fanciful theories of its origins. Pliny the Elder, in his monumental "Natural History" offered a version that, whilst not entirely accurate, clearly reflects some indirect knowledge. "The larva [of the 'bombyx'] then becomes a caterpillar, after which it assumes the state in which it is known as 'bombylis', then that called 'necydalus', and after that, in six months, it becomes a silk-worm. These insects weave webs similar to those of the spider, the material of which is used for making the more costly and luxurious garments of females, known as 'bombycina'." He then went on to less accurately attribute its very origins to Kos itself. "Pamphile, a woman of Kos, the daughter of Platea, was the first person who discovered the art of unravelling these webs and spinning a tissue therefrom; indeed, she ought not to be deprived of the glory of having discovered the art of making vestments which, while they cover a woman, at the same moment reveal her naked charms[38]."

Problematically, if we seriously wish to make a significant link between ancient Greece and China from this single fact, there is a total absence of contemporary evidence of any direct contact between the cultures. The earliest known potential direct influence from China into the Mediterranean basin was a full two centuries later – in the second century BC, when the intrepid Chinese ambassador and

---

[37] E M Craik 2004 "Knife and fire: medical practice of east and west" in *Proceedings of COE* meeting held at Kyoto November, 2003 (published as *Globalization*, Kyoto, Iwanami Shoten) pp 227–43

[38] Pliny the Elder "The Natural History" XI, 26

adventurer Zhang Qian spent more than a decade in the Near East retrieving information (including amassing data on drugs).

Quite early Mediterranean references exist, however, relating to the "Seres", the ancient name in both Greek and Roman for the inhabitants of the eastern parts Central Asia. It is a name which is also indelibly linked to silk itself. "Seres" literally means "of silk" or "the people of the land where silk comes from". The name itself is even thought by some to actually derive directly from the Chinese word itself for silk – *si* 絲. It should not be assumed, however, that these people were the Chinese themselves; it can be reasonably surmised, however, that they were the people who brought the silk out through Central Asia to trade it in Persia and even in Asia Minor itself.

The earliest known reference to the Seres, albeit of disputed authenticity, comes from Ctesias in the 5th century BC, contemporary with Hippocrates, and he mysteriously referred to them as being of "portentous stature and longevity[39]." Ctesias was a physician and historian from Caria (close to Kos) who had certainly travelled at least as far as Persia.

Pliny the Elder actually referred to them in terms of the Tarim Basin, an area just north of the Himalaya range which we will discuss in much more detail shortly. He wrote: "that beyond the Emodian Mountains (the Himalayas) they look towards the Serae (Seres), whose acquaintance they had also made in the pursuits of commerce; that the father of Rachias (the ambassador) had frequently visited their country, and that the Serae always came to meet them on their arrival. These people, they said, exceeded the ordinary human height, had flaxen hair, and blue eyes, and made an uncouth sort of noise by way of talking, having no language of their own for the purpose of communicating their thought[40]."

Early Trading across Central Asia and the Persian Empire

Any reasonable consideration of the circumstantial evidence suggests that a direct connection between China and Greece or Rome was not in any way critical for trade to have taken place. A less direct link through traders or nomads would have sufficed, from region to region, or tribe to tribe, and there is plenty of evidence of this in the archaeological record. Cowry shells, for instance, were used in Shang Dynasty China as the earliest forms of currency centuries before the earliest

---

[39] David Christian 2000 "Silk Roads or Steppe Roads? The Silk Roads in World History" (Journal of Word History, Vol 11) pp 1-26

[40] Pliny the Elder "The Natural History" XXIV http://www.perseus.tufts.edu/hopper/text?doc=Plin.+Nat.+6.24&redirect=true#note-link17 retrieved 3/1/2010

references to either moxa or acupuncture[41], and these shells are understood to have originated from as far afield as the Maldive Islands in the Arabian Sea[42]. In the same period, wheat seed arrived in China from Europe or Asia Minor. Bronze technology also percolated eastwards, as did the use of chariots in warfare.

Kos, of course, is today commonly associated with the world of the Greeks, but just before the time of Hippocrates, Kos was not part of the Greek world at all, but found itself at the Western end of the vast Achamaenid Persian Empire, only coming under Hellenic influence just before Hippocrates was born. Kos fell to Greece in 479 BC and the father of modern medicine was born only around twenty years later. The Hippocratic corpus was undeniably written in Ionic Greek, but the island of Kos actually lies close to the mainland of Asia Minor and far from the centre of Hellenic civilisation, only around five kilometres from the coast of modern Turkey and ancient Caria. So it is quite reasonable to suggest that most of its earlier cultural influences would have been from the neighbouring mainland rather than from the wider Aegean. Prior to and during Persian rule, this area was in fact recorded as being Carian controlled. The ancient city of Halicarnassus (now Bodrum) was close by on the mainland, complete with its famous mausoleum which was one of the Seven Wonders of the Ancient World. Local coastal cults and cultures may therefore have actually provided the immediate seeds of what was to become recognised as early Greek or "Hippocratic" medicine.

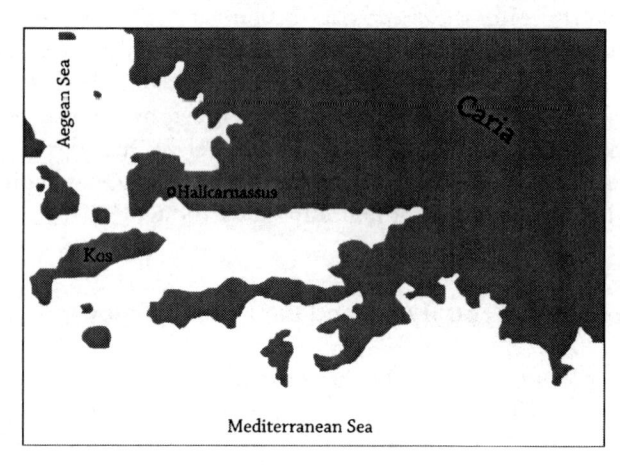

Map showing the proximity of Kos to the mainland of Asia Minor and Turkey

---

[41] Wang Yu-Ch'uan 1980 "Early Chinese Coinage"(Sanford J. Durst Numismatic Publications, New York)

[42] "The Cowrie Shell as Money" Colin Narbeth. Cowries were used as currency around the world for millennia, mostly originating from the Maldives. Europeans used them in Africa to trade for slaves. At one time in Uganda a single shell could purchase a woman slave. http://www.conchsoc.org/pages/MW_6_p19-21a.pdf retrieved 3/1/2010.

Part 1 – the Roots

During Persian domination, this area was controlled by the subjugate Carian dynasty, the most famous of whose "satrap" rulers was (by almost unbelievable co-incidence given the Latin appellation for mugwort) a warrior queen named Artemisia the First. Her fame has been passed down to us for some quite dubious reasons, however. The historian Herodotus, a local himself, recorded her escapades in the naval attack on the Greeks at Salamis in 480 BC, noting that it involved the cynical and ruthless sinking of one of her own companion ships with the loss of all hands on board in a desperate but successful measure to ensure her own ship's escape.

This rather startling coincidence in this cruel queen's name amazingly does not even end there: it was another later Carian queen with the same name (Artemisia the Second) who subsequently built the even more famous mausoleum in Halicarnassus in honour of her husband King Mausollus – a husband who was also rather shockingly her brother. It was an edifice which became known as one of the Wonders of the Ancient World. Artemisia herself grieved quite literally to death, dying two years later herself. She is said that to have mixed some of her husband-brother's ashes into her drink on a daily basis[43]. Mausollus himself had been the satrap of Caria under Persian domination between 377 and 355 BC. He ruled both the area and the neighbouring islands –even including, for a short while, wresting Kos itself back from Greece.

The Carians had a longstanding reputation as mercenary soldiers, and were recognised experts in warfare. Their prowess, for instance, had been highly valued by the pharaohs who employed them as mercenaries. When Alexander the Great conquered the Persian Empire, he is recorded as having encountered a Carian settlement close to Baghdad far to the East, and it is speculated that this was a military colony which may have been guarding the end of the trade route into the Asiatic interior (see the map of the Persian Empire and the routes of the Royal Road). The city of Opis was an ancient Babylonian city close to modern Baghdad, although its exact location today remains uncertain. It was where the road forked, the main route south-east heading to Susa, the winter capital, and the secondary road heading eastwards deep into the heart of Central Asia. Opis was therefore effectively the western end of any East-West trade route in the sixth century BC. Carian mercenaries can thus be assumed to have been well travelled all over this part of the ancient world. Whether this would have brought foreign and indeed curious influences back to their homelands (including perhaps the medical practices of central Asian nomads as we will soon suggest) remains, however, purely a matter for speculation.

The road running East from Opis ran through Ecbatana, a summer residence of the Persian kings, on to Rhagae which was a centre of Zoroastrianism (the

---

[43] Pliny the Elder suggested that the name *artemis* in connection with the plant genus is actually partly derived from this queen Artemis II – as well as from the goddess Artemis herself.

principle religion of the Achamaenids), and from there to Merv the capital of Bactria, the major oasis city at the end of the main road in what today is Turkmenistan.

This great Persian Empire was at its peak under the rule of Cyrus the Great who died around 530 BC. It stretched from the Aegean right through to the Indus, extending east into Bactria, today comprising part of Turkmenistan, Afghanistan, Tajikistan and Kirghizstan. Stability, trade and communication were key characteristics of this culture, so the idea of direct connections between Kos (or at least mainland Caria) and ancient Kabul or Samarkand in its North Eastern frontier regions can hardly be viewed as controversial.

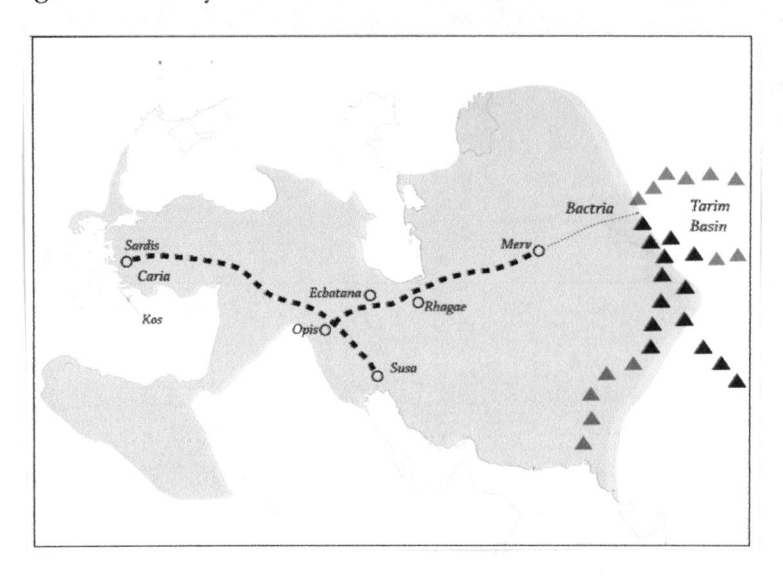

Map of the Persian Empire c. 500 BC showing its full extent from the Aegean to the Himalayas.
(The route of the "Royal Road" is shown by the dotted line)

The "Royal Road" had both postal stations and relays at regular intervals along its route. Using fresh horses, royal couriers were said to be expected to cross the entire empire from Susa to Sardis in an astonishing nine days (a distance of nearly 3,000 kilometres). Beyond Merv, however, the possibilities for trade and good communication become increasingly more tentative.

This area in the heart of Asia has since time immemorial been both link and barrier between East and West, acting as geographical, cultural and technological watersheds. It is an area which we will examine in more detail shortly. First, however, we must switch our focus further to the East.

Ancient China and its Furthermost Western Reaches

China at the time of Cyrus of Persia was much smaller in extent than later in the Han dynasty when its outer frontiers extended right out into this border zone. For centuries before the Han, however, this same Central Asian area had been well known to the Chinese for its jade. In Han times, it was also the legendary horses from what is now Kazakhstan which drew its military adventurers to the region, but the area's jade had been equally valued as much as a thousand years earlier. We can be sure of this because it is beyond dispute that the major consumers in the early jade trade from the Tarim basin were the ancient Shang rulers of agricultural China[44].

For more than a millennium jade was used in China primarily as a sacred material for religious purposes. This ancient jade was found on the surface of the soil or in riverbeds, but it was rare even then. The idea had evolved that somehow it had originally fallen from Heaven, and therefore that it had some special power imbued into it, particularly so when it was shaped into symbols which represented the deities themselves, or when it was used for funerary purposes as a preserver of previous life. In earlier times, for instance, small pieces of jade had been shaped into cicadas (the emblem of spring) and placed on the tongue of the deceased[45]. By the time of the Han this practice had developed into the magnificent jade funereal suits which have more recently been found in tombs from this period. At least since Shang times this jade was being recovered from the Tarim basin, the very desert corridor where traders, travellers, nomads or migrants from Central Asia would have completed any eastward crossing from Eurasia over the Pamir Mountains. Whether it was ever collected in such earlier times by people who might be identifiable as being Chinese or not is debatable and possibly unlikely as we shall see, but the material collected was clearly traded or taken right into the heart of early China itself.

The watershed itself is composed of a mighty range of mountains, the Pamirs, which constituted the ultimate mountain passage for travellers making their way from ancient Merv, Kabul or Samarkand over this cultural and geographical Great Divide. Coming down from the plateau, they would have found themselves at the Western end of the immense Tarim Basin itself, and would then have had to find their way north or south around the lethal Taklamaken Desert. This desert comprises the heart of the Tarim and had to be safely skirted round if they or their goods were to proceed further eastwards. The Taklamaken desert acts as an effective sink hole for the huge amounts of water flowing down off the northernmost mountains of the Himalayan Range, the Kunlun Mountains. Most

---

[44]Liu, Xinru 2001 "Migration and Settlement of the Yuezhi-Kushan. Interaction and Interdependence of Nomadic and Sedentary Societies" (Journal of World History*)* 12 (2): 261–292

[45] "China's Three Thousand Years" 1973 (Times Publications)

of the water coming down from the northern aspects of this huge range of mountains never makes it even close to an ocean, evaporating in the wastes of the desert itself or pooling into oases.

Schoolchildren in China misleadingly today learn that the "opening" of this East-West trading route popularly known as the silk road occurred in 139 BC when Zhang Qian, the Chinese ambassador-adventurer, travelled westward across the Pamirs, the first Chinese known to do so. The term "silk road" was actually first coined late in the nineteenth century by a German geographer, Baron Ferdinand von Richthofen (1833-1905) and his more accurate use of the plural form *Die Seidenstrassen* far better reflects the shifting network of routes which was used for many sorts of trade and exchange between East and West, not merely for silk. Materials passing along these routes are known to have included ceramics, glass, precious gems and livestock[46]. It is actually also quite incontrovertible that these "roads" were being regularly trodden centuries, probably millennia, earlier than Zhang's expedition.

In Roman times Pliny the Elder reported a "stone tower" which he said existed on the Pamir Plateau, a place where goods had been traditionally exchanged between traders from the East and the West. In the early second century Maës Titianus, an ancient Roman-Macedonian traveller, actually reported reaching this famous Stone Tower, but its exact location and even its existence remains uncertain. According to one theory, it was at Tashkurgan in the Pamirs. (The word Tashkurgan actually means "stone tower" or "stone fortress" in Uyghur). Scholars today, however, more generally favour somewhere in the Alay Valley, on the pass directly west of Kashgar, since Tashkurgan itself is on another high mountain pass from Kashgar southwards into what is now Pakistan[47].

Whatever the true provenance of the Stone Tower may have been, it would seem positively naïve to believe that some form of mutual exchange was not taking place in this region millennia before more formal recorded exchanges were begun, though unfortunately we have frustratingly little in the way of direct evidence of it. What does exist, however, as we will shortly see, is actually very persuasive.

Challenges to this ideado remain, however, and one of the most cogent lies simply in the scale of the geography. Travelling from West to East, the trader first had to cross the Pamirs, through their 20,000 foot high mountains. The word Pamir

---

[46] David Christian 2000 "Silk Roads or Steppe Roads? The Silk Roads in World History" (Journal of World History, Vol. 11) pp 1-26

[47] John E Hill 2009 "Through the Jade Gate to Rome: A Study of the Silk Routes during the Later Han Dynasty, First to Second Centuries" (BookSurge)

beguilingly means "wide, high grassy valleys between mountains" - but these mountains are some of the highest in the world. This name has been adopted, it would seem, because of the importance of their valleys and passes, rising to over 13,000 feet in height, rather than in relation to the mountains themselves. It provides vital clues as to this range's usefulness to nomadic herders who would have seasonally exploited this exact type of high altitude meadowland for summer pasturing; but these valleys were just as important, of course, for the traders.

If the weather in the mountains had been kind and the journey undertaken in the right season, the eastward-bound traveller would have descended thankfully into the Tarim basin, in expectation of finding welcome and sustenance at Kashgar, the ancient oasis town at the Western end of the desert.

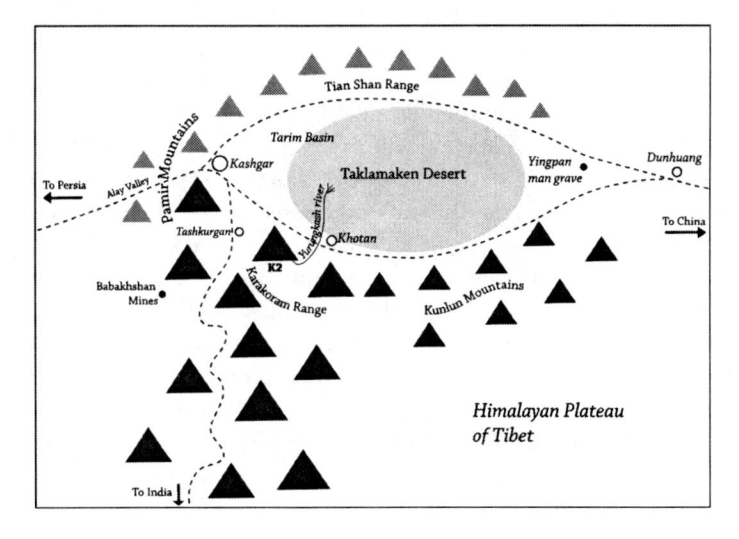

Map showing the Tarim Basin with the Pamirs and Persia to the West, the Tian Shan to the North, the Kunlun Mountains to the South, China to the East, and with the Taklamaken Desert at its heart. The key trade routes are shown in dotted lines. Key place names mentioned in the text are also identified.

Kashgar, for many travellers who had crossed the Pamirs, would be their logical turning point – the place to trade and rest, and to exchange horses or camels before a return journey back over the mountains before the winter snows set in – certainly more logical than a stone tower somewhere up in the mountains. But if the trader or traveller was to continue eastwards from Kashgar, his caravan could have only continued by skirting north or south around the deadly Taklamaken Desert. In contrast to the relatively benign literal meaning of *"pamir"* describing the summer passes through the lofty range of mountains, the name of this desert leaves no room at all for doubt – because "Taklamaken" literally means "Go in and you won't come out". The only way onwards was and still is around its edges, skirting between the searing desert heat and the northern or southern slopes of the Kunlun Shan or Tian Shan ranges respectively.

Travellers still rely to this day on the oases fed by the streams which come down from the snow fields of these mighty mountain ranges. And beyond this desert, there still would have remained eight hundred miles of perilous journey before the first true signs of Chinese civilisation might have been encountered at these earlier times.

What is of interest not only to the story of this trade route but also possibly to the story of moxibustion is that mummies have been found well preserved in this arid region dating from as early as 1000 BC and they have been profiled through DNA to be clearly of Western Eurasian origin, despite their final internment in what is definitively dry East Asian soil. Even more remarkably, the textiles found on one of them are actually suggested as having originated from Celtic civilisations in central Europe – a plaid fabric, similar to that of a modern Scottish kilt. Elizabeth Barber, a professor emeritus and leading expert on ancient textiles, analysed the cloth and went so far as to suggest that these mummies may have shared Celtic ancestry with the Scots, and specifically identified that the cloth was almost identical to samples found in ancient salt mines in Hallstatt, Austria, an area once inhabited by early Celtic tribes[48]. Professor Victor Mair of the University of Pennsylvania has led much of the investigations on these mummies since the 1990s, investigations which have included their genetic mapping. He suggests that they link up eastern and western Eurasia in the Bronze and early Iron Age in a much closer way than had been previously considered possible. It is **entirely** plausible therefore that trade of valuables and exchanges of ideas between the ancient Chinese and the far west of the Persian Empire – including the coast of the Mediterranean – did indeed filter piecemeal back and forth across these vast tracts through the auspices of intermediary peoples wandering seasonally along this corridor well before this route had been officially "opened" by Zhang Qian.

There is telling further supportive evidence in the archaeological record. The lapis lazuli found in the tomb of Tutenkhamun in Egypt (c.1300 BC), for instance, has been identified as originating from its only known source at the time, from Badakshan in what is now north-eastern Afghanistan (at the approach to the Pamirs in what is now known as the Wakhan corridor). Lapis lazuli has been profitably mined there for a staggering six thousand years. In just the past few decades, in fact, its profits have been used to fund both anti-Soviet Mujahideen fighters and the anti-Taliban Northern Alliance army.

So with jade being traded eastwards and lapis lazuli going westwards, precious minerals were moving simultaneously in either direction with only the Pamirs in between, and this was happening at least from as early as 1200 BC and quite possibly earlier.

---

[48] Elizabeth Barber 2000 "the Mummies of Urumchi" (W.W.Norton & Co)

There is even one startling instance of evidence of early trade across the Pamirs which actually specifically links ancient Egypt with China itself. An Egyptian mummy dated from 1070 BC has astonishingly been identified as having vestiges of silk in its hair. It was discovered in a tomb in the village of Deir el Medina in the Valley of the Kings. This tiny sample represents the smoking gun of cross-continental trade in silk all the way from China to Egypt – a full eight hundred years before the silk route was said to have been "opened"[49].

Did this trade include the silk moth itself with a cocoon perhaps being carried across the continent in a pack on the back of a camel arriving in some unlikely fashion on the island of Kos? We just do not know, but it actually seems a remote possibility. Even more intriguingly, and perhaps more realistically, such traders may even have been exchanging knowledge of early nomadic medicine.

The Nomadic Peoples of Central Asia

A characteristic of these central areas of Asia right up to recent times is the preponderance of nomadic peoples who occupy them, most of whom followed their herds through seasonal pasturelands. Population pressures, weather changes or wars might take them far from their usual seasonal ranges, and there can be no logical reason to dismiss the possibility that some type of early moxibustion might have been used by these people, particularly if one subscribes to the view recorded in the *Suwen* that moxibustion came "from the North", the very areas where such tribes, so troublesome to the Chinese through the centuries, dominated the landscape. When one considers that mugwort when dry makes an ideal material for tinder, and is a plant of the wayside, it becomes more than a probability that any nomadic community familiar with it would have been carrying a sack of dried mugwort with them throughout their seasonal migrations so that they could light their fires easily. Mugwort would most certainly have been a prized material for them, regardless of any other therapeutic or shamanistic purpose they might have put it to.

Perhaps it was these very nomads who acted as the mysterious intermediaries in medicine, technology and trade between East and West. Or perhaps it was simply through more mundane percolative trading between oasis towns.

Such a suggestion, that moxibustion may have travelled from the centre of Asia not only eastwards but also westward, at first may seem ridiculous. But an intriguing suggestion for exactly just such a possibility unexpectedly but strikingly reveals itself in one of the core texts of Hippocrates and his followers, specifically in "Of the Places of Man". In this text, (which Craik identifies as possibly the earliest surviving piece of Greek prose as well as probably the earliest of the Hippocratic corpus) Hippocrates specifically identifies points indicated for cautery

---

[49]http://www.silkroadfoundation.org/artl/silkhistory.shtml retrieved 3/1/2010

for eye problems (an early echo here of Louis Frois' thousand-cone treatment on his back for eye problems mentioned previously). From their descriptions, the locations for these treatments seem pretty closely equivalent to GB1, Bl1, GB12 and "behind the head on either side at the occiput" at GB20 or possibly Bl10[50]. In the Mawangdui texts, which may be of similar age or slightly later, we should note that moxa cautery is also clearly discussed and indicated for treatment of eye problems. Importantly, the Greek verb *kaiein* (καιειν), which is the word that has been subsequently generally translated as "to cauterise", actually means just "to burn" (coming from the verb καίω – "to burn or set alight") rather than "to brand" as implied would occur with the heated iron "buttons" in cauterisation. There is an interesting resonance between this word with its association of setting light to something, and the ideogram "*jiu*" for moxibustion containing the image of a fire burning something, and indeed the word *mogusa* meaning a herb which can be set alight.

The Tinder Fungus

Craik also takes pains to identify that Hippocratic cauterisation, while clearly often meaning aggressive penetrative burning of tissue with heated irons, also sometimes meant no more than warming of the skin. As importantly, she further identifies that in another text, "Of Internal Affections", the use of a vegetable matter as a fuel for cauterisation is clearly alluded to. *Mykes* (μυκης), a word normally translated from the Ancient Greek as mushroom or fungus, is the word which was used in this Hippocratic text to describe the burnt vegetable matter used in the cauterisation process.

Might a ball of moxa nap look as much like a puffball of fungus as a ball of wool which was how the Jesuits described it centuries later? Actually there may be more to this than such a simplistic suggestion. There is a fungus, *Fomes fomentarius*, which has been commonly used as tinder, and which is in fact understood to have been a standard method for starting a fire since at least 3000 BC. Even today it is commonly known as Tinder Fungus, and it grows on the side of trees, beech in northern Europe and oak in the south. This fungus was ground to a fine powder and then ignited with flint and iron pyrites. The flint was struck against the pyrites creating a spark which was carefully directed to land in the prepared fungus and then blown into an ember. If the fungus was hammered flat, it could be turned into something resembling felt, and in this state it could then actually be kept smouldering, allowing the user to transport fire easily from one place to another in a limited area.

---

[50] E M Craik 2004 "Knife and fire: medical practice of east and west" in "Proceedings of COE" meeting held at Kyoto November, 2003 (published as *Globalization*, Kyoto, Iwanami Shoten) pp 227–43

Lorraine Wilcox offers us another extraordinary connection in a report she posted on the internet in 2010. She records an account given to her concerning a traditional cautery therapy used until recent times in Finland, using exactly this same fungus, *Fomes fomentarius*, the Tinder Fungus. It is called Taulakääpä in Finnish. Kääpä is the Finnish word for tree-fungus, whilst Taula is the name of the cauterisation therapy. The fungus was first boiled in sodium hydroxide (which itself was made from birch ash), then cut in pieces and dried. Small pieces of it were then used in some kind of moxa-type scarring treatment, being stuck to the skin at the required location by moistening the base of each piece and then igniting and burning them until they dropped off. Taula was reportedly used for treating tumors and growths, but we should not interpret this too literally perhaps. Her report also even recounted that an old chart was used for the therapy which has been likened to a Chinese chart of the back *shu*-points, although frustratingly no surviving chart is known to exist. If this **was** the case, however, it suggests that, like moxibustion, Taula may have been commonly and efficaciously used on the back.

We can even add a little more flavour to this curiosity, by introducing into our story the prehistoric "iceman" whose frozen body was discovered in the Alps in 1991. He was found with two walnut-size lumps of tree-fungus in a pouch on his person. Ötzi, as he has since become known, has been identified as a native of alpine Italy, and is thought to have been been attacked and mortally wounded whilst crossing a high frozen alpine pass, taking himself off to die on an icefield – an act which preserved him for discovery and exhumation around 5,300 years later. These pieces of fungus had a consistency somewhere between cork and leather (suggestive of the process of being hammered into a felt as was decsribed above). Each lump was pierced and tied to a leather thong. Initially scholars assumed the fungus to be tinder, something which would seem eminently sensible for him to have been carrying given where he was journeying in such cold conditions. However, given also that it has been suggested that he had some form of meridian lines tattooed on his body, it is also rather tempting to offer an alternative and more radical suggestion – that the tattoos and the fungus together might provide a clue that this ancient Italian might have been familiar with some form of early Taula-type moxibustion therapy. Certainly he had groups of short, parallel, vertical lines tattooed on both sides of his lumbar spine, a cruciform mark behind the right knee, as well as various marks around both ankles, all located where important acupoints exist, but no further evidence for this early acupuncture idea has as yet been provided, and (regrettably for us) no burn scars have been identified on his body.

It should also be added however that, in the last decade, Austrian microbiologists have identified that the lumps of fungus he was carrying, if ingested, can also act as a natural anti-parasitic medicine. Since Ötzi's digestive tract was revealed to have been infected with whipworm, it has recently become more generally suggested that he was carrying these lumps of fungus for use as a medicine and not as a tinder, and definitely not, in that case, for some early form of moxibustion. Since he also had traces of iron pyrite particles in his pouch along with the fungus, however, it cannot be suggested that the jury is absolutely unanimous on its current conclusions.

Certainly it is indisputable that connections between certain fungi and material for tinder do exist. Is it possible that some form of moxibustion, using a tinder fungus on points which are at least similar to traditional acupoints, existed empirically in the very earliest parts of the Hippocratic canon of medicine? It is probable, unfortunately, that we will never know, but, based on the isolated allusions in the Hippocratic corpus, it is clearly possible.

But we now need to switch our focus back to Central Asia and to these prehistoric traders between East and West. Just who were these mysterious trading intermediaries, if that's what they were, and might they help tell us more?

The Trade of Jade

To find out, we need to sweep back to ancient China, a full millennium before the Han, to the unlooted tomb of Fu Hao, a female warrior queen of the Shang dynasty. Her tomb was discovered and excavated in 1976. It contained more than 750 jade pieces (as well as over 7,000 Maldive cowry shells). All of this jade has been traced to Khotan in modern Xinjiang, deep in the Tarim Basin far from known Shang control. Fu died and was interred about 1200 BC, a full millennium earlier than the Han who are known to have been the first Chinese who actually extended their direct control this far westwards.

It is documented in the earliest Chinese records that the trade of jade from this area at the time was controlled by the *Yuezhi* people. These people remain nebulous and largely forgotten today, but their influence in the history of central, southern and eastern Asia, as we shall see, can hardly be sniffed at. Their name literally means "Moon people" but the suffix "zhi" (氏) was used in Chinese to denote those who were considered western barbarians. They were, in fact, almost certainly more western than the ancient Chinese could have imagined. Remarkably, the *Yuezhi* are recognised today from DNA remains as being a people of Indo-European origin – not East Asian at all – who must have somehow settled in the regions of the Eastern Tarim basin in pre-historical times. They were also quite clearly largely nomadic. Sima Qian, who knew nothing of their Indo-European origins when he was writing his histories in the Han dynasty, simply recorded their beginnings (as far as the Han Chinese were concerned) as follows: "The *Yuezhi* lived in the area between Qilian and Dunhong." Dunhong is now understood to be a mountain in the Tianshan range, and Qilian is the northernmost range of the Kunlunshan range – the two ranges to the north and south respectively of the Tarim Basin.

It seems likely therefore that Sima Qian, based on the historical evidence he had at his disposal, considered this area to be their natural homeland in the heart of Central Asia. In addition they were elsewhere recorded as being the prime traders of the prized jade. The most valued "mutton fat" jade, named because of its opalescent whiteness and the slight greasiness in its sheen, originated from exactly this area where the *Yuezhi* were said to have been living.

Khotan, where Fu Hao's jade originated from in the thirteenth century BC, is an oasis town on the southern edge of the Taklamaken desert at the foothills of the Kunlun Mountains, well beyond the farthest western reaches of ancient China. Even today this area is still known for its *yangzhi*, or "mutton fat" jade. This *yangzhi* or white jade (*baiyu*) is still a valuable commodity. In 2008 it was used as the backing material of the gold medals in the Beijing Olympic Games; two millennia earlier it was being sent as tribute to the imperial court in Beijing. One carved piece in the Forbidden City weighs in at a staggering five tonnes.

White nephrite mutton fat jade can still be found in the deposits of the Yurungkash (otherwise named "White Jade River") in its wide flood plains of sand and gravel outside Khotan's city boundaries. This appropriately named White Jade River (*Baiyu He* in Mandarin) flows down straight out of the Kunlun Range, disappearing out into the arid vastness of the desert.

The *Yuezhi*

Before we turn our attention specifically to the repeated appearance of the word "white" (*bai*) in our story, we need to further look into the story of the *Yuezhi* themselves, these Western barbarians who were trading the local jade with the Chinese during the first millennium BC. What transpired in the second century BC for them is a little known migration, but one which had consequence for the development of civilization and religion in the whole of Asia. It was a migration which took this nomadic people back westwards across the Pamirs to Bactria, then later south into India. In the process, its people transformed themselves into one of the greatest empires of the era, becoming the famed Kushan dynasty of India. And it was one of the greatest Kushan kings, Kanishka the Great, who was subsequently largely responsible for the promotion and dissemination of Buddhism from India across the world, including, of course, to China itself.

This *Yuezhi* migration westwards had been initially triggered by pressures from another nomadic people, the *Xiongnu* (often written and referred to as the Hsiung-Nu). They came from further north and had displaced the *Yuezhi* from their eastern homelands in the second century BC. The *Xiongnu* have become far better known in the story of Chinese civilisation because, for a millennium or more thereafter, they continuously harried the north-western flanks of the Chinese empire, giving sufficient cause for the Chinese to conceive the immense project of building their Great Wall to try to keep them out. The *Yuezhi*, these jade traders from earlier times, had by then withdrawn completely from the story of China, moving back to the western side of the continental divide – back to what might be seen as the "West", conquering and then settling in Bactria (Daxia as it was known as by the Chinese), or modern day northern Afghanistan.

This migration by the *Yuezhi* took place in the second century BC, and, remarkably, the event was picked up at the time by chroniclers in both East and West.

Strabo, the Greek chronicler, called them the "Asioi". "But the best known of the nomads are those who took away Baktrianē [Bactria] from the Greeks; the Asioi and the Pasianoi, and the Tacharoi and the Sakaraukai, who originally came from the other side of the Iaxartou [Jaxartes or Syr Darya river][51]," he wrote.

Zhang Qian, meanwhile, spent a year with the *Yuezhi* in Bactria in 128 BC as part of his extraordinarily extensive travels. His stay with them occurred only a few years after they had settled the area. "The Great *Yuezhi*" he wrote "live 2,000 or 3,000 *li* (500-750 miles) west of Dayuan (Ferghana)…They are a nation of nomads moving from place to place with their herds, and their customs are like those of the *Xiongnu*. They have some 100,000 or 200,000 archer warriors[52]."

So we have at least two separate definite instances in which this single people crossed this great range of mountains to settle on the other side – the first unrecorded in prehistory when they had originally travelled eastwards from their Indo-European homelands for reasons unknown, and the second after their violent displacement by another nomadic people when they moved back to the west. As importantly, we also know that these people were regarded as natural and well-respected traders because they were described as such in contemporary records.

What happened to them over the subsequent two centuries makes for an irresistible story, one that is known throughout Asia, but is little known in the English speaking world. It tells how this little known people came to dominate the three major trade routes of the then known world. One was the sea route from India to the West, a sea route which crossed the Arabian sea and into the Persian Gulf; another was the sea route from India to East Asia, to Java, Sumatra and Indochina; and the third was the vital land route across Asia both East and West, and up through northern India into the Himalayas, to Kashgar, Khotan and beyond into the hinterland of the Chinese empire. "The land of this is not easy of

---

[51] Strabo's "Geography" 11.8.2

[52] Burton Watson 1993"Records of the Grand Historian of China: Han Dynasty II"- Translating from the *Shiji* of Sima Qian (Columbia University Press) p 234

access"[53] wrote the author of the *Periplus*[54] around 70 AD, but the key people who truly opened up this massively lucrative trade route were originally the *Yuezhi*. The empire they developed has become known as that of the Kushans, one of the names the Chinese themselves used for them – one of the four tribes of the "Great *Yuezhi*."

Their first stop was Bactria, where one of their great leaders, Kujula Kadphises, unified what were known as the "great *Yuezhi*" tribes. He then invaded the territory to the south, the Kabul valley and Kashmir. His son added Northern India to the realm, to make the Kushans effectively a world power in their own right. Within two further generations they had crossed the Punjab and overran northern India as far as the Jumna River.

But that is only the beginning of the more important part of the story of their empire. Their greatest ruler is still remembered today in China, Mongolia and Tibet. In Japan he appears as an evil genius in one of their most famous *manga* comic books. In Sri Lanka and Southern India he is remembered as the third of the four pillars of Buddhism, and he is seen as being responsible for the spread of Buddhism right around Asia. Despite this, relatively little is known about the man himself, but we do know his name – Kanishka the Great. An inscription on a tablet found in 1993 in Afghanistan has finally revealed for us a little more of the legend. "Architect of the great salvation, Kanishka the Kushan, the righteous the just, the autocrat, the god, the worthy of worship…In the Year One it has been proclaimed unto India, unto the whole realm of the ksatriyas…and he had submitted all India to his will." The empire extended from the Pamirs and Afghanistan (and at one stage as far as Khotan in the Tarim Basin), down to Peshawar in Pakistan (their summer capital), into the plain of India and the Indus, and round down the Ganges to the edge of Bengal – an extent of around 3000 miles.

The stamp of this empire remains indelible in India to this day. Possibly in 127 AD the Kushans inaugurated their new era ("the Year One"), a dating system which is still used on the front page of some Indian newspapers alongside the AD dating of the Christian era.

But it is in two other fields that their influence has been most felt in the world – those of religion and of commerce.

---

[53] From the translation by William H. Schoff 1912 "The Periplus of the Erythraean Sea: Travel and Trade in the Indian Ocean by a Merchant of the First Century" (New York: Longmans, Green, and Co). Retrieved online http://depts.washington.edu/silkroad/texts/periplus/periplus.html 3.1.2010

[54] The *Periplus Maris Erythraei* (or 'Voyage around the Erythraean Sea') is an anonymous work from around the middle of the first century CE written by a Greek speaking Egyptian merchant.

The time of Kanishka was a time of Eurasian stability and peace – the time of Hadrian and Antonius in the West, and of the Han in the East, a time described by Edward Gibbon as "the happiest time in the history of the world". The Kushans exploited this time of vast peaceful empire, becoming "very rich indeed" in the process, as one Chinese chronicler put it. They inherited a run down economy, but began to supplement the silver and copper coins with gold ones, astutely struck to the weight standard of the Roman Empire, something which offered them the widest possible circulation. They were aiming high, at a currency that would facilitate large scale wholesale commerce across a vast region.

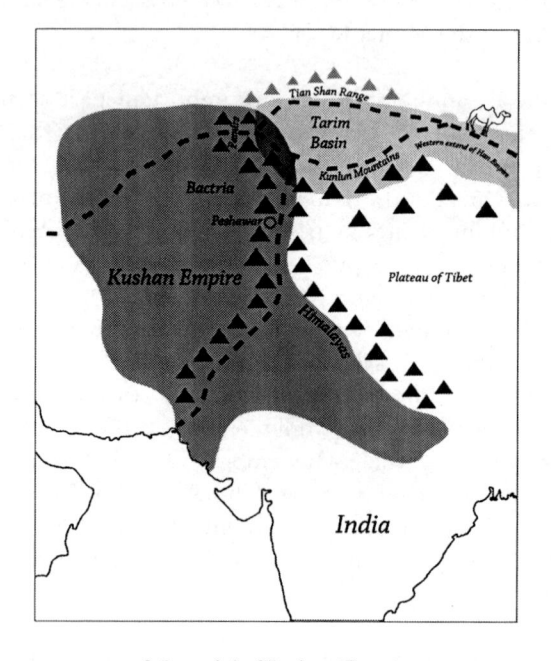

Map of the Kushan Empire

Recent estimates have suggested that Kushan wealth in terms of gross domestic product at the height of their empire added up to nearly 30% of the wealth of the world – more even than either Rome or Han China – all essentially because of their empire's position, and because of the acumen of the empire's rulers. In a sense, their enterprise marked the very beginning of a global economy. In the second century BC, the Greek historian Polybius(ca. 200-118 BC) wrote: "Previously the doings of the world had been, so to say, dispersed, as they were held together by no unity of initiative, results, or locality; but ever since this date history has been an organic whole, and the affairs of Italy and Africa have been interlinked with those of Greece and Asia, all leading up to one end[55]."

---

[55] W. R. Paton 1922 "The Histories of Polybius, Book 1" (Loeb Classical Library Edition) – retrieved online
http://ancienthistory.about.com/library/bl/bl_text_polybius_i.htm 3/1/2010.

But it was not just in commerce that their influence told. In Ayurvedic traditions, one of its founding physicians, Caraka, is said to have been Kanishka's guru - in a slightly reminiscent relationship of the one between the legendary Qibo and Huangdi in China. This may of course also be legend, but the spread of Buddhism across the East is undeniable fact, and this was specifically triggered when Kanishka took the decision to officially support Buddhism.

This was Mahayana Buddhism, as is practised by most Buddhists today. Mahayana was itself a recent development. It differed from the more ascetic Buddhism that preceded it in India in that it strongly stressed the miraculous life and personality of the Buddha, an idea officially sanctioned by Kanishka himself. Before this, the Buddha had been represented by non-personal symbols – by a wheel, a riderless horse, or a footprint. From this time on, the Buddha became humanized into the iconic image which has survived to this day, anomalously attired in a Greek toga[56].

Kanishka himself is reputed to have had built a Buddhist stupa in Peshawar that was, if Chinese eye-witnesses are to be believed, the highest building in the world before the age of sktscrapers.

The influence of the Buddha may have failed to spread to Greece and the Mediterranean as may have been intended, but it most certainly spread eastwards, with the Kushan monk Lokaksema becoming the first translator of the Buddhist scriptures into Chinese, establishing a translation bureau in the heart of China, at its capital Luoyang. The spread of Buddhism essentially depended upon the widespread peace that existed at the time across Asia, but, as importantly, it was inextricably linked with the commerce which followed directly behind it which in turn depended upon the religion's ethics and ethos. Trade thus followed religion in an almost inevitable process, and vast wealth accrued for the Kushans as a consequence. In further consequence for mankind, the Buddhist religion arrived first in China, then Korea and South-East Asia, finally appearing in Japan two centuries later.

So who exactly were these Kushans, these *Yuezhi* before they went west across the Pamirs and ultimately founded their massive empire?

As has been previously mentioned, they are today recognised as being of Indo-European origin. It is tempting to speculate a little here on account of some curious descriptions in another early Chinese text. The *Shan Hai Jing* (the "Classic of the Mountains and Seas") is a largely fabled geographical and cultural account of pre-Qin China dating from around 200 BC. Similar to the *Nei Jing*, it appears to have been multiple-authored. In its script it enigmatically describes a "white

---

[56] It is tempting to wonder whether the prime intention of clothing the Buddha in this fashion was that Buddhism should spread west as much as east based on the anomalous adoption of the toga for the Buddha's apparel.

people with long hair" – the *Bai* people living to the West of China. And as curious as this description may appear to us today, these people really did exist.

The Mummies of Central Asia

Tempting as it may be to dismiss this record along with much of the rest of the text as being fanciful, we have evidence today of blond hair found on mummies excavated in the Tarim Basin dating from as long ago as 1800 BC. Typically, they have been revealed with broad noses and Caucasoid features, and, furthermore, we now know from their DNA that these people were essentially Indo-Europeans and not East Asians. These same mummies also endorse Pliny's descriptions of the Seres as being of "great height" and of Ctesias as being of "portentous stature". The best preserved of all the mummies found to date is the so called "Yingpan Man"[57], believed to have been interred in the 4th or 5th centuries BC. A full two metres tall, he was both brown-haired and bearded with his face covered with a gold foil death mask, itself a Greek tradition. He also wore magnificently elaborate red and maroon wool garments embroidered in gold and decorated with images of fighting Greeks or Romans. He was certainly a man of great wealth, no doubt accumulated from trading, almost certainly with both East and West. More bodies from this early period were discovered in 2009 and they further suggest that a mixture of peoples have lived in the Tarim Basin since at least the start of the Bronze Age[58]. Even today, in fact, blond hair is not unknown among the Uyghur people of the Tarim basin.

And right up to the present, the effects of these non-Chinese "white" ethnicities provide discomfort for the Chinese political status quo. The modern Chinese historian Ji Xianlin, wrote the preface to the book the "Ancient Corpses of Xinjiang"[59] which is a modern Chinese study of the mummies written by Wang Bighua. In it, Ji writes that modern China "supported and admired" the research by foreign experts into the mummies. "However," he writes, "within China a small group of ethnic separatists have taken advantage of this opportunity to stir up trouble and are acting like buffoons. Some of them have even styled themselves as the descendants of these ancient 'white people' with the aim of dividing the motherland. But these perverse acts will not succeed."

---

[57] This mummy was found at the eastern end of the Tarim Basin near Lop Nur which is where the PRC have more recently been conducting undergound nuclear tests.

[58] Li, Chunxiang. "Evidence that a West-East admixed population lived in the Tarim" (BMC Biology) http://www.biomedcentral.com/1741-7007/8/15#IDAH0OBH retrieved 17 February 2010.

[59] Wang Binghua (Editor) 2001 "The ancient corpses of Xinjiang" translated by Victor Mair (Xinjiang People's Press)

In 2011 the mummy of the famous "Beauty of Xiahe" was peremptorily withdrawn from viewings while on tour in museums in the US along with other Chinese ancient artefacts. No official reason was given, but it can be surmised that it was because of the growing interest in the figure which was exacerbating regional political sensitivities and tensions on account of the self-evident hair colour and facial features of the mummy which were not Chinese.

"Mister White"

A key clue for all of our respective speculations seems to converge on the word "*bai*" or "white", the adjective which Ji Xianlin was applying to the mummies, and which was additionally applied not just to the *Yuezhi* people, but also to the jade they traded, and to the river from which their jade was collected. It is an adjective as well which appears in the history of acumoxa in the eponymous name of the little known but nebulous "Mister White" or "*Baishi*" whom we mentioned earlier in the lists of the chroniclers of the Han Dynasty as one of the primary authors of the then-still-surviving medical texts. He is one of the forgotten fathers of East Asian medicine, and it is in connection with this mysterious figure that we tentatively return from the history of the wider region to the story of moxibustion itself.

The early Han chronicler librarians recorded what appear to us today as three separate schools of medicine – the Yellow Emperor (*Huang Di*) School, the *Bian Que* School, and the "Mister White" *Baishi* school. These records appear in the *Qi Lue*, which was a catalogue of the holdings of the Han court in 26 BC, almost immediately before the break between the end of the Western Han in 9 AD and the slow recovery of the later Eastern Han between 25 and 74 AD. In it, there are definitive references to seven separate compendia on medicine, one of which is referred to as the *Huang Di Nei Jing*, which suggests that it might be the original text of the one which exists today. What is intriguing to our investigation is that, of these seven compendia, two are attributed to our mysterious "Mister White" (*Baishi*). Even more interestingly, the *Nei Jing* is recorded as being of eighteen *juan* (volumes) in total length, whilst the two works attributed to Mister White comprise a comparatively massive total of seventy-four volumes (in other words potentially containing four times as much material). The list of the contents of the *Qi Lue* is a sobering one if only because it tells us how much must have been lost, presumably in the cataclysmic period between the Western and Eastern Han:

Huang Di Nei Jing	18 volumes
Huang Di Wai Jing	37 volumes (lost)
Bian Que Nei Jing	9 volumes (lost)
Bian Que Wai Jing	12 volumes (lost)
Baishi Nei Jing	38 volumes (lost)
Baishi Wai Jing	36 volumes (lost)
Pang Pian	25 volumes (lost)

By the time of Huangfu Mi, the author of the Systematic Classic in around 260 AD, nearly all of this can already be confirmed as having been lost, to the extent that it is not entirely possible for us even to be completely certain that the text we know today as the *Lingshu* was even then part of the Han *Huang Di Nei Jing* compilation at all. This loss in the records of early Chinese medicine was almost certainly due to the turmoil at the end of the Western Han period which was itself almost certainly more catastrophic to the early medical literature than the earlier Burning of the Books may or may not have been. This short period of fifty years included massive flooding as the Yellow River changed its course, consequent widespread starvation, a civil war, and a change of capital (from Chang'an/Xian to Luoyang). A general hiatus of civilization of around sixty-five years ensued, so it is perhaps hardly surprising that so much of the labours of the early Han scribes seem to have been lost in this period.

At around 200 AD, for instance, the author of the preface to the *Shang Han Lun* also made no reference to this Mister White (although he does make reference to both the *Suwen* and the *Nan Jing*), providing further evidence that no further record of this tradition had survived. Nothing further has emerged in the centuries since, and as yet unfortunately no archaeological findings have revealed anything further either. The Yellow Emperor School is assumed today to have simply superseded or subsumed the others to have become the dominant surviving school, with the *Nei Jing* classics effectively becoming its textbooks. Bian Que, who was associated with the second school of medicine, has at least passed into the mythology of Chinese medicine as a legendary physician and may well have been directly or indirectly associated with the *Nan Jing*, but absolutely nothing at all survives to tell us more about the mysterious Mister White.

This lack of record has some similarity, of course, to the lack of surviving moxa texts beyond what has been found interred in tombs in the second century BC and discovered in the twentieth century, despite their clear seminal influence on the development of acupuncture *jingluo* channel theory. It is quite tempting, therefore, for us to speculate whether, whoever Mister White might have been, it may have been more than accidental that his story was so completely lost. In the same way that we have already speculated that the moxa texts did not survive because they failed to suit the new emerging medical *Zeitgeist*, it actually may not have suited the creators of this same new more scientific Chinese medicine for Mr. White's influence to have survived either.

For a second, we must step back, and look again at *Suwen* 12 which introduces us to the only extant clue in the surviving literature to the origin of moxibustion. "Moxa burning originated in the North" it states. The North, of course was also the region from where the ever hostile Xiongnu rode in from in their raiding parties, taking hostages and exacting tribute for their return. The North was synonymous for the Chinese with horse-riding nomads, people who, according to the *Suwen*, "find joy in living in the wilderness and consuming milk".

It was not, of course, just the more northerly *Xiongnu* who lived this way. There were also the mysterious nomadic *Yuezhi* people, who may very well have been those very same "white people with long hair" as described in the *Shanghaijing*. Whilst these people were described as "white", the Han themselves were often described as the "black haired" people. There certainly was frequent interaction between these two distinct white and black peoples, since the *Yuezhi* had enjoyed longstanding trading relations with the Chinese for centuries prior to their displacement by the *Xiongnu*. So could our mysterious Mister White have actually been one of these people, or at least might he have had some sort of close association with them?

It is clearly quite possible that moxibustion originated somewhere in Central Asia amongst the many nomadic peoples spread across its vastness. Today mugwort is still a plant of the wayside, a plant of both highway and byway. It is also quite self-evident that it requires little in the way of technology to convert it into a usable therapeutic medium, and its application is extremely low-tech. Such a resource would have been an attractive resort for the nomad whether travelling in the high plains of the Himalayas or in the Siberian steppes. In both places it would also have been readily identified as useful tinder in the vital practice of starting a fire.

Whether the imaginary ambassador (if one existed of course) for this heat therapy was a member of the *Yuezhi* or even Mister White himself must remain, at least until further archaeological discoveries are made, a matter of pure speculation. The same holds true, of course, as to whether this curious heat treatment might have similarly percolated westwards through nomadic traders and found another less enduring home in Kos.

Based on the dates of these Hippocratic texts, and the probably slightly later texts of Meng Zi and Zhuang Zi referred to shortly, if there are connections between Greek and Chinese medical practices, as far as moxibustion is concerned, it remains merely a matter of speculation. The possibilities are fascinating nevertheless.

Further Thoughts on the Origin of the Word "moxa"

In the late seventeenth century, nearly two thousand years after Hippocrates had lived and died, those self-same ancient Greek medical texts just might in fact have provided a plausible alternative source (or at least a supplementary one) for the modern word "moxa" itself. We will even shortly suggest that its etymological origins may actually be as much Greek as Oriental, and we will even speculate whether these origins might be connected as much with the Germanic languages of the low countries of Europe as with the Japanese.

As described earlier, the Reverend Busschof returned from Batavia/Jakarta and invented this word which he selected supposedly because of its Japanese origin.

We have already pondered on the curiosity of his choice, given that he stated that the best moxa came from China, and that he was taught the treatment by the "doctress" from Vietnam thousands of miles distant from Japan. Perhaps there were other factors that led to his selection of this particular Japanese word in addition to those which may have related to its use at the time in Japanese.

We might speculate that he experienced suppurative moxa treatment at St36 (he recorded it as both "on my feet and knees") for his gout with this woolly material, and if he was familiar with Greek (he was a post-renaissance clergyman after all and he actually referred to Hippocratic medicine in his *Het Podagra* tract seven times), he might well have consciously favoured coining the word "moxa" because of its resonant connections to Greek as much as its relationship to Japanese. He may have been struck by its similarity to the Greek word *myxa* (μυξα), meaning mucus or suppurative discharge. But given that he specifically denied that large blisters are formed at the site of the burn, just tiny *escars* as he called them, this seems unlikely.

The Greek word *myxa* itself, however, comes from the very same root word as *mykes* (the word used in the Hippocratic text to define the combustible vegetable matter or fungus for cauterisation)[60]. If he were using solely the Japanese as his source, he might far more likely have coined the word "*jaxa*", from the apparently more widely used contemporary Japanese words *yaito* or *yakikusa*[61]. The similarities between the three words moxa, *mogusa* and *myxa* (μυξα) are very striking. So did he choose the word because of his knowledge of the Hippocratic corpus? This is far from improbable since he serially referred to Hippocrates in his tract.

(Another odd co-incidence occurs here, incidentally. The same Greek word *mykes* supplies the prefix to *mycobacterium*, of which **tuberculosis** is the most notorious– an ancient disease that will cross the path of our explorations on several occasions – with leprosy another *mycobacterium* not far behind it. Tuberculosis, like other mycobacterial infections, is extraordinarily difficult to treat. The "fungal" connection in this case refers to the way that such bacteria are observed to grow on the surface of liquids when they are cultured.)

An even more intriguing possibility exists, however, concerning the choice of this word "moxa" – which is that the good Doctor Busschof actually **did** know the plant that provided the woolly matter he despatched back from Batavia but chose not to reveal it for commercially sensitive reasons. There are possible grounds for

---

[60] E M Craik 2004 "Knife and fire: medical practice of east and west" in "Proceedings of COE" meeting held at Kyoto November, 2003 (published as *Globalization*, Kyoto, Iwanami Shoten) pp 227–43

[61] Some interesting semantic pedantries occur here: the verb *mueru* from which *mogusa* derives has an intransitive sense ("a herb which burns"); the verb *yaku* from which *yakikusa* derives has a transitive sense ("a herb which one burns").

making such a suggestion because of another uncanny co-incidence which relates to the etymology of the actual word for mugwort. As we will find out soon in Part 2 the Stalk, in Northern Europe the mugwort plant has long-established associations with its ability to repel insects. The English word "mugwort" is in fact derived from the Saxon word "mycgwyrt" meaning "insect plant". Alternative versions of the word "mycg" for mosquito or midge are scattered right across European languages, all seemingly related and therefore ultimately most probably all derived from the same more ancient Indo-European source[62]. Some trace the word merely to the Latin ("mosca" or "fly" from which the word "mosquito" derives). The same word derivation occurs in Germanic as well as Romance languages, however, and in Scandinavian (mugge), Russian (moschka), Middle German (Muecke), Dutch (Mug), and Old French (mosche). But the one that is the most bizarrely similar to the word moxa itself is in Walloon – a Romance language from a region in modern Belgium. In Walloon, the tiny fly at the root of the word for mugwort is actually known as **mochse**.

Since Busschof was a man from the Low Countries, if he was not actually aware of the plant source of the moxa he sent back to Holland, the word he chose to describe it contains an extraordinary assonance to a functional word as it is still used today in his native country.

Such explorations conclude nothing, however, merely adding suggestions to suggestions. If any conclusion at all can be drawn, it might simply be that the origin of the Western term "moxa" may not be as straightforward as has generally been assumed.

One last interesting connection remains on this topic. A full five hundred years after the time of the Reverend Busschof, in the mid-twentieth century these same iron "button cautery" techniques still survived in isolated instances as part of Europe's own inherited canon of traditional medicine, and may actually have provided the stimulus in France for Dr Paul Nogier's initial investigations into auriculo-therapy with needles. In the early 1950s, he discovered that two of his patients had areas of their ears cauterised by a local lay healer with therapeutic effects on their sciatica. His own subsequent investigations into what have come to be understood as the micro-systems of the ear arose directly from this discovery[63]. This tiny anecdote provides another interconnected side-shoot in the story we are investigating.

As intimated above, in Chinese there are no similar sounding words to "moxa", the word *jiu* being the equivalent to the Japanese *kyu* for moxa therapy, whilst for the plant itself the word *ai* or *aiye* is equivalent to mugwort and is roughly

---

[62] The Proto-Indo-European stem MU- is in fact most probably onomatopoeic in origin.

[63] Nigel Oleson 1996 "Manual of Auriculotherapy" (Churchill Livingstone)

equivalent to *yomogi* in Japanese. The processed nap in Chinese is referred to as *airong* 艾絨, literally meaning "velvet of mugwort". The Japanese *mogusa*, meaning "herb for burning" seems to fall somewhere in between these two later Chinese terms, and any attempt to equivocate by comparison of Han style characters used in both languages merely serves to compound confusions.

What follows is a simplified attempt to match some of the terms used across the three languages:

English	Chinese	Japanese
Moxibustion/cautery	*jiu*	*kyuji, yaito, yaihi*
Moxa nap	*airong*	*okyu, mogusa, yakikusa*
Mugwort plant	*ai, aiye*	*yomogi, ooyomogi*

The Ultimate Origins of Moxibustion

Leaving aside the possibility that moxibustion had some connection with an important island in the Aegean, legends also have it that the origins of moxibustion were associated with the Brahmins of India in the 8th to 6th centuries BC[64], but there seems to be no strong evidence to support this. Newman-Turner and Low quote Wang Xuetai, who postulated: "In primitive society, when people were warming themselves by fire, they accidentally discovered that by applying heat to the abdominal area they could relieve symptoms of abdominal pain, distension and fullness[65]." They suggested that this might well explain how moxibustion began, doing so in terms which resonate with the records of the origins of moxa in *Suwen* 12. Such a view can in fact also be supported by one of the fourteen medical scrolls found in Mawangdui which hints at a more localised heat therapy – the "Therapeutic Treatments for 52 Diseases" (*Wu Shi Er Bing Fang*): "When treating a patient with dysuria, ignite grass or firewood. Position the patient's back towards the fire and roast, while two people massage his buttocks[66]."

Another reference to moxibustion can be found in this text offering a contrasting and quite striking description of a treatment for a case of an inguinal hernia, however, quite different from the simple "roasting" described above. In this instance an incision is made with a stone in the scrotum, after which medicinals are placed on the incision and "then cauterisation is performed on the wound".

---

[64] U.A.Casal "Acupuncture, cautery and massage in Japan". (www.nanzan-u.ac.jp/SHUBUNKEN/publications/afs/pdf/a136.pdf)p 226 - retrieved 3/1/2010

[65] Wang Xuetai 1986 "A brief study of the history and ancient literature on acumoxibustion" Journal of Chinese Medicine.

[66] Roger Newman Turner and Royston Low 1987 "Moxibustion, its Principles and Practice" (Thorsons) p13

Three cases of treatment with moxibustion for leprosy are also mentioned, so if simple roasting by a fire was the original spark for the treatment it appears to have developed into something quite different quite quickly.

Elsewhere in the Mawangdui scripts other references to cautery occur using alternative materials including cattail (reed mace) burnt on a wart, and a cigar of hemp wrapped in mugwort leaves being burnt over the vertex of the head to create a blister in a person with inguinal swelling.

A further Mawangdui text, the *Mai Fa* or "Model of the Vessels" also refers to cauterisation at or above the waist if "vapour ascends and does not descend". But Donald Harper, who is an expert on these texts, is quite convinced that cauterisation with any material, mugwort or otherwise, far from constituted a major part of general therapeutic practice at the time these texts were written. Other heat therapies are also mentioned, including roasting, hot-pressing (or ironing) and balneotherapy (hot bath treatment). Intriguingly, given the discussion we entertained on European fungus cautery, mugwort mixed with willow mushrooms is also referred to as being used as a fumigant in another text, though this was (according to modern scholarship) almost certainly a part of an exorcist practice.

It seems more likely that the origins of this therapy go back far earlier, and as such are most certainly lost in pre-history. As a result, it is impossible for us to draw any sort of conclusion of exactly what the origins of this practice might have been, but we can take a stab at it nevertheless based on the story we have weaved so far.

The willow mushrooms mentioned above perhaps offers us the best clue. Burning tinder fungus (from birch and oak trees) on the skin, it will be recalled, appears to be a strand of early European traditional medicine which has survived literally up until yesterday in Scandinavia. We now can be fairly sure that something similar also formed a small part of the Hippocratic corpus 2,500 years ago, and would have almost certainly come to Kos from mainland Asia Minor. A similar practice may even go back a further 2,800 years if the fungus in the alpine iceman mummy's pouch is in any way connected with cauterisation. The clue for us is in the use in both East and West of materials for tinder – ones that were invaluable to the nomadic pastoralist and herdsman alike and which were vital for survival. Any tinder had to be widely available but it was also, almost by definition, only in seasonal supply and would therefore have accrued some inherent value of its own from its having to be stored and preserved. We can imagine that somehow its use became adapted to being burnt on the skin. The probability would be that its usage in this sense would have been originally shamanic – and, as we will see when we look deeper into the nature of mugwort, such ideas have survived right into the modern era. The materials used differed in different regions: in western Eurasia, it seems to have been tinder fungi; in eastern Eurasia it was wayside mugwort – the materials differ, but the application seems in some sense uncannily similar. Was there one single origin of the practice, or were there two – one eastern and one western? Did the practice start out, for instance, somewhere in a wilderness and then spread east and west, adapting itself to differing tinder pactices along the way – or was it one of those human phenomena that pops up in different places at some not dis-similar time?

Like so many things in our anthropological past, we will never know.

The Development of *jingluo* Channel Theory

Of the fourteen medical scrolls interred in 168 BC which were found at Mawangdui in Hunan in China, the two which deal specifically with moxibustion and channel pathways are today known as the *Zu Pi Shuyi Mai Jiu Jing* ("Eleven Vessel Foot-Arm Moxa Classic") and the *Yin Yang Shuyi Mai Jiu Jing* ("Eleven Vessel Yin-Yang Moxa Classic"). Neither scroll was found thus entitled; they were given these titles by modern scholars. Both scrolls were written on silk, and a further copy of one of them written on bamboo slips was subsequently found in 1983 in Hubei province which suggests that the therapy they represent may have been known quite widely.

Both scrolls include descriptions of the origins and pathways of eleven unconnected mai, or vessel/meridians. This contrasts with the twelve interconnected meridians described in the *Lingshu*, but the descriptions of the pathways of those that are described are strikingly similar. Of the eleven Mawangdui meridians, there are six channels to the leg and five to the arm, of which six are *yang* and five *yin* (the *jueyin* Pericardium meridian of the arm is effectively missing). The two texts also systematically record a list of symptoms associated with disease or dysfunction of each channel. There is, however, some variance in the directionalities of the channels between the two texts. Finally, it is not even completely clear whether mugwort was the material of choice for treatment of these *mai* in these texts, although it is generally accepted that this was the case.

What is also quite intriguing concerning the content of these two *jiu jing* "moxa classics" is the absence of any reference to points for treatment or any types of description of point locations. After a description of ailments associated with each particular vessel, the "Eleven Vessel" classic particularly repeatedly and formulaically prescribes "in all cases of ailments from these things, cauterise the [respected] vessel" – but it never goes beyond this. There are never points or specific loci on the channels described for such treatment, only the vessel or *mai* itself. Where on the vessel or exactly how it should be cauterised is not specified, as a result of which we literally know nothing today of the approach and techniques used in these cauterisations.

The channels of the foot are described in much more detail than those of the hands. Yamada speculates that this might be because the foot channels were revealed first or perhaps because the foot channels were considered to be more important. These speculations are particularly interesting given the contrasting relative absence of channels on the legs of the Shuangbaoshan figurine described previously, on which seven of the nine lines run on the trunk and arms. Clearly we have a huge gap of understanding still to fill.

Mugwort and Moxibustion – the Very Earliest References

But why choose mugwort anyway? Mugwort is certainly not the only plant that has been or is currently used in moxibustion – peach stem, mulberry stem, bamboo skin, or *Deng Xin Cao* also receive comparatively more modern references. Particular qualities, though, make mugwort especially suitable. It grows wild in a wide variety of climates so is readily available; and it can also be easily processed into a woollen nap which burns easily and evenly. These qualities are exemplified in the Japanese word *yomogi* which is generally used to denote mugwort. Etymological resonances in this word indicate both that it is a plant which grows well "all over", and which also burns with ease.

We have already suggested that it was a plant that would have been readily available as effective tinder. Perhaps as importantly, mugwort also had certain esoteric attributes in the East Asian herbal canon which may have given it an extra edge over other combustible plants which grew just as abundantly. We must bear in mind traditional East Asian medicine's undeniable roots in demonic medicine, and theculture's observations of ancestor worship and beliefs in ghost affliction which survive to the present day[67]. In both East and West, the mugwort plant itself has been traditionally regarded as having specific properties for warding off evil spirits and associated afflictions, and it is still used in Japan as a combustible for Buddhist purification ceremonies. The therapeutic use of needles has been suggested by some scholars to be micro-representations of the spears which were known to have been thrown by the *wu* shaman of ancient China when chasing off demons. This theory proposes direct connections between the exorcism of evil spirits by *wu* shamen and acupuncture as we have inherited it today. In similar vein, mugwort, traditionally used to ward off evil spirits, was most probably burnt ceremonially for the same reasons, but when burnt in much smaller quantities on the body it may have become culturally transformed into a proto-medical procedure. Mugwort was sometimes hung by the Chinese from the waist as a demonic deterrent, a habit that is, rather remarkably, exactly reflected in a medieval European tradition apocryphally ascribed to St John when in the wilderness who was mythologised in the Middle Ages to have worn a belt of mugwort for this same purpose, a phenomenon which we will examine further in Part 2 the Stalk.

---

[67] See Paul Unschuld 1985 "Medicine in China, a History of Ideas" (University of California Press)

The Moon over Matsushima

The earliest recorded surviving descriptions of moxibustion and mugwort in ancient China are actually found separately in poetic texts from the Spring and Autumn Period and from and philosophical ones from the middle of the Warring States.

The earliest description of all occurs in the *Shi Jing* or "Book of Odes. These poems comprise the oldest surviving collection of Chinese poetry and are thought to date from as long ago as 1000 BC, although they were not formally collated until the time of Confucius, and, centuries later, still had to be reconstructed from memory after their destruction in the Burning of the Books.

Ode number 72 contains the following lines:

彼采艾兮一日不見、
如三歲兮

James Legge[68] translated them as follows:

> "There he is gathering the mugwort! A day without seeing him
> Is like three years!"

We cannot be certain as to exactly what purpose this gathered mugwort might have been intended for, but it was clearly being gathered for something. There is a distinctive direct echo, however, from this verse in the next surviving reference which is from Meng Zi (379-272 BC). This second description definitely does allude to the use of mugwort for curative purposes – to the timescale of three years which is still the traditional timespan required for the maturation of mugwort for moxibustion. It seems unlikely that this is mere coincidence.

Meng Zi (Mencius in Wade-Giles transliteration) in Book 4 chapter 9 wrote about the importance of a Confucian ruler "storing up" his benevolence. To illustrate his point he wrote:

> "The case of a prince who might want to be king today is like someone with a seven year old illness needing three year old mugwort to cure it."

今之欲王者，
猶七年之病求三年之艾也

The meaning implied by this is clear. Mugwort can help cure chronic illness. Given the relatively anarchic age of competing nation states in which he was writing Meng Zi was recognising the importance of benevolence in a ruler. For

---

[68] James Legge's translation 1898
http://etext.virginia.edu/chinese/shijing/AnoShih.html retrieved 3/1/2010.

him, benevolence was as necessary as having some matured (three year old) mugwort in a medicine chest ready to help cure a chronic (seven year old) illness. Without it, Meng Zi implied, the health, whether of the state or the body, would simply deteriorate, leading to decay and ruin. It is important for us to note, however, that he never actually stipulated that the mugwort should be **burnt** to cure this chronic illness although the likelihood does exist. That link, however, is quite definitely made, however, in the writings of Zhuang Zi.

Zhuang Zi[69] (370-301 BC) wickedly satirises Confucius in chapter 29 of "the Robber Zhi", "quoting" him as saying (immediately after his bruising encounter with the Robber):

"My case has been like that of the man who burnt moxa on himself without being ill. I rushed off to stroke the tiger's head, played with his whiskers, and I narrowly escaped his mouth!"

丘所謂無病而自**灸**也，
疾走料虎頭，
編虎須幾不免虎口哉

(The characters both for mugwort and for moxibustion where they each occur in these three texts have been separately highlighted in bold.)

Reviewing these three sources together, we can sketch out a bigger picture.

The extract from Meng Zi implies that mugwort may have already been the material of choice for moxibustion, and also that a three-year maturation process to enhance its effects was already considered essential, a tradition which survives to the present day. This ageing of mugwort (which may, as we have already discussed, be in the heart of the etymology of the ideogram *jiu* for moxa itself) is an interesting topic which will be revisited later when we examine the plant's chemistry. We can further surmise that it might already have been a tradition already hundreds of years old by the time of the Mawangdui texts if the coincidence found in Ode 72 is significant. It also possibly suggests that moxa was already being widely used to treat chronic disease (i.e. a "seven year old illness").

Yamada believes that Zhuang Zi's phrase "burning moxa on oneself without being ill" was a country proverb, referring to someone doing something stupid. If this is the case, apart from implying that moxibustion was in widespread use, it also suggests that it was not yet being popularly used as a preventative method of treatment in the way that it did later, at least by Tang times. But in the same way that we cannot be absolutely certain that Meng Zi implied that the threeyear old mugwort was necessarily for use in cautery therapy, we can neither be certain,

---

[69]Commonly referred to as Chuang Tsu when using Wade Giles transliteration.

unfortunately, that Zhuang Zi was definitely implying that it was mugwort that was to be used for cauterisation. The two clues are circumstantially strong enough nevertheless to suggest that both were true, although it would certainly be a step too far to assume from this that any treatment being alluded to depended on any sort of channel or vessel system.

These two latter quotations, however, do suggest that both aged mugwort and some kind of moxibustion therapy would have been familiar enough to the literate classes of the time to have been used in two complex metaphors, both clearly expected by their authors to be readily intelligible to their anticipated readership – certainly more so than they are today to a modern reader of these texts.

It should also be added that these two august philosophers had not that much in common with each other in their interpretations of life, Meng Zi being very much a Confucian, and Zhuang Zi identifiable as a Daoist of a particularly impishly anti-Confucian bent. More recent scholarship suggests that the distinctions between these two schools of Confucianism and Daoism may not have been quite as clear as they appeared to earlier scholars, but differences do quite clearly exist, with Zhuang Zi's writings being one of the more obvious examples. Overall, the fact that references to moxa and mugwort occurs in the literature of both philosophies must at least suggest that moxibustion was quite widely used across contemporary Chinese literate society, which is not something necessarily evident at all from the Mawangdui texts.

The History of Moxibustion through the Centuries

After the Mawangdui texts[70], which could well of course actually have been contemporaneous to both Meng Zi and Zhuang Zi, the next reference to moxibustion which can be considered in any way credible is in the biography of Cang Gong (the "Master of the Granary" whose given name was actually Chunyu Yi) in the *Shi Ji*("Historical Records") of 90BC[71]. This biography describes twenty-five medical case studies, dated approximately between 186 and 154BC. Fifteen of these were recorded as being cured, two with moxibustion and two with something which might be considered as proto-acupuncture. Neither acupuncture case, however, in any way accords with the application of any recognisable treatment using channel theory: one merely describes the insertion of a needle at

---

[70] Unless otherwise noted, the information concerning the "classical texts" comes from the work of Birch and Felt 1999 "Understanding Acupuncture". Almost all these texts are not available in English. The references to the *Suwen* come from Maoshing Ni's 1995 translation (Shambhala), the *Lingshu* from Wu Jing-Nuan's 1993 translation (University of Hawai'I press), and the "The Systematic Classic of Acupuncture & Moxibustion" translated by Yang Shou-Zhong and Charles Chace 1994 (Blue Poppy Press).

[71] Bai Xinghua 2001 "Acupuncture, a Visible Holism" (Butterworth Heinemann)

the back of the head of a prince (which apparently resuscitated him); the other cured a case of hot and painful feet by inserting needles in three locations probably on the sole or arch of the foot. In contrast, the moxibustion cases conform to the principles outlined in the Mawangdui texts in both diagnosis and treatment, strongly confirming the idea that acumoxa medical practice in China was in transition at the time, with moxa still dominant as a practice. This cautery therapy was seemingly based on a seminal channel theory in contrast to a basic form of acupuncture which had yet to condense into any sort of theoretical model which might be recognisable to us today, or even a little later by the authors of the *Nei Jing* or *Nan Jing*.

The *Huang Di Nei Jing Suwen* and *Lingshu*, which together are widely regarded as the classic seminal canons of East Asian acupuncture, are our next waymarkers. The idea that these are truly **the** seminal canons is of course an arguable assumption since we will never know the exact provenance of the therapeutic traditions collated in the *Nei Jing*, and can only make scholastic best guesses, aware that other source texts have been lost and that the surviving literature represents a compilation of separate traditions any one of which may have been more venerable in age than the others. Additionally, it is accepted that these early surviving texts were widely corrupted, edited and added to over the ensuing centuries. However, in these particular *Nei Jing* texts it is acupuncture and not moxa which incontrovertibly emerges into the limelight, something which pretty much sets up their relationship for the next two millennia right up to the present day.

It is actually quite arguable that the *Suwen*, which is more often accepted as the earlier of the texts, reveals as much about bloodletting as it does about acupuncture, giving respect in its references to stone needles (*bian*) as much as to metal ones (*zhen*), and paying less attention to *qi* manipulation than to simple "piercing" (*ci*) which has strong echoes of piercing to release blood or pus.

In fact Donald Harper identifies a passage of text in *Lingshu* 7 which closely resembles an ancestral passage in another Mawangdui text – with revealing differences: it neatly substitutes both the *bian* (needle, often of stone for puncturing) with *zhen* (the metal needle), and the word *nong* (pus) with *bing* (ailment). If evidence is required of what Harper describes as a "rapid transition" of ideas in Chinese medicine at this time, this is perhaps one of the most telling.
The *Lingshu* is widely accepted today as initiating a more complete picture of something which we might recognise as acupuncture *jingluo* channel theory. Chapter 10, one of its less controversial chapters and certainly one of its most important, is particularly significant in this respect, since, similarly to *Ling Shu* 7 it seems to quite shamelessly borrow the Mawangdui moxa channel texts as its basic descriptive template. In the two Mawangdui texts and in *Lingshu* 10, the authors follow the identical formulaic pattern to describe each channel: first comes a description of the origin and pathway of the channel, which is then followed by a description of the symptoms if the channel is either "moved", diseased or

dysfunctional. No such echoes from those earlier moxa texts exist in the *Suwen*. The author(s) of the *Lingshu*, however, then offer up two extra factors of the most significant added value – a vital connection between each channel to create a larger circuit of *qi*, and an idea of excess of pathogenic *xie qi* and deficiency of upright *zheng qi* as being the two causative factors of illness in each channel. The idea of reinforcing deficiency and reducing excess was in fact mooted in two of the other Mawangdui texts, but there is no real evidence that this idea relates to the use of moxibustion. Unschuld, moreover, considers the chosen terminology implicit within these two terms (*zheng* and *xie*) as being as much political as medical, an idea which reflected a part of a paradigm shift in the way health and illness were being viewed[72]. *Zheng* (meaning upright), for instance, can quite plainly be seen as an idea which is firmly rooted in Confucian ideology.

With these simple additions, along with the iconoclastic additional application of *qi* manipulation with fine metal needles, the basic theoretical framework for acumoxa is set for the next two millennia – with needle therapy being promoted to a clear state of dominance.

Further evidence of a direct connection with *mai* of the Mawangdui texts exists elsewhere in the descriptions of the *jingmai* of the *Nei Jing* and is illustrated in the chart below which demonstrates the variations in channel direction as identified within various passages in the Mawangdui texts, the *Suwen*, and the *Lingshu*.

Clear inconsistencies occur between chapters in the received text in terms of their descriptions of channel direction and circulation. Such anomalies create frustration to the modern reader looking for completeness and coherence, something which apparently was not viewed with such importance by the collators of these early texts. Perhaps we do not as yet have enough information with which to make any clear sense of these differences, but the directional anomalies which have survived in these chapters actually present what might best be described as precious fossilised tracks in the sand, and they suggest how channel directionalities may have ultimately evolved from these earlier moxa texts.

Lingshu 1 and *Lingshu* 17, for instance, both identify channel directions identically to the specific Mawangdui text which also identified the *mai* by their relationships to the legs and arms. *Lingshu* 10 and *Lingshu* 16, however, describe their directionalities as they are still accepted today.

---

[72] An Interview with Paul Unschuld. 1994. European Journal of Oriental Medicine 1:4; p 9.

Part 1 – the Roots

	Lu	LI	St	Sp	Ht	SI	Bl	Ki	Pc	TB	GB	Liv
	Arm taiyin	Arm yang ming	Leg yang ming	Leg tai yin	Arm shao yin	Arm taiyin	Leg tai yang	Leg shao yin	Arm jue yin	Arm shao yang	Leg shao yang	Leg jue yin
Ma wang dui 11 Yin/Yang	In	In *tooth*	In	Out *Stomach*	In	Out *Shoulder*	In	In	-	In *ear*	In	In
Ma wang dui 11 Foot/Arm	In	In	In	In	In	In	In	In	-	In	In	In
Ling shu 1 & 17	In	In	In	In	In	In	In	In	In	In	In	In
Suwen 29	Out	In	In	Out	Out	In	In	Out	Out	In	In	Out
Ling shu 5	-	In	In	In	-	In	In	In	-	In	In	In
Suwen 45		In	In	Out		In	In	Out		In	In	Out
Suwen 59	?	?	?	?	?	?	?	?	?	?	?	?
Suwen 79	In	Out	In	Out	Out	In	Out	In	Out	Out	In	In
Ling shu 16	Out	In	Out	In	Out	In	Out	In	Out	In	Out	In
Ling shu 10	Out	In	Out	In	Out	In	Out	In	Out	In	Out	In
Nan Jing 23	In	In	In	In	In	In	In	In	In	In	In	In
Nan Jing 24	Out	In	Out	In	Out	In	Out	In	Out	In	Out	In

Chart showing various channel directionalities in the different texts

The pervasive centripetal model, described in the Mawangdui Eleven Vessels of Foot and Arm text, and picked up both in *Lingshu* 1 & 17 and also in *Nanjing* 24, offers us the first suggestions of the clinically important *jing-ying-shu-jing-he* (spring, brook, stream, river, sea) classification of points of *Lingshu* 1, of course, as well, incidentally, as the directionalities of the Divergent Channels as described in *Lingshu* 11.

Harper proposes that the locations on the pathway of a vessel which were realised as being more efficacious than others were initially identified through cauterisation, but that this process then culminated with the identification and naming of acupoints where needles were inserted[73].

The Mawangdui moxa texts can thus be seen to have supplied the seminal template for acupuncture *jingluo* channel theory – and as importantly, we can suggest that it was the practice of moxibustion which catalysed the transformation of "needle therapy" from one that was primarily focused on localised lancing and bloodletting into something which used needles to promote health in a way which today might be described as holistic. If this indeed happened, it appears to have done so by adapting and developing the earlier *mai* vessel concept into a more involved and sophisticated circulating channel system through which *qi* over the whole body could be regulated by exploiting and accessing the newly identified acupoints by needles or indeed by moxa itself.

The Role of Technology

One further development was taking place at the time which was also a vital part of this story and it cannot be ignored. In contrast to other technologies, the Chinese had been initially slow in their general development of metallurgy. Whereas bronze was in widespread use in the Mediterranean basin around 2000-1200 BC, it failed to arrive in China until near the end of this period. In fact even when it did arrive its use was comparatively limited although it was indisputably worked with unique and extraordinary skill. Stone tools, for instance, remained the standard in agriculture throughout this period. Copper and tin were in short supply in comparison to the Mediterranean basin, and perhaps as well there was such hierarchical control by the ruling elite that no-one gave any creative thought to easing the toil of the peasants who were producing the food. If this was true, it serves to remind us that contemporary medical thought was similarly very much the domain of these same elite classes, and it is a matter of speculation as to what sorts of therapies were actually available to the general population at this time.

Iron working similarly appeared in China later than in the West, making its first inroads during the Warring States period. Iron certainly offers a superior raw material for swords and it was first put to this use in China at this time. Wars invariably stimulate technological (as well as medical) innovations, and it may even have been the incorpation of iron into their swords which gave the Qin the technological edge to conquer the other competing nation states.

Once this iron technology finally arrived, the inventiveness of the Chinese mind caught on quickly. There is evidence that within a mere couple of centuries the Chinese developed ploughs and ploughshares which were superior to any in use

---

[73] Donald Harper 1998 "Early Chinese Medical Literature - The Mawangdui Medical Manuscripts" (Keegan Paul)

elsewhere in Eurasia at the time and which remained unsurpassed in equivalent technological design in Europe for a further thousand years.

The tomb of Prince Liu Sheng, where those earliest examples of metal needles were found, was also found to contain more iron objects than bronze ones, something which may well have been significant.

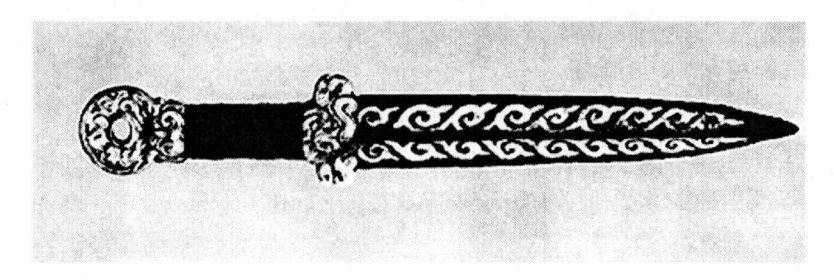

An iron dagger found in Liu Sheng's tomb

Iron (and even more so, of course, steel) is much harder to forge than bronze, certainly in terms of a quality product. Iron's melting points are much higher than that of bronze, and that of steel is even higher. It is also clear that the inherent brittle fragility of cast iron, whilst perhaps satisfying the demands of larger agricultural implements or larger weapons, would hardly suit those of an acupuncture needle let alone those of a serviceable sword. As discussed earlier, those earliest needles which survive were made of gold and silver, but they may well have been merely symbolic because of their thickness. Fine steel needles, if they were used at all so long ago, would almost certainly have perished into a rusty dust.

Iron working appeared first in Xinjiang in the North West (doubtless through the percolative trade from the West as this area lies on the eastern end of the silk route). It took a few centuries, however, for ironworking techniques in China to have developed sufficient for iron to be considered a superior product to bronze. Copper and tin, the constituents of bronze, were in even shorter supply in the south of China, and it may well have been because of this that the world's first blast furnaces for smelting iron appeared in this region rather than further north or west. It may also be coincidental and fanciful, but (as every acupuncturist knows from *Suwen* 12) needling was supposed to originate "from the south", in the same way as moxa was supposed to come "from the north". Perhaps in this sense it really did.

These earliest known blast furnaces appeared in Southern China at around 100 BC, a date which places their development at much the same time as the first acupuncture case study in the *Shi Ji* mentioned above, as well as placing them later than the Mawangdui moxa texts and almost certainly before the *Suwen*. So, however much the authors of the *Nei Jing Suwen* and *Lingshu* may have alluded to older needling texts, those innovations in therapeutic techniques which involved fine needle insertions would have been only recently technologically possible at the time when these same texts are estimated to have been compiled. In fact, certainly as far as fine needle therapy is concerned, those even earlier texts which were repeatedly alluded to in the canon seem unlikely to have been much more than romantic notions. The many references to them may have been added to inlay authenticity and Confucian respectability into the main text.

Such technological developments in metallurgy, occurring as they were at the same time as the birth of acupuncture and at the dawning of the idea of *qi* manipulation, might also serve to explain the apparent relative "downgrading" of moxibustion as the needle therapists made their impact upon the medical practices of their time. Here was the most modern technology of its age, epitomised by the skilled use of these finer needles by refined physicians. Furthermore, this needling must have acquired a cachet in its therapeutic application, requiring skill and dexterity which is beautifully evoked in some of the more eloquent chapters of the *Lingshu*[74].

Acupuncture was thus initially dependent upon two interdependent skills, one of metallurgy, and the other of needle dexterity. No such skills were required in the processing of mugwort nor in the practice of moxibustion – no furnaces or forges, and no particular technical dexterity. It was low-tech in every respect of this new arrival, and thus perhaps had diminishing appeal to the wealthy ruling elite.

One can imagine a conversation in a bath house in the early Han dynasty – "How are those blisters on your back healing up? From that moxa cautery? I thought so…Have you heard about this new *Zhen* thing? So much classier than that *Jiu* stuff which hurts so much and leaves those horrible blisters. Are they still weeping? So unnecessary! My new physician's trained in needling, you know – he's so clever and skilful with his *Zhen* needle. You hardly feel it, no more than a mosquito bite even when it goes quite deep – but my back pain vanishes almost instantly. And there's no blood – not like those butchers with their *bian* stone – not like them at all! You should try it out for that shoulder of yours – I'll give you his address."

Moxibustion in other Early Texts

Also of relatively unexplored significance in the history of moxibustion is the Five Phase classic the *Nan Jing*. This text is understood to follow on behind the *Nei Jing* and offers us the earliest surviving relatively homogenous Chinese medical classic. One of its unexplored significances lies in the fact that it fundamentally fails to mention moxa at all, something which effectively seems to complete the story of

---

[74] For an excellent exposition of this eloquence, the reader is referred to Charles Chace's essays in the Lantern journal – "The axes of efficacy" and "On greeting a friend" - Volume 6, issues 1 & 2.

the early tensions between the two therapies and their inter-development – between the "practice" of moxibustion, and the "art" of acupuncture. In completely ignoring moxibustion, the author of the *Nan Jing* may be inadvertently but helpfully highlighting for us the ultimate supremacy of delicate needling techniques over the cruder smouldering of mugwort.

Further circumstantial evidence exists for this idea, because another facet of the earlier medicine is also entirely absent from the chapters of the *Nan Jing*. We discussed earlier how the roots of Chinese medicine are intertwined with ideas of magic, demonology and sorcery. Texts containing spells and incantations were unearthed along with the moxa texts at Mawangdui, and occasional references to similar rituals are encountered here and there within the chapters of the *Nei Jing*, suggesting that they were still surviving if only vestigially. Nothing of the kind, however, exists in the *Nan Jing*. The absence of any reference to magic or demonology along with the absence of any reference at all to moxibustion strongly suggests that the author of the *Nan Jing* was writing the text book for a new systematised medicine on a far blanker page than any that had gone before.

One further idea concerning the *Nan Jing* is proposed by David Keegan[75]. He actually hypothesises that the *Nan Jing* emerged from a separate tradition to the dominant *Huang Di* school. He suggests that it may have been originally a part of the *Bian Que* school, although he does not provide a conclusive case for this. Certainly a tradition has persisted that this text was written by Qin Yueren, the supposed real name of Bian Que himself, so it is hardly unreasonable to suggest that the text may be associable with a school of medicine of the same name. Based on the language and structure of the *Nei Jing* texts and that of the *Nan Jing*, however, Keegan is explicit that the text of the *Nan Jing* is distinct from the *Nei Jing* tradition: "The more we examine the *Nan Jing* the less it looks like an explication of the *Nei Jing*" he writes, and it is difficult to disagree with him.

If the *Nan Jing* was indeed reflective of the *Bian Que*s chool, it also strongly suggests, of course, that this school had little or no truck with moxibustion, being as its eighty-one chapters so completely ignore it.

The *Lingshu* already contained many beautiful passages suggesting that needling should be performed with the utmost dexterity and care. In contrast, moxibustion texts from both earlier and later seem generally directed towards the lay practitioner rather than the scholar or sage physician, suggesting that moxa may have rapidly become the resort of the lower classes, whilst acupuncture became the fashionable therapy for the cultural and ruling elite. Classical acupuncture was never promoted in the more basic terms used in these moxa texts, though over the centuries of course there may well have been many illiterate acupuncturists.

---

[75] David Joseph Keegan 1998 "The Huang-ti Nei-Ching: the structure of the compilation; the significance of the structure" (Unpublished Doctoral Thesis)

Right into the current period, in fact, moxibustion is frequently performed only by the acupuncturist's assistant or apprentice, or is prescribed for application at home by a family member as an adjunct to the needle therapy. Today in the West, many of us would have no trouble at all describing acupuncture as a therapeutic "art", but few would be willing to make such a grandiose claim for basic moxa treatment. By the time of these classics of early Chinese medical thought, there may already have existed some scholastic snobbery towards the practice of moxibustion from which it has suffered ever since.

Paul Unschuld observes that no actual **methods** of cauterisation were actually described at all in the *Suwen*, whilst needling techniques are described and alluded to frequently in its chapters. He concludes from this that the compilers of the *Suwen* regarded moxa as a "popular, trusted and effective remedy", a fact which obviated a requirement for any written instruction on its application in the "manual". This indeed may be true, since so much is assumed of the modern reader when encountering these opaque early texts today – something which is often only helped with the aid of the anthropological and linguistic spotlights provided by sinologists and scholars.

Unschuld's conclusion is at least debatable, however, precisely because one of the strongest conclusions we can draw from the similarities and differences which reveal themselves in these early texts is that moxa cautery may have provided the catalyst for the channel theories on which these very early classic acupuncture texts depended. If this was so, moxibustion lay at the very heart of the medical practices described and we would expect to find it alluded to in more detail – unless, of course, there was a motive for not doing so. It does not necessarily follow at all that descriptions of its application should have been so totally omitted – even if it were indeed as popular as Unschuld suggests. There may have been other reasons, one being that moxa was becoming consciously relegated to a lower status as a more primitive or basic form of treatment. Some isolated technical references to moxibustion techniques do exist in the *Lingshu*, although we can unfortunately be far from certain whether they were contained in the original text. We will examine these references later in Part 3 the Stems.

Unschuld, however, also persuasively suggests that the *Nei Jing* texts reflect a deliberate break with older traditions which have failed to survive, and it seems likely that this fact above all others might be the decisive factor in the mere "marginal recognition" of moxibustion in these texts[76].

In tune with this, the *[Zhen Jiu] Jia Yi Jing* (Systematic Classic [of Acupuncture and Moxibustion]) of circa 280 AD also pretty much ignores moxibustion despite its name, even in its discussions of cold-type illnesses. In Book 3, however, it does

---

[76] Paul Unschuld 2003 "Huang Di Nei Jing Su Wen – Nature, Knowledge, Imagery in an Ancient Chinese Medical Text" University of California Press pp 315-317

helpfully list the number of moxa cones (*zhuang*) applicable to each and every acupoint for the first time alongside the needling depths. In some sense this fills an important missing gap in the record. It also lists some contra-indicated points. Since the *Jia Yi Jing* purports to be a distillation of three earlier texts, the *Suwen*, the *Zhen Jing*[77] and the *Ming Tang* (the last of which was subsequently lost and the received texts of the other two containing no recognisable references to this particular topics), these specific inclusions must offer us clues as to the possible content of this missing classic. In other words, the *Ming Tang* might actually have included more early information on moxa use than the other texts.

The word "*zhuang*", incidentally, contains an interesting implicit connotation. It is the word used for moxa cones but is actually a counting word, literally referring to numbers of anything that are "strong, able-bodied, or healthy". To quote a point as requiring three "*zhuang*", therefore, implies that the patient will not just receive three cones of moxa but will also benefit from "three strengthenings"[78]. This choice of the word "*zhuang*" must have been deliberate and suggests a contemporary understanding that moxa could be used as a way of strengthening the constitution of the patient. It furthermore provides us with a prelude to its later application for disease prevention and longevity.

The Systematic Classic also contains a somewhat less systematic section which contradicts the listing of points and the numbers of cones applicable to each in Book 3. This occurs in a section discussing illnesses of "cold and heat" (Book 8, Chapter 1, Section 6). The text clearly describes constitutionally deficient patients and sees them as being particularly susceptible to such illnesses and then lists specific indicated points for treatment. The number of cones, however, is at wide variance to those listed elsewhere, suggesting it might have been from a different source altogether. Huangfu may have seen it as important to include this section, wherever it may have originated from, despite it clearly eluding his valiant attempts at systemisation.

This section also identifies for the first of many times in the literature the usefulness of moxa in the case of rabid dog bites[79].

In the third century, Ge Hong wrote about moxa in the "Emergency Prescriptions to keep up your Sleeve" (c.341 AD). He focused particularly on its use in emergency treatment, and was also the first recorded physician to use intermediary

---

[77] The *Zhen Jing* is generally accepted for the sake of expediency and convenience to have been retitled the *Lingshu* sometime before the Tang Dynasty, which may or may not be correct.

[78] Lorraine Wilcox 2008 "Moxibustion, the Power of Mugwort Fire" (Blue Poppy Press) p9

[79] Yang Shou-Zhong and Charles Chace 1994 "The Systematic Classic of Acupuncture & Moxibustion" (Blue Poppy Press)

substances between the moxa and the skin, using garlic, dough with pepper, and salt, and was also the first, in fact, to recommend using salt moxa on Ren8.

In the seventh century, the venerable Sun Simiao, in his description of extra points in the *Qian Jin Yao Fang* ("Formulas worth a Thousand Ducats"), specifically mentions that some points are especially powerful when treated with moxa. Here moxa is highlighted for the first time in the surviving literature as a preventative treatment both for longevity and as an agent against infectious diseases. Sun also identified the "pressure-pain" *ashi* phenomenon at these and other points. These ideas will resurface later in our investigations. In the *Qian Jin Yi Fang* (the "Supplement to the Thousand Ducat Formulas") of 682 AD, he also stipulated the use of fewer and smaller moxa cones to produce more tonifying effects, although elsewhere in his writings he usually advocated large numbers of cones.

In the same period the "Moxibustion Method for Consumptive Disease" (written by Cui Zhidi in 670 AD) described the use of moxibustion for what was unquestionably tuberculosis. This text was subsequently lost, but is referred to repeatedly in later centuries.

A little later in 752 AD, Wang Tao wrote the *Wai Tai Bi Yao* ("Important Formulae and Prescriptions revealed by a Governor of a Distant Province"). It was a herbal treatise with many references to moxibustion but not to needling because of Wang's cautionary attitude to the risks implicit in acupuncture. "Acupuncture can kill living people", he wrote, "but cannot revive the dying. If one desires to record this [technique], then I'm afraid one will harm life. [Therefore]...I only adopt moxibustion". For some physicians earlier forms of acupuncture were thus apparently regarded as being just too dangerous. In some sense this text might even represent a reaction to the dominance of the needle therapist, but nevertheless it did not have a major influence on the development of medicine in China.

Quite soon after this printing was invented in China, and the availability of medical texts changed forever.

In the twelfth century, the moxa stick was invented and the associated *Shi Zhen* tradition began, a school which possibly pushed Chinese moxibustion more towards indirect treatment. Also in the twelfth century the *Huang Di Ming Tang Jiu Jing*, an important moxa-only text, was written – a text which latterly influenced modern moxibustion in Japan, particularly Isaburo Fukaya.

In 1127 Zhuang Chuo wrote the *Gaohuang Shu Xue Jiu Fa* "Moxibustion on Gaohuang shu Bl43" and he described the wonderful effects of applying moxa to Gaohuang shu or Bl43.

"The Book of Bian Que's Heart" the *Bian Que Xinshu* of 1146 described moxa extensively. Its author, Dou Cai, endorsed moxibustion both for preventative medicine and for longevity as well as for emergency use. His treatments were characterised by the use of huge numbers of cones, and he ascribed enormous importance to moxa treatment: "A doctor's use of moxibustion to treat disease is like the use of fuel to cook a meal," he wrote – a powerful simile in a culture so suffused with the culinary arts as the Chinese.

In the next century, the *Bei Ji Jiu Fa* ('the Moxibustion Methods for Use in Emergencies") of 1226, a moxa-only text, was published but was subsequently lost in China. Fortuitously, it had by then been exported to Japan where it sowed its own particular seed, and it is to Japan that we need to go to pick up the story and subsequent developments.

Acumoxa in Japan

Acupuncture and moxibustion is said to have come to Japan with Buddhist monks in the sixth century. Some stories suggest that it arrived with the legendary Buddhist saint Kobo Daishi, about whom legends abound. Daishi had studied Buddhism in depth in China before returning to Japan, bringing with him all he had learnt. How true this version of events is is debatable, particularly since it appears to have occurred (in 806) well after Chinese medicine had already arrived in Japan – particularly since, as is suggested by Casal, it so suited the "money-loving priesthood"[80]. A more reliable version of events actually describes acumoxa arriving even earlier – in 562 with another monk, Chiso, who definitely brought the first texts on acupuncture to Japan. What can much more reasonably be claimed is that both acupuncture and moxibustion truly flowered into something which can be recognised as Japanese somewhat later in the seventeenth century, although to some degree they also separated at the same time. This separation has import on our later investigations into the relevance of moxibustion today.

At this time the unique Japanese tradition of acupuncture practice by the blind was initiated by Waichi Sugiyama's unsurpassed mastery with the *hari* needle and by his successful treatment of Shogun Tokugawa's serious illness. No matter how skilful and refined the blind "*hari*" acupuncturists might have become, however, it was obvious that the associated practice of burning a highly combustible herb on a patient's skin could never be as safely or effectively practised by the non-sighted; at best it could only be done by sighted assistants under their direction. Moxa-only texts had been appearing in Japanese almost a century before Sugiyama, but it may well be possibly as a consequence of this novel appropriation of acupuncture by the visually impairedthat several texts appeared at this time in Japan which

---

[80]U.A.Casal "Acupuncture Moxibustion and Massage in Japan".http://nirc.nanzan-u.ac.jp/publications/afs/pdf/a136.pdf - retrieved 3/1/2010

specifically refined the traditions of general moxibustion. Such texts (*Mokyu Susetsu, Ipon Do Kyusen, Kagawa Kyuten*, and *Meika Kyusen*) effectively established a tradition of discrete moxa practice which utilised empirical treatment points for specific diseases. Goto Gonzan (1659-1733), who was an innovative scholar-physician and the author of *Mokyu Susetsu*, reframed contemporary thinking on pathology by teaching that all illness was basically caused by stagnation of *qi*. He used moxibustion as a basic tool for re-activating its movement because it "has the ability to reach the stagnation of coldness in the earth immediately because it has the active qi of the sun"[81]. As a result of his work, even physicians who specialised in drug treatment began to incorporate moxa into their practice. This in turn led to greater use of moxa amongst ordinary people with different regions developing their own characteristic styles of practice.

It was around this same time, of course, that Busschof and Cleyer were reporting about moxa to their European readership. In 1690 Engelbert Kaempfer arrived in Japan and began studying Japanese culture. Kaempfer wrote a treatise entitled "Moxa in China and Japan" in which he described its practice with some wonderment. Interestingly he described the size of moxa cones used then as being the size of half a grain of rice, so this minimalist approach in terms of cone size has hardly varied in at least the last three hundred years. It is quite clear from his writings that the use of moxa at the time was widespread in Japan: he noted that he found it impossible to find a single Japanese person who did not show some signs of scarring from moxa.

Gonzan developed what he termed the "Five Pole Moxibustion Method" which he used to treat most diseases, although he was clear that its application should be varied between four basic approaches. The locations he advocated were all on the back: at the "upper pole" – at the spinous process of the first thoracic vertebrae; at the "lower pole" – at the coccyx; at the "middle pole" – midway between the upper and lower poles; at the "left pole" – 1.5 *cun* left of the middle pole; and at the "right pole" – 1.5 *cun* right of the middle pole.

He identified four main causes of disease, but creatively recognised that it was rare that only one of these might be involved on its own. As such, using a set of basic principles, he could adapt his simple treatment approach to suit each and every patient he encountered. We look at this treatment in another context in more detail in Part 3 the Branches. For now it is enough to identify that the numbers of cones per treatment would today be considered beyond excessive, but one other part of his approach in particular has survived to become a fundamental part of the approach in the treatments of Sawada and Fukaya in the twentieth century, and thus to have particular influence on us today. This is in the treatment of palpatory findings in the abdomen and back, particularly in terms of knots and muscular stiffness.

---

[81] Peter Eckman 1996 "In the Footsteps of the Yellow Emperor" (Cypress Book Company)

It is probable that this deepening understanding in Japan of the use of moxa, along with possible better strains of mugwort and the development of refinement and processing techniques which resulted in a purer final product, has concertedly influenced the way moxibustion has been practised in Japan right into the current era when it remains a specialism in its own right.

It is ironic that it may have taken the supremacy in skill of the blind *hari* practitioners of acupuncture to ignite and kindle a more appropriate scholastic and investigative approach to moxa by sighted practitioners, something which had been largely missing from East Asian medicine since the times of the *Nan Jing*.

Later Chinese Texts

Meanwhile, back in China in the Yuan dynasty, Zhu Danxi had published the "Heart Methods of Danxi" in 1347. Its modern significance lies in the controversial fact that it describes the use of moxibustion for treating heat conditions. This was echoed in the work of Li Chan in 1575 ("Entering the Gate of Medicine").

Moxibustion was praised as a sexual stimulant before intercourse in the seventy-eighth chapter of the renowned erotic novel the *Jin Ping Mei* (published in 1610 and later described by a critic in theQing dynasty as "the most incredible book under the heavens"). Unfortunately this is a huge book, and the translation into English (currently in three volumes) has only reached chapter fifty, so those who might be interested will have to wait to know what was going on in this chapter[82]. This text, incidentally, directly echoes a passage from one of the Mawangdui texts of fifteen hundred odd years earlier in which a man who has over-indulged in sexual activity could "cauterise his body to bring forth his *qi*." In "the Seven Losses and Eight Profits of the Techniques of Sex", the exhausted male is recorded as being re-invigorated by "giving medicine and performing moxibustion, then supplying it to the body by serving food[83]."

This time was also a period of importance for the development of acumoxa generally, it coinciding with the end of the Ming Dynasty. Until recently, the significance of this period in relation to the development of moxibustion has been largely unknown in the English language literature. Thanks to the work of Lorraine Wilcox, however, real insight can now be gained into the practice of moxibustion during this period through her distillation of the following works –

---

[82] Wolfram Eberhard 1983 "A Dictionary of Chinese Symbols" (Routledge and Keegan Paul)

[83] Vivienne Lo 2005 "Imaging Practice: Sense and Sensuality in Early Chinese Medical Thought" in "The Warp and the Weft: Graphics and Text in the Production of Technical Knowledge in China" Leiden (Brill) p396

The Moon over Matsushima

Yang Jizhou's "Great Compendium of Acupuncture and Moxibustion", Zhang Jiebin's "Illustrated Supplement to the Categorized Classic" and "Jingyue's Complete Works", and Li Shizhen's "Great Pharmacopoeia". Each of these original texts has provided Wilcox with a rich source of material from which to review the contemporary conceptions of moxibustion therapy. No modern study of moxa in English can garner any respect without acknowledging the value of her work.

Of significance, Zhang went against more recent theories and opposed the use of moxa in heat conditions, but this view remained a far from unanimous one at the time, since Gong Juzhong endorsed its use in all conditions including heat in his floridly entitled work "A Spot of Snow on a Red (hot) Stove".

Further moxa texts were still published in China subsequent to these texts, one of which was the *Shen Jiu Jing Lun* ("Miraculous Moxibustion Classic") of the nineteenth century, so it is self-evident that moxa was still being practised medically, but its use as a primary therapy may well have already become less widespread, as it has certainly latterly become in the modern era with the resurgence of interest in traditional medical techniques. Texts from the Qing dynasty and later are generally characterised only by repeated focus on the moxa pole or by simply repeating ideas from earlier texts.

More Current Use of Moxa

Anyone who has attended an acupuncture department in a TCM hospital in China will be well aware of moxa's copious use as part of the repertoire of techniques in *Zhong Yi* TCM if for no other reason than because of the attendant pervasive smoke. Generally it is used as an adjunct to acupuncture treatment. It performs little or no function as a primary treatment, becoming almost exclusively composed of indirect techniques, particularly the application of the moxa stick or pole. Nevertheless, its widespread usage has prompted Radha Thambarijah (whose early training in China in the 1970s included methods which were pre-TCM) to provide the unequivocal advice that if one should approach an acupuncture clinic and not smell moxa smoke, one should simply run away in the opposite direction.

What seems to have happened is that, as far as "modern" TCM acumoxa is concerned, the use of "direct moxa" (the application of the smouldering mugwort directly on the skin) seems to have fallen into relative disuse. There are pre-TCM exceptions to this, however. James Tin Yao So, a Christian minister in China, reportedly became a more modern advocate of aggressive direct moxibustion treatment after seeing and taking part in its use in China in the 1930s as a way of saving cholera patients during an epidemic[84]. As a result of this experience, he developed a lifelong passion for acupuncture and moxibustion.

Here in the West, its use generally conforms to that of modern China and *Zhong Yi* TCM, described below. In Europe, where there were earlier influences from Vietnam and Taiwan particularly, it is probable that more direct moxibustion is used than in the USA, but its use is hardly systematic, and any treatment in hospital-type clinical environments is totally precluded because of its smoke.

The most common application of anything approaching "direct" moxa in the UK is when relatively small cones are placed on acupoints, lit with a taper and then swiftly lifted off as the patient indicates that she feels the heat. It has been aptly termed "snatch moxa" by Peter Eckman and is described more fully in Part 3 the Branches.

In Japan, the practice of moxibustion has become established very much in its own right, and the two practices (acupuncture and moxa) have come to be separately licensed in the country. This separation may have placed further demands on the moxa therapist which have resulted in further specialisms and applications in the practice of moxibustion which seem not to have developed elsewhere. So the search into the deeper intricacies of the treatment takes us, not back to the country of its birth, but rather to the very one which seems to have given us its common westernised name.

In 1895, as a direct reflection of Japan's dramatic modernisation process, the Medical Practitioner's Law was passed by which acupuncture, moxibustion and massage were no longer officially recognised as medical therapies[85]. In response, Professor Kinnosuke Miura led a movement to attempt to investigate acumoxa using the serological and immunological investigations available at the time. As a result of these early studies, moxibustion particularly became recognised as producing clear and significant changes in the body chemistry, something which will be examined in much more detail in Part 4 the Branches.

Two names popularly dominate the development of moxa therapy in early twentieth century Japan – Isaburo Fukaya and Takeshi (Ken) Sawada[86]. Though

---

[84] Birch& Felt 1999 "Understanding Acupuncture" (Churchill Livingstone)

[85] Manaka et al 1995 "Chasing the Dragon's Tail" (Paradigm Publications)

[86] There seems to be some confusion as to the given names of Sawada. Sawada Ken is often referred to as an acumoxa specialist, while Sawada Takeshi is generally referred to as a moxibustion specialist. Actually, the two names refer to the same man (1877-1938). He was apparently never officially licensed as an acupuncturist, only as a moxibustionist. The differences in the given names most probably reflect two different readings (on-yomi and kun-yomi) of the same name. On-yomi reflect Japanese

neither was involved in research, both men developed their own particular styles of practice and adopted protocols for treating all sorts of disease and disorder including psychological ones. In the 1930s, for instance, before the advent of antibiotics, Sawada was reported as both treating and curing TB (both pulmonary and the more intractable renal variety) with his specialist techniques. Fukaya comprehensively studied ancient moxibustion texts, particularly the *Huang Di Ming Tang Jiu Jing*, and from these texts and from his widespread clinical experience he developed his own unique effective protocols and approaches, thus further popularising the therapy.

Another less well-known name in the West, but one of equal importance, is Shimetaro Hara, a doctor who became fascinated by the actions of moxa and spent a lifetime researching it including in the treatment of tuberculosis. He also actively endorsed its health promoting properties.

Other perhaps better known names of twentieth century Japanese acumoxa also commonly used moxibustion as a primary part of their treatment: Kobei Akabane corrected his left-right heat-perceived channel imbalances with the application of moxa on the back *shu* points; Sorei Yanagiya explored moxibustion; and Dr Yoshio Manaka actively investigated and encouraged its use particularly with difficult cases, developing his own root treatment protocols and symptomatic prescriptions.

The most common form of direct moxa technique in Japan is "*toonetsukyu*" (penetrating moxa) or "*okyu*", in which small pieces of moxa, anything from rice-grain sized to thread-like, are placed on and burnt to the skin. Indirect techniques include "*chinetsukyu*" heat-perception moxa, in which relatively large cones are placed on the skin and removed when or before the patient feels warmth or heat, and "*kyutoshin*" moxa-on the-needle-head, in which a loose clump of the nap is placed on the handle of an inserted needle and burnt. Akabane himself wrote a book exclusively on this subject [87]. Other commercial preparations provide alternative ways of applying indirect techniques particularly for self-treatment at home.

It is the first type, however, the "*okyu*" direct moxa treatment which has attracted the most interesting research results, and in varying degrees is the most commonly used technique by the acumoxa therapist in Japan. It is applied in a wide range of ways: musculo-skeletal *ashi* type treatment, root treatment protocols (*ben* and *biao*), targeted treatment of intractable visceral and organic disease, for psychological problems, for both health maintenance and disease prevention, in traditional treatments (using Eight Extraordinary Vessel Opening and Coupled Points, for

---

pronunciation of Chinese words at the time of their adoption as *Kanji* (written characters from the Chinese) – kun-yomi generally reflect native Japanese words.

[87] Akabane "*Kyutoshin Ho*" or "Moxa-on-the-Needle-Head Method"

instance), in "emergency" protocols, in microsystems treatment, and in home supportive treatment. In the development of these techniques, new empirical points have been discovered, and some variations to standard point locations have also been revealed which seem to be particularly indicated with these approaches.

But we are moving clear of a discussion of the "roots" of moxibustion as it is practised today, and are clearly already above ground. More details on these matters follow in subsequent sections.

The Moon over Matsushima

Part 2 – the Stalk

> "HAVE IN MIND, MUGWORT, WHAT YOU MADE KNOWN
> WHAT YOU LAID DOWN, AT THE GREAT DENOUNCING
> UNA YOUR NAME IS, OLDEST OF HERBS
> OF MIGHT AGAINST THIRTY, AND AGAINST THREE
> OF MIGHT AGAINST VENOM AND THE ON-FLYING
> OF MIGHT AGAINST THE DEMONS WHO FARE THROUGH THE LAND"[88]

The Nature of Mugwort

All *Artemisia* belongs to the botanical tribe *Anthemideae* of the *Asteroideae*, a subfamily of the *Asteraceae* or *Compositae*. There are over 550 species of *Artemisia* alone.

Mugwort itself is a weed which flourishes on poor, dry and sandy soil, such as exists on roadsides or wasteland, particularly on soil which has been disturbed. It likes sunny positions, grows 1 to 1.8 metres high, and tends to be found in distinctive stands. Often extensive stands of plants can be seen randomly scattered alongside roads and motorways in late summer. On autumn and early winter evenings, after the plants have died back, they are prone to stand out grey and ghostlike along the roadside when lit up by cars' headlights.

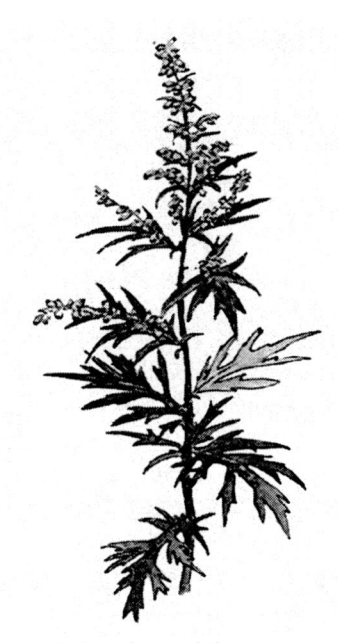

The plant seems to be selective in where it grows, rarely in what might seem to be more promising or fertile places, and often even in the downright difficult –

---

[88] From an Old English pre-Christian lay about mugwort, preserved in the Lacnunga, a Wessex herbal from the 10th century. Mugwort is listed as the first of nine sacred herbs which possibly reflect a shamanic tradition already in the process of being lost as the lay was being written down for posterity. The "on-flying" might be understood best as a metaphor for infectious disease, although it was literally perceived culturally as some form of transmittable poison. It is unclear what is being referred to by "the great denouncing".

(The watercolour painting of the mugwort plant shown above is by Jenny Craig)

growing between cracks of concrete in disused carparks, or on marginal soil alongside roadways, buffeted by the slipstream or spray of the lorries rushing past, suffering both their diesel emissions and the salt washed off the road from the previous winter. All of this suggests that it chooses not to bother with the rough and tumble of competition with its neighbours in established soil, preferring for itself locations which are less desirable for plants than the norm.

Mugwort might thus be seen to be a more wilful and perhaps contrary member of the Artemisia family.

Strains of the plant which are bushy and have thicker and more downy or flocculent undersides to their leaves are considered the best for moxibustion. These downy strains are not generally encountered in Europe, although Culpepper in the seventeenth century described it nevertheless as "very hoary white underneath". The hairs on the underside of the leaf (often referred to as the "nap") contain the volatile oils which are particularly essential for direct moxibustion techniques.

There are around two hundred strains of mugwort. Whilst the type *Artemisia vulgaris latiflora* is widely considered the usual type for moxa production, other types are utilised and often preferred. These strains include *Artemisia montana (yama yomogi* or "mountain mugwort" in Japanese), *Artemisia princeps (ooyomogi* or "big mugwort" in Japanese), *Artemisia argyii* (regarded as the superior strain in China), *Artemisia indica*, and *Artemisia chinensis*.

Certain locations in both China and Japan have been traditionally favoured for growing or collecting mugwort for moxa production. In China these are near Huanggang and Qizhou close to the Yangtze in Hubei (reputedly because of climate and soil), Guangdong (the source of most moxa rolls), and also in the Changbai Mountain Range in Jilin. According to Li Shizhen, one of the most renowned figures in the long history of East Asian medicine, and a native himself of Qizhou, this area's moxa could "penetrate a wine jug", so (for Li) its qualities of penetration seem to have been what made it most valuable.

In Japan, the traditional prime growing area is frequently quoted as being around Mount Ibukion the frontier between Gifu and Shiga prefectures. Other prefectures, however, namely Niigata (Echigo), Toyama (Etchu), Ishikawa and Nagano now account for the majority of moxa production in the country. It is said the the *yomogi* with the best down on the underside of the leaves is grown where there is good snow in winter.

The traditionally favoured locations in both countries, however, are confusing. If the *yang* properties of the sun's rays are the essential factor for the premium mugwort nap, which is an idea that has been proposed for centuries, all locations listed above would seem improbable, since none, apart from Guangdong, is at the more southerly regions of either country. The Changbaishan range, an area of some mystique with its very own mythical monster, is actually quite close to China's north-easterly border with North Korea, but it is also well known for being in an area full of a variety of medicinal herbs. Huanggang in China is famous for its local medical specialities and is the traditional and cultural home of the "Four Treasures" (snake, turtle, bamboo, and moxa).

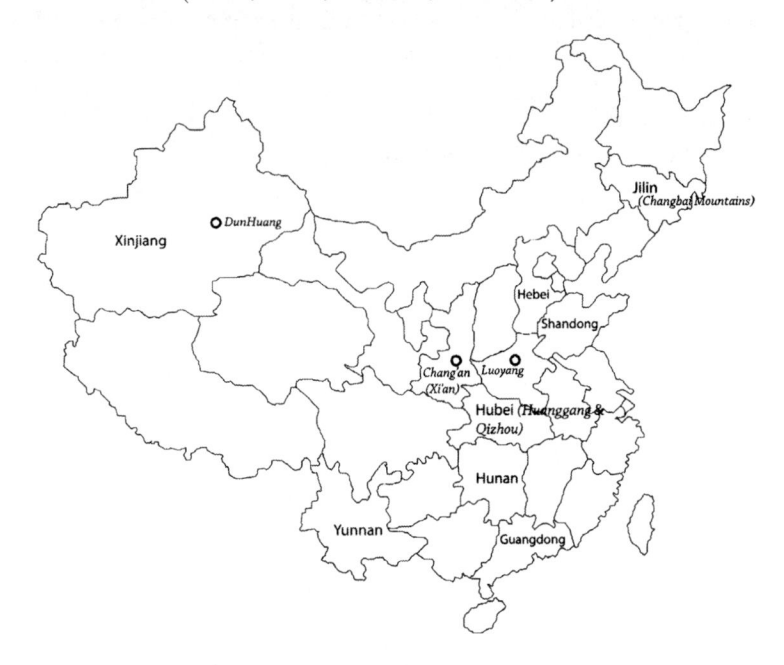

Map of China showing favoured locations for mugwort for moxa, and also showing some key locations mentioned elsewhere in the text.

Like Changbaishan in China, Mount Ibuki in Japan also holds a reputation for its medicinal plants, and is even mentioned as such in Japanese Buddhist mythology. In its very name incidentally, Ibuki contains a subtle play on words, containing the word for *ki* or "breath of life" in Japanese and the verb *iburu*, "to smoke".

At best we can initially conclude that there may be both complex and varying reasons for the favoured status of these areas for the cultivation of mugwort for moxibustion, some of which will re-emerge later in this section.

Since Mount Ibuki is so often mentioned in the same breath as references to good quality Japanese moxa, a little more information about it would seem warranted[89]. In fact, rather confusingly, two separate Ibuki mountains exist in Japan and actually both have been recorded in different eras as being famous for their moxa. One Ibuki mountain is in Tochigi prefecture, and the other is in Shiga. In the

---

[89] Most of the subsequent information on the geography of moxa production and its production comes from Ryuzo Oda's "Studies of Moxa" published in ten parts in the Journal of the Japan Society of Acupuncture and Moxibustion between 1983 and 1998.

earlier records of the use of Japanese moxa, it is quite clear that Mount Ibuki in Tochigi was being referred to, but this preference seemingly switched after the Azuchi period at the end of the seventeenth century. Adding to this confusion is the fact that each mountain also even has its own area called Shimejigahara, a special place name associated with mugwort occurring on occasions in ancient *Waka* poems in connection with moxa. A typical example occurs in "*Komizu no Goei*" a prayer to the Buddhist deity *Merofu Kannon* from the *Shashekisu* of 1289:

"We earnestly look to you for salvation while we are living in this world – the moxa-mugwort (*sashimogusa*) of Shimejigahara[90]."

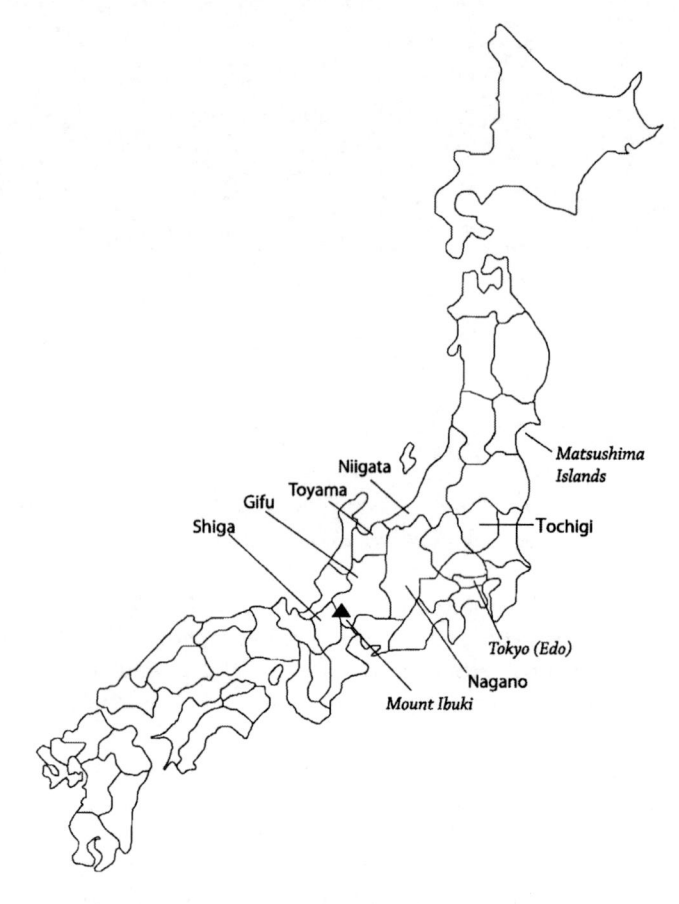

Map of Japan showing favoured locations for mugwort for moxa

Mugwort in this instance is apparently being used as a metaphor for human kind – albeit not immediately an obvious one to a casual reader. The metaphorical likening of the mugwort to the human is in fact not confined to the Japanese. In

---

[90] Fister P "Merofu Kannon and her Veneration in Zen and Imperial Circles in Seventeenth Century Japan" Japanese Journal of Religious Studies 2007 34-2: 436.

China, Li Shizhen endorsed selecting mugwort plants "in the shape of a human form" for increased efficacy, an idea somewhat similar to symbiotic relationship with the human figure which is still ascribed to ginseng roots.

In fact neither of the two Ibuki Mountains has more recently been the prime growing areas for production of mugwort for moxa in Japan, and two separate factors have probably been determinants. Firstly, alternative locations of abundance of the better strains needed for refined nap may have been discovered. Secondly, since the processing of moxa largely takes place during winter months, the existence of an available local workforce may have been a critical factor. Seasonal weather conditions may well have exerted a decisive commercial influence, offering distinct commercial advantages for local production because of associated seasonally lowered wages in particular rural areas. This certainly seems to have been the reason for the subsequent supersession of Shiga prefecture as the prime production area, firstly by Toyama prefecture, then in the nineteenth century by Fukui and Ishikawa prefectures, and ultimately by Niigata prefecture in the early twentieth.

This issue of workforce economics may yet still play a role in moxa production today in the context of the wider global economy in which we live. Whilst trekking in Nepal recently, a friend encountered a Japanese-run moxa processing plant flourishing in the mountains, harvesting and processing quality moxa which is being exported back to Japan. This location is exploited partly no doubt because of the quality of the mugwort found there, but also almost certainly partly because of the local economy and the country's low wages: the profits from the processing plant are in fact being creatively used to help finance a well-run Japanese acupuncture project in the country .

Notwithstanding all of these factors, the influence of the sun does still play a contributing role. Research confirms that mugwort leaves grown in sunlight do have more flocculence in the down on their underside than those grown in shade[91]. Such scientific findings confirm the sorts of traditional associations we find when we review the subject of moxa: moxa is *yang*; and the sunny side of the mountain, of course, is also *yang*.

The very etymology of the ideogram for *yang* contains an image of flags fluttering in the sunshine on just such a mountainside where mugwort might be found and collected. So we can extrapolate that mugwort grown on a sunny south facing slope must by definition be imbued with that little extra *yang*-ness. Another interpretation of the right hand side of the character suggests that it is a lizard basking in sunshine, as they are wont to do on the warmth of south-facing stone or wall.

---

[91] Aizawa S, Sakamoto S, Yoshihama I, Sakamoto K 1981 "Comparison with Artemisia vulgaris grown in the Sunlight and Shade" Journal of the Japan Society of Acupuncture and Moxibustion; 31(1): 27-33.

陽

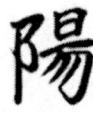

The character for "yang" – on the right, the image of the sun is positioned over an image of flags, fluttering in the wind

Mugwort Processing for Moxa

In Japan, the mugwort for prime moxa production is traditionally collected from lower slopes on exactly these sunny southern sides of mountains, the best coming from areas with good winter snowfall. The smaller leaves are preferred for superior moxa and are selectively individually picked from the harvested plants, then allowed to bleach in the sun for three or four days, perhaps to absorb still more *yang* energy, being turned over every day. It should be born in mind that Japanese summers are intensely humid, so this process is surely important to avoid mould growth. Next they are force-dried in hot rooms of over 100° C to reduce the water content to as little as 2%, after which they are stored in darkness until winter, when the real refining finally begins.

It is important to bear in mind that early winter in Japan is normally very dry, and this may be a vital factor in the final quality of the product, since the refining is all done in a dry environment. Certainly it is accepted that the best quality moxa can only be processed in very dry conditions.

The leaves are processed to separate the fibrous material from the woollen – the purer the resultant woollen down becomes the more refined is the final product. Traditionally this is begun by first pulverizing the leaves with rotating stone-grinders turning at speeds of 30-50 rotations per minute. This process may be repeated two or three times.

The residue is then sieved to remove the initial impurities, typically in large almost horizontal cylinders of up to four metres in length called *nagadoshi*. These cylinders are divided into separate sections by increasingly finer meshes of wire and bamboo wicker. These massive cylindrical sieves are tilted at a very slight angle with their ends a little lower than their mouths, and are then rotated rapidly at around 30 rotations per minute. A vibrating sieve may also be used. With these processes completed, the relatively pure nap is finally tossed in special rotary grading winnowers (known in Japan as *tomi*s). Again, the rotation is done at high speed – this time up to two rotations per second which results in the remaining impurities exiting through the gaps in the winnowers' sides leaving high-grade moxa inside, with the nap being rendered increasingly purer at each step of the process.

Coarser grades, which come from the earlier stages of the process, are more suitable for indirect techniques, particularly moxa stick use, and the finer grades are reserved for direct techniques. With super pure Japanese moxa, as little as 2% of the original leaf weight remains at the end of the refining process. By contrast, fine Chinese moxa generally retains as much as 20% of the original weight, although recently some Chinese products are being refined to similar standards as the Japanese. The traditional differences in refinement between the two countries are not insignificant and may well explain some of the differences of approach. One Japanese study goes so far as to suggest that the selection of leaf is critical. The raw plant material selected for the most refined moxa (smaller younger leaves selectively picked) include less extraneous matter on the individual hair surfaces, more uniformity in the individual thickness, flatness and crookedness of each hair, and a general uniformity of smoothness of the hair surfaces themselves[92].

When ignited, moxa smoulders rather than burns with a flame, and does so at a temperature which is frequently said to depend on its degree of refinement. Generally also, the more refined it is the quicker it burns, allowing scope for variation in technique as we shall see later. Refined moxa is also traditionally aged for two or three years, as has clearly been the case since the Warring States period in China, at least according to the text from Meng Zi as discussed in the last section – and possibly from even earlier. We can guess that something specific occurs in this drying and maturation process which adds to the moxa's effect, similar to the laying down of fine wine or the ageing of whisky, but it has proved impossible to be completely clear about this. As we will see later, we can, however, consider the strong possibility that this ageing creates a softer heat when the moxa is burnt, something which is facilitated by an altered balance between the various chemicals originally contained in the mugwort leaves due to the prolonged evaporation of oils.

Less debatable is the fact that older moxa is more yellow in hue. This change in colour also suggests an alteration in the proportions of chemical constituents in the nap. Even in this current scientific age of biochemical analysis, however, this remains far from completely clear, and the essential mystery as to how the founders of the therapy might have stumbled upon the apparent importance of this supposed essential ageing process remains. Whilst it might at first seem unlikely, it is actually quite possible that such a long ageing process would have been something originally discovered by nomadic peoples who may well have been the first to develop the basic therapy. Mugwort harvesting, after all, would have been an annual seasonal event done in midsummer and a little later, and quantities would have needed to have been kept safe and dry at least throughout the ensuing year. Colour changes would then have been quite evident between the previous year's batch and the next year's. Furthermore, since lighting and keeping

---

[92] Aizawa S, Sakamoto S, Yoshihama I, Sakamoto K 1982 "Morphological Changes in the Producing Stage of Moxa/Morphological Differences in the Quality of Moxa";; Journal of the Japan Society of Acupuncture and Moxibustion; 32(3): 242-249.

a fire would have been such a vital business to any nomadic community, it would hardly be improbable that stores of mugwort would have been carefully cached and secured at or near traditional campsites in case the mugwort that was being carried might be ruined by rot or damp ingress – something which could result in effective disaster. In this way, stores of mugwort which might be several years old could have been recovered and then practically compared in terms of their combustibility. In this way it may well have been first noticed that aged mugwort was simply more effective as a tinder, catching alight faster and more easily.

Super pure and aged moxa is said to burn at a much lower temperature – claimed by some commercial literature to burn at around 75° Celsius – whilst slightly less pure (*wakakusa*) moxa for *kyutoshin* moxa-on the-needle-head technique is claimed to burn at around 135°[93]. In contrast, raw unprocessed moxa for indirect use such as moxa sticks is said to burn as hot as 400°. The differences claimed are popularly seen as being as important as they are substantial. In fact, experimentations in this area suggest that there are nothing like the temperature differences claimed in the literature, but the differences are of significance nevertheless, and do allow for very different approaches as well as variety of effect.

The results of these experiments and investigations of temperature led by Jenny Craig are recorded in some detail in Part 4 the Branches. We were unfortunately unable to ascertain or confirm the exact impact on combustion temperature that was achieved by ageing although some of the original oils clearly do evaporate over time and this may well have some impact. One other result from this ageing, however, as well as from any extra refinement, is that the smoke is unquestionably rendered more acceptable. With refinement and ageing, as well, the original colour of the floss lightens and yellows, and the ash residue also reduces, most probably because some of the volatile oils are lost in the ageing process. The moxa becomes easier and more cohesive to handle, and it is also more easily ignited (something which would have been a noticeable boon for the nomads). Generally the ash also tends to tighten up whilst burning, thus holding its shape rather than falling apart, though this has probably less to do with the ageing and more with the level of its refinement. This tightening up is an important factor, of course, whenever moxa is burnt on the handles of needles, since it considerably reduces the risk to the patient-practitioner relationship from moxa falling off onto the patient's skin.

More highly refined samples of moxa tend also to leave a jet black ash behind when burnt, whilst less pure samples leave incrementally greyer and whiter ash. It is quite easy, therefore, to visually assess the purity of a moxa sample simply by burning it.

---

[93] "Waka-kusa" literally translates as "young herb". The relative freshness of the herb when compared to more refined types for direct use is almost certainly designed to exploit its slower burning nature.

One further important possibility may result from the ageing – that the spectrum of infra-red radiation which moxa emits on burning shifts in its profile. This shift may result in a spectrum of radiation which is more resonant with that emitted by the human body itself, something which is a fascinating possibility that is also looked at in some detail in Part 4 the Stems.

The Arcana of Mugwort

In terms of mugwort's more esoteric associations, a glance at its associated Western etymological derivations gives interesting food for thought.

Firstly, any plant with the suffix "wort" almost certainly has a history of use in herbal medicine.

Mugwort was in fact known as one of the nine healing herbs of the Anglo-Saxons[94], and its original old English name ("mycgwyrt") means literally "insect plant", indicating one of its uses in both the West and the East as a natural insect repellent, particularly when the flesh of the plant is rubbed. Eric Brand, reporting on the internet after a visit to China to inspect moxa production there, observed that the "Encyclopedia of Chinese Medicinals" by Zhao and Xie notes that one of the reasons that moxa was considered sacred in ancient China was because it is never infested by pests – it appeared to have an inherent power which meant it could dispel both pests and evils[95].

Its flowers are known, incidentally, to create one of the principle pollens involved in post mid-summer hay fever, so it is clearly not just insects that the plant can irritate.

There is, however, unfortunately quite little written about it in the Western Herbal canon – it mainly figures as an appetiser and digestive, or as a herb to regularise menstruation. Culpepper endorsed the use of the fresh herb to counteract "the overmuch taking of opium", though exactly how this may have been affected or effective remains a mystery, most probably through smoking. This application may have, in fact, originated in China where this use has also been recorded. It was additionally widely used as an ingredient in beer before the widespread adoption of the hop, a fact which has led to a common misinterpretation concerning the origin of its name – reduced erroneously by this association to its "mug-" prefix, being assumed to be directly related to the eponymous drinking vessel. In cooking it was also often used as a flavouring ingredient in stuffing for

---

[94]The others were: chamomile (*Chamaemelum nobile*), crab apple (*Malus baccata*), fennel (*Foeniculum vulgare var. dulce*), greater plantain (*Plantago major*), stinging nettle (*Urtica dioica*), thyme (*Thymus vulgaris*), watercress (*Nasturtium officinale*) and wood betony (*Stachys officinalis*).

[95]http://www.bluepoppy.com/blog/blogs/blog1.php/moxa-grading retrieved 1/7/11

duck and goose, and is in fact used in some seasonal Japanese, Korean and Chinese dishes to this day.

One curious property ascribed to the plant in both East and West relates to its ability to deter unwanted visitors. In the West this amounted to putting some mugwort under the threshold with the intention that annoying friends and relatives (or maybe just the odd bible salesman) might decide not to bother knocking. In Japan it was put to similar but slightly different use. The unwanted visitor was assumed to have already been welcomed into the home – but could be encouraged to leave by discretely burning a little mugwort in the back of the person's shoe which would have been left at the door as is customary in Japan. As a result of this the visitor might suddenly become noticeably restless and decide he needed to be on his way.

A somewhat similar idea existed relating to identifying a thief: a large cone of moxa would be placed and burnt in any impression left by the thief's foot. This burning was believed to render the thief instantly incapacitated by pain or at least readily identifiable as a result of it – something which might best be described as sympathetic magic.

The theme of mugwort and feet persists elsewhere as well. Roman soldiers were reputed to line the soles of their sandals with mugwort to reduce fatigue. Pliny the Elder optimistically wrote that a "wayfaring man" with mugwort tied about his person would neither feel tired, be struck by the sun nor be attacked by a wild beast.

It has actually been suggested that mugwort was actually planted along the verges of Roman roads for this very purpose. Seeing how commonly stands of the plant appear alongside motorways today, one has to wonder whether this was true – it is far more probable that the plant just establishes itself by seeding itself along roadsides in the disturbed soil. A thousand years later than the Romans, however, in *De Vegetabilus* (which was an early text on the plant kingdom of around 1250) Albertus Magnus similarly described how mugwort "tied to a traveller's leg" could relieve weariness. In medieval times a Latin invocation was used when picking the mugwort for the purpose of increasing these powers: "*Tollam te artemisia, ne lassus sim in via*". A translation of this is: "I shall pick you mugwort, so I will not be tired on the road". This interesting common theme persists, repeating itself across many centuries[96]. In the "Art of Simpling" of 1656, William Coles claimed that a person could walk forty miles before noon without tiring with a sprig of mugwort placed in the shoes.

The German word for mugwort is *beifuss*, the Dutch is *bijvoet*. Both can be traced back to the Old High German *bibōz*, the exact literal meaning of which remains unclear, but which in turn was modified to *bivuoz*. "*Bei Fuss!*" in modern German

---

[96] Anna Pavord 2005 "The Naming of Names" (Bloomsbury Publishing)

is a term used to instruct a dog to walk at heel, implying something next to the feet. Its use as the word for mugwort is thus often similarly assumed to be derived from its association with reducing fatigue in the legs or feet, but actually the origin may be a little more complex still, being possibly derived from an older germanic word meaning "to beat" – which has been suggested to imply that it was considered to be able to beat off evil.

Other European names resonate in similarly mysterious ways. Most Slavonic languages have similar names for mugwort and its relatives: Polish - piołun, Belarussian - palyn [палын], Slovak - palina, Czech - pelyněk, Slovenian and Croatia - pelin and also Bulgarian - pelin [пелин]. These names are derived from a common Slavonic root PAL, to burn, or bright, or clear. Such etymological associations suggest it has been used for burning, either practically as tinder or shamanistically since the dawn of history.

In other Slavonic languages (of the Western and Eastern branches), mugwort has another unrelated name which is said to mean black stalk or dark grass, and it is a name that recently has become well known throughout the world for disturbing reasons of modern history. In Czech this is černobýl, in Ukrainian chornobyl [чорнобиль], and in Russian chernobyl [чернобыль]. These all derive from another similar Proto-Indo-European root: KER – to burn or fire, which has representatives in many languages including the Latin *cremare* – to burn – from which the English word cremation derives. These "KER-" names are less common than the more common "PAL-" derived words but they cast a very different shadow on the subject, something which we will come across in Part 3 the Branches when we will encounter a wholly unexpected connection between this Slavonic word and moxibustion treatment following the nuclear disaster at the Ukrainian Chernobyl nuclear power station.

The plant does also feature quite prominently in some of the more esoteric literature of plant lore. Mugwort "pillows" were reputed to stimulate restless sleep with vivid dreams, often of an uncomfortably vivid nature. There also exists a tradition in several cultures, doubtless of shamanic origin, of its ability to protect at quite an arcane level. The following quotation from an Anglo-Saxon herbal of 1050 opens in similar vein to those referred to above, but develops towards its end into somewhat stranger territory:

"Let him take in hand this wort *artemisia*, and let him have it with him, then he will not feel much toil on his journey. And it also puts to flight devil sickness; and in the house in which he hath it within, it forbiddeth evil leechcraft and also it turneth away the evil eyes of evil men[97]."

---

[97] Anna Pavord 2005 "the Naming of Names" (Bloomsbury Press) p122. This originally comes from the Anglo-Saxon herbal entitled just "Apuleius" of circa 1050.

Even the word *"Artemisia"* itself may be suggestive of another deeper universal understanding. Artemis was the Goddess of Hunting, of Progeny, and of Life and Death and Longevity. Her name is usually believed to have been derived from *artemês*, meaning uninjured, healthy, vigorous; as such she would have been seen to be the goddess who is herself inviolate and vigorous, and who might grant strength and health to others. According to the original Herbarium of Apuleius Platonicus (which was said to originate from the second century), the mugwort plant was originally "found" by Diana (the Roman name for the Greek God Artemis): "Of those worts that we name Artemisia, it is said that Diana did find them, and delivered their powers and leechdom[98] to Chiron the Centaur." Chiron the Wounded Healer, of course, was believed to be responsible for teaching human beings the art of medicine.

The Chinese "equivalent" mythological character to Artemis/Diana (an archetypal Goddess whose origins may go back as far as paleolithic times) was *He Xian Gu* (*Ho Hsien Ku*) or *Kosinko* in Japan. She has been described as an eternally young woman who by strange coincidence is sometimes clad in mugwort[99] – offering more mysterious hints of ancient understandings and further hints at mugwort's contribution to longevity which we will discuss later in more detail.

The aboriginal *Ainu* of Japan also held mugwort as one of their oldest and most sacred herbs, using it to scare the "devils of disease" who were said to dislike its smell. Mugwort is still used ritually by both Shinto and Buddhist priests in Japan as tinder for sacrificial fire.

In North America it is said to have been widely smoked by Native Americans for the purpose of driving away evil, though whether this was done in pipes or in smudge sticks in sweat lodges is a little unclear. It may well have included both, since it has been described elsewhere as providing a smooth smoke with a mild "hit" which has been more recently used to help withdrawal from nicotine addiction.

Strictly speaking the plant used in North America was not *Artemisia vulgaris*, which is not native to the continent, although it has thrived since being inroduced. For the Dakota tribe of the Great Plains, it was *Artemisia gnaphalodes* or Wild Sage. They invoked the *"to"*, or spirit, of the plant to protect against malevolent powers. The leaves were also used as the bed of the sacred pipes of the Omaha in ceremony at the installation of a new chief[100].

---

[98] "Leechdom" is an archaic term for medicine.

[99] U.A.Casal – "Acupuncture, Cautery and Massage in Japan" www.nanzan-u.ac.jp/SHUBUNKEN/publications/afs/pdf/a136.pdf - retrieved 3/1/2010.

[100] Gilmore MR 1914 "Uses of Plants by the Indians of the Missouri River Region", republished 1977 (University of Nebraska Press)

The Kiowa tribe of the central plains used the plant in their peyote rituals during which they underwent hallucinatory shamanic experiences whilst under the influence of peyote cactus alkaloids. They stuffed its leaves in cushions which were either sat or lain on by those submitting to the ritual, a habit which has a familiar resonance with the habit of mugwort being used in dream pillows in Europe.

The Miwok tribe living in what is now Northern California set store in mugwort's protective powers in ways which also resonate with European traditions. They believed that ghosts could be kept at bay if the leaves were rubbed on the body or if the plant was worn as a necklace, especially if the wearer had been handling a corpse.

The Chumash of Southern California were said to have used some form of moxibustion with mugwort or *Artemisia Douglasiana* (another local variant), but it is uncertain whether this was a traditional practice, or something they learnt from Chinese railway workers.

Mugwort has been known by several other names in folklore in English. One of these is "St. John's Plant", a name which was used in different languages throughout Europe. This should not, of course, be confused with St. John's Wort (*hypericum perforatum*). St. John the Baptist reputedly wore a garland of mugwort as a defence against evil spirits when in the wilderness, though when this non-biblical apocryphal tradition arose is uncertain. In his gospel St. Mark actually described John as being clothed in camel's hair with a girdle of skin or leather around his loins, eating locusts and wild honey with no mugwort in sight. It is probable that this adoption of mugwort into the medieval mythology of St. John is an instance of a transformation of a pre-Christian tradition into another resonant tradition of a later age. It is suggested that St. John's assertion that "He must increase, I must decrease"[101] is the root of this connection, by its association with the transitions of the sun before and after the summer equinox. By the Middle Ages, the myth seems to have become firmly rooted as a popular Christian tradition, with the plant becoming known as *Cingulum Sancti Johannis*, or belt of St. John, an association that has survived to this day with the French and Portuguese.

Mugwort's protective powers appear to have even extended to the architectural design of Christian churches in the 13th Century. An example survives in the roof bosses of Exeter Cathedral (in the English West Country) which are carved with sprays of mugwort.

What is quite certain and equally fascinating is mugwort's association with the Festival day in honour of St. John (June 24th) and (as we will soon see) with the proximity of this festival to midsummer. Mugwort was clearly intimately associated with this feast day when it was draped on the roofs of buildings as a

---

[101] Gospel of St. John. 3:30.

means of protection against demons and disease. Banckes' Herbal of 1525, the earliest surviving printed herbal manual in English, advocated that it should be hung on the house to keep out ghosts and ill-spirits, a habit surviving in the Isle of Man right up until the 19th century.

In Holland and Germany a strong belief persisted that, if the plant was collected on St. John's Eve, it had particular enhanced powers of protection. In some traditions it was worn around the waist and the wearers would dance around the fire before casting the mugwort belts symbolically into the dying embers.

Extraordinarily, in an uncannily similar fashion, bunches of mugwort are hung up in doorways and windows in Japan, China and Taiwan in observation of the festival of the Fifth Moon. This festival, on the fifth day of the fifth moon of the Chinese calendar, is the *Duanwu* or Dragon Boat Festival in China. The fifth moon of the Chinese calendar occurs in June, its exact date each year being dependent upon the date of Chinese New Year which is lunar dependent, but more often than not it falls a few days before midsummer, and not long therefore before the Festival of St. John in the West. In southern China this would have been a time when summer illnesses and epidemics would have begun to appear.

When we consider the plant's ubiquitous widespread use as an insect repellent it is no great conjectural leap to wonder whether this practice of hanging the plant over windows, doors or roofs would have unwittingly repelled mosquitoes carrying malaria, yellow fever or encephalitis, although the connections between these diseases and the mosquito astonishingly have only relatively recently been made.

A single recorded exception to this exists in the literature of Indian medicine. In the 6th century BC, an apparently unique connection was made between malaria and insect bites in the *Sushruta Samhita* but the idea was evidently rejected by later generations. Apart from this one instance, it appears that literally no human-being of any influence considered the lowly mosquito to be so lethally dangerous until 1877 when the first positive connections were made with elephantiasis in India. Finally in 1894, the case was finally proven against the mosquito regarding malaria. Dr Patrick Manson, who later founded the London School of Tropical Medicine, captured a batch of mosquitoes in Rome and rushed them back to London in a diplomatic bag by train via Paris. On arrival back home he was warmly welcomed by his family, and, after tucking his son up in bed, he surreptitiously released the mosquitoes before quietly closing his son's bedroom door and leaving events to take their course, as of course they did[102]. A dose of quinine administered

---

[102] Medical research ethics have certainly been revised since this important discovery was made. Manson was knighted and made a Fellow of the Royal Society, and his collaborator Ronald Ross won the Nobel Prize for Medicine in 1902. Today, they would have been struck off as physicians and probably ended up in prison!

immediately after his son broke out with malaria saved the boy, and the case has been effectively closed against the mosquito ever since. Today mosquitoes are known to potentially carry any one of as many as a hundred fatal diseases and are estimated to have been responsible for the death of as many as 45 billion people. There is an African proverb: "If you think that you're too small to make a difference, try sleeping in a closed room with a mosquito" – which is something of an understatement given this astonishing estimated death toll.

The possible consequent reduced occurrence of observable lethal disease (which we now know to be insect-borne) in households whose apertures were draped with mugwort would certainly be a simple explanation for one of its perceived powers of protection. The same may well have been true in its similar use in Europe during the Festival of St. John.

U.A.Casal in his fascinating study of moxa usage in Japan[103] identified this co-incidence himself in a slightly different way, recognising that "among the Central European Peasantry we equally still find chaplets made of mugwort worn at the summer-solstice festival." There exists, however, one potent dissimilarity between these traditions – which relates to how the plant was collected. Whilst mugwort is seen in the East as being particularly *yang*, with its association with the power of the sun and its being picked from south facing slopes, a curiously opposite tradition appears to have evolved in the West. Instructions for harvesting the plant in Europe suggested that the mugwort with most magical power should be picked "just before the waxing moon, preferably from a plant facing north". In relation to the interpenetrations of *yin* and *yang* one might interpret this endorsement to be a maximising of the *yin* (the moon and the northerly aspect) within the *yang* (the height of summer). This connection of mugwort with the moon in fact may simply be down to the god Artemis being sometimes interpreted as a moon goddess.

The day of the Dragon Boat Festival is also described by many sources (particularly Chinese) as the traditional time to harvest mugwort for moxa. It is quite possible that there have been some confusions here – mugwort *is* indeed traditionally harvested at this time, but this may have been as much for hanging over doorways to ward off illness and evil spirits as it might have been for processing into material for moxibustion. It may, however, be the last time in the year that the leaves can be harvested for good quality moxa, as the quality of the down on the underside of the leaves changes after the plant flowers. In southern China, the period for harvesting for moxa actually traditionally spans between the third day of the third moon (when the plant is large enough) and the fifth day of the fifth moon (after which it soon flowers).

---

[103] U.A.Casal "Acupuncture, cautery and massage in Japan" p.226. www.nanzan-u.ac.jp/ publications/afs/pdf/a136.pdf - retrieved 3/1/2010

Once again, a look at the roots of a Chinese character provides potential further speculative insights into its cultural history in China. The Han character for mugwort 艾 utilises the "cut grass" radical. Culturally and etymologically this surely implies that mugwort was seen as a plant that was scythed. It is quite possible that, at this ancient time when mugwort was being represented cryptographically, the plant may not have been used primarily as a medicinal plant in the way it is used today, but rather it may have been employed in more shamanic ways; it may well be that it was being primarily used in these ways that still survive to this day – by hanging over doorways, etc. for the deterrent of evil spirits, for which purpose it would have readily been scythed whole.

Incidentally, Li Shizhen in the Ming Dynasty would have fundamentally disagreed with this analysis. He quoted Wang Anshi's "Character Explanation" *Zi Shuo*, saying: "Mugwort can cut out illness like cutting weeds, and this is why the character is as it is." Li specifically endorsed the idea of harvesting mugwort for moxa on the day of *Duanwu* and does not seem to have been struck by some of the more esoteric traditions. He was quite clear that, at least in Ming times, mugwort should be cut stalks-and-all at the time of the fifth day of the fifth lunar month, and actually quotes a song from his father Li Yuechi that illustrates this:

> "It is produced on the sunny side of the mountain,
> And picked at the Dragon Boat Festival.
> It treats diseases and is applied to illness as moxibustion.
> It results in benefits that are not small[104]."

Both father and son were clearly adopting an earlier tradition, since Wang Dao and Sun Simiao, both Tang physicians who wrote on moxa, were saying much the same thing a millennium earlier. What was the quality of the processed moxa they were using? We have no way of knowing, unfortunately.

It is impudent to challenge the scholarship of one of the most authoritative historical figures in Chinese medicine, but it may just be that interpreting from old texts and characters is no more than a gift for the creatively inclined of **any** age, a conclusion which would suggest that all such interpretations should be treated with discrimination and caution and not necessarily be accepted as fact.

What is beyond debate is that at least one of the premium moxa producers at Mt. Ibuki in Japan (and arguably therefore one of the premium producers worldwide) nowadays collects the plants selectively on the mountains lower slopes through May and June and is quite specific that, once it has flowered, it is too late for harvesting for high grade moxa. The plant flowers around midsummer, triggered, we can guess, by the stalling of the day-to-day change in daylight around the solstice. Picking in May and June means that the harvest of prime mugwort for

---

[104] Lorraine Wilcox 2008 "Moxibustion the Power of Mugwort Fire" (Blue Poppy Press) p99

medicinal use is best seen as more of a rolling process, one which, at least today in Japan does not necessarily involve the scything of the plant on a particular day at all.

The reason for this current practice of careful selection of leaves becomes clearer with the help of a microscope. The hairs in the nap of the younger leaves are denser, thicker and shorter with a rounder cross-section than those in the nap of the older leaves. This is the fundamental reason, it would appear, for their selection. The careful selection of leaves in the picking process clearly affects the quality of the final product since the individual hairs are cleaner, smoother and more uniform.

These differences in perceptions with regards to harvesting (either scything the plant whole in mid-summer or selectively picking the particular plants throughout the early summer) may actually characterise a key difference in moxa production which in turn serves to explain some of the differences in final moxa product coming from either China or Japan. We have previously discussed the possibility that the origins of the word "moxa" from the Japanese word "*mogusha*" may illustrate the fact that Japanese moxa was being distributed across the China Sea for centuries as the premium material in the orient for moxibustion. Whether or not this was true, today it is indisputable that the finest product coming from Japan is refined to a far higher degree than most of the premium grade coming from the PRC. There may, in fact, be identifiable morphological and elemental differences in composition between samples of *Artemisia* from the two countries which, when analysed, may also explain some of the difference in quality[105]. The variations in approach to harvesting and differences in processing, however, are almost certainly the prime factors in these perceived differing grades of quality.

Mugwort's Chemistry

So much for moxa's more magical attributes. What of its chemical constituents? Some interesting research has been carried out on *Artemisia princeps* (one of the strains used in Japan for purer moxa) in California[106]. Two methods of extraction were employed after steam distillation – dichloromethane extraction and simultaneous purging and extraction. A total of 192 volatile chemicals were identified in the resultant residues. The most abundant of these were borneol (which has both antiseptic and analgesic properties and is almost identical chemically to camphor), cineole (eucalyptol), artemisia acetate and alpha thujona. Borneol, as we shall see in a later section, may have a particular role on the

---

[105] "Comparative Study of Artemisia princeps pamp. Grown in Japan and China"; Journal of Japan Society of Acupuncture and Moxibustion. 1997; 47(1): 6-13.

[106] Department of Environmental Toxicology, University of California, Davis 95616, USA

promotion of immune response through its chemical activation of heat shock proteins. It is difficult to be certain, however, how much the particular chemistry of moxa bears on its final quality and particularly on its therapeutic effect when burnt; nor can we be certain how many of these 192 chemicals remain in the matured nap since the ages of the samples tested were not specified. It is probable, however, that they were not aged samples.

Extracted by DRP	*ppm*	*Extracted by SPSE*	*ppm*
borneol	10.27	1,8-cineole	8.12
alpha-thujone	3.49	artemisia acetate	4.22
artemisia alcohol	2.17	alpha-thujone	3.20
verbenone	1.85	beta-caryophyllene	2.39
yomogi alcohol	1.50	bornyl acetate	2.05
germacren-4-ol	1.43	borneol	1.80

A chart showing the main component chemicals of mugwort

Certainly, with regards to indirect moxa use, the effects of the chemical constitution may not be as important: the most likely biochemical effect apart from the effect of the heat would be from secondary inhalation of the smoke. With direct techniques, of course, there is contact between the heated volatile oils and the pores of the skin, and it can be realistically assumed that some absorption takes place. We can envisage this as a kind of localised thermo-aromatherapy, and we shall see that this may measurably add to the immune response.

Some further research from Japan adds a slightly deeper perspective to the above. By adding moxa to a mixed solvent of chloroform, methanol and water (in the ratio 5:5:1) two primary components were identified. The hydrophobic solid found in the separated chloroform solution was established as $C_{37}H_{76}$ (heptatriacontane). The hydrophilic solid found in the separated methanol and water layer, however, was found to primarily contain tannins[107]. Particular focus was then paid to these two components, the heptatriacontane (which is an alkane[108]) and the tannins and also to their relative proportions, as a result of which further conclusions were drawn.

---

[107] Tannin compounds are widely distributed in many species of plants, where they play a role in protection from predation, and perhaps also as pesticides, as well as in plant growth regulation. The astringency from the tannins is what causes the dry and puckery feeling in the mouth following the consumption of unripened fruit or red wine.

[108] Alkanes are also known as paraffins or saturated hydrocarbons. They are chemical compounds consisting only of hydrogen and carbon. They are not very reactive and

The most refined moxa samples investigated clearly contained the highest proportions of heptatriacontane and the lowest of tannins, whilst the cruder samples contained the opposite proportions. Actually these differences were proportionately far more significant in the proportional quantities of the tannins found in the different samples, suggesting that the proportion of tannins significantly reduces (reducing to around a fifth of the initial weight of tannin found) through maturation and refinement.

From the data in this research it is quite possible to suggest that the higher relative proportion of heptatriacontane to tannin contributes to the faster speed of burn generally observable in more refined and aged moxa as well as to some of the attributed therapeutic effects, and that this increased speed of burn in turn keeps the temperatures lower in small cones, thus attenuating the peak temperatures at a cone's base[109]. It is also reasonable to suggest that those plant strains in which the non-volatile tannins naturally occur less might be preferable for higher grades of moxa nap.

Some further interesting complementary information regarding the plant's constitution is provided in some research published by the Japan Society of Acupuncture and Moxibustion which investigated the relative qualities of two varieties of mugwort – *Artemisia montana* (*Yamamogi*) and *princeps* (*Ooyomogi*)[110]. Both of these strains are used in Japan for higher grade moxa. The report asserted that, by tradition, the quality of the mugwort is initially judged by evaluating the thickness of the down beneath the leaf and by the strength of its fragrance. This fragrance is thought to be proportionate to its cineole content which must therefore be assumed to survive the ageing process. Interestingly, the cineole content was analysed to be more abundant in the Montana samples, and the fragrance was correspondingly confirmed as being stronger as well, although, with samples from differing locations this was clearly also affected by the material's origin. This research may well explain Ibuki Mountain's claim to fame as the home of the best moxa plants – it provides perhaps both the most conducive soil and the best strain of plant with the most cineole, the most heptatriocontane and the least tannin.

Further hints at the properties of different types of moxa appeared in another article published by the same journal – "A Study on the Radical Scavenging Effects of Moxa" – in which it was shown that different moxas produce different

---

have little biological activity being viewed as a molecular tree upon which can be hung the more biologically active/reactive portions of the molecule.

[109] Dr Kazuko Kobayashi (Meiji College of Oriental Medicine). American Journal of Chinese Medicine, Vol XVI, Nos. 3-4, pp. 179-185.

[110] Journal of the Japan Society of Acupuncture and Moxibustion 1997; 47(1)6-13.

effects and differences in radical scavenging activities [111]. But this touches particularly on a theme relating to the immunological effects of moxibustion, something which we will explore in much more detail in in Part 4 the Stems.

---

[111] Journal of Japan Society of Acupuncture and Moxibustion. 1990; 40(4): 377-379.

Part 3 – the Branches

"THAT TORTUROUS, BARBARIC PRACTICE, THE USE OF THE MOXA, IS CLOSELY RELATED TO THIS PLANT"
Charles Millspaugh[112]

"THOSE DISEASES THAT DRUGS DO NOT CURE, THE KNIFE CURES; THOSE THAT THE KNIFE DOES NOT CURE, FIRE CURES; THOSE THAT FIRE DOES NOT CURE MUST BE CONSIDERED INCURABLE."
Hippocrates[113]

"HOLY SOULS, YOU CANNOT MOVE AHEAD UNLESS THE FIRE HAS STUNG YOU FIRST"
Dante [114]

Tonification and Dispersion in the Classical Texts

Suwen 12 states that "the method of moxibustion comes from the North, the land of winter, cold and snow, of nomadic people living off meat and milk products, prone to invasion of cold, excess and distension". Whilst this makes some sense, it also bears a small challenge – the high altitude tundra of Inner Mongolia (which is apparently being described here and lay beyond the northern borders of the Han Empire) is hardly a good growing area for mugwort, whilst the "roasting" of a patient's back by a fire side (described in the third Mawangdui scroll referred to in Part 1 the Roots) seems much more likely to be fitting inside a Mongolian nomad's tent than some fancy moxa technique. What was being described here in the Suwen might more truly echo the traditional origins of heat therapy rather than anything specifically related to the combustion of mugwort or similar herbs, or indeed the origins of discrete *jingluo* channel therapy. We can recall, furthermore, that in the texts found in the Mawangdui tomb there were references to heat treatments which involved materialsother than simply mugwort. But we clearly cannot discount the idea that this major reference in the *Suwen* might well allude to the introduction of moxibustion in at least some prototypical form from the nomadic tribes of central Asia.

What is also interesting, however, is that *Suwen* 12 goes on to specifically describe the associated disease and disorder from living in this "northern" environment as being those of fullness generated from the coldness of the *zang* internal organs.

---

[112] Charles Millspaugh "American Medicinal Plants" 1892

[113] Hippocrates "Aphorisms" 7.87 (c. 400 BC)

[114] Dante "Purgatorio Canto" 27 - Mandelbaum Translation (early 14th century)

This offers clear indicators of its possible early applications – if moxa treatment was much used by these people, it implies that it was understood to have some capacity to disperse this fullness as well as to warm the cold.

Suwen 28, however, describes moxa in slightly differing terms: "When the network (*luo*) vessels are full while the conduits (regular meridians) are depleted, cauterise the *yin* and pierce the *yang*. When the conduits are full while the network vessels are depleted, pierce the *yin* and cauterise the *yang*." Unfortunately, it remains far from clear as to how we might confidently be able to diagnose either condition since no further clues remain for us in the text. It seems unlikely that it was from the pulse, and much more likely to be from either symptoms or wider palpation. What does seem probable, however, (and potentially very important) is that the author(s) of this particular chapter were working from a tradition or an understanding that saw moxibustion as being useful for tonifying or supplementation, and needling as being more useful for dispersion. Such an idea seems, superficially at least, to convey a quite different concept from what was introduced to us in *Suwen* 12. This apparent diversity of tradition is of course far from a unique occurrence in these texts, and in fact neither of these two initial interpretations of mechanisms turns out to be a universal understanding or interpretation of the mechanics of either technique in the rest of the received *Nei Jing* texts.

Lingshu 51, discussing cold "entering the middle", advocates moxibustion "if needling does not reach it" – although it then goes on to imply that this cold should be particularly dispersed at the *he* sea points. Here we may have a more developed reflection of the initial idea proposed in *Suwen* 12. The cold, having entered the middle, generates the fullness which requires dispersion by moxa at the *he* sea points. These particular points, in the context of the more developed *jingluo* channel theory, are where the channel flow is said to flow deeply into the interior of the body, so this makes some clinical sense for us today. Warming such points of deeper divergence might even seem an ideal way to route the warmth of the moxa deep into the interior, where it may then naturally disperse the stuck coldness in exactly the fashion that is hinted at in *Suwen* 12.

Lingshu 73, however, takes moxa in a slightly different direction again, endorsing its use "when yin and yang are both empty" which clearly is a pre-terminal vacuous condition. In this case there seems to be an implicit comprehensive restorative tonifying action being proposed, although frustratingly it is not made clear at this point in the text as to how or where the moxa should be used in this respect. Shortly after, however, it states that moxa should be used "at the points.. when the channels are depressed and sinking" implying tonification at deficient points along the channel in question,identifiable, we must assume, from palpation.

Other scattered references in the *Lingshu* seem to endorse this idea of general tonification: when the pulse is "sinking and depressed, use moxibustion only" (*Lingshu* 48); or that, when "there are depressions along or in the course of the meridian", moxa should be used (*Lingshu* 10). It seems quite reasonable to interpret such depressions as palpably deficient acupoints. In these latter cases, in clear contrast to the *Suwen* 12 reference, a warming and supplementing action to the regular channels seems to be being described with nothing specifically occurring in relation to cold or fullness stuck in the interior. It should be noted here, however, that some chapters of the *Lingshu* are considered to be apocryphal, written possibly as late as the 8th century AD, and the seventy-third chapter may be one of them. If so, we can only guess what the original seventy-third chapter may have consisted of.

Lingshu 51 (which may also possibly not be an original text)[115] gives us a useful clue to this possible dual action of dispersion and tonification by getting right down to a nitty-gritty description of technique, one which has survived to this day as the only example of moxa technique which appears in any of these texts. It begins by echoing the idea expressed in *Lingshu* 73 that, for some conditions, moxa may be more effective than acupuncture. "Moxibustion can be effective when needling is not effective," it states. This is a telling statement, being as it is buried so deeply in the heart of what has been regarded across the centuries as a needle classic (*zhen jing*) or canon of acupuncture. It is particularly telling in terms of its minimalism, just slipping such an idea in without any further elaboration. If this is an original chapter and not apocryphal, it suggests itself to be the first instance in the surviving literature from the time that moxibustion was regarded as being essential in the treatment of intractable disease.

The author(s) of *Lingshu* 51 next go on to describe discrete techniques.

> "When the *qi* is full, disperse; when hollow, tonify."

So far so good, since this clearly conforms with perhaps **the** fundamental idea at the heart of the *Nei Jing* texts. The text then goes on to develop these different treatment approaches.

> "When using fire to tonify do not blow on the fire. In a moment it will go out by itself. When using fire to disperse, quickly blow on the fire to propagate the action of the mugwort, then extinguish the fire."

---

[115] There is no corresponding text in Huangfu Mi's "Systematic Classic" (which was said to have distilled the texts of the *Suwen*, the *Lingshu*, and the *Ming Tang* into one homogenous classic text). Since detailed descriptions of supplementing and dispersing needle techniques exist in this classic with none at all concerning moxibustion, it begs the question whether the techniques of tonifying and dispersing with moxa existed at all in Huangfu's time. It is also quite possible, of course that Huangfu was working from a different edition or version to the one which Wang used to complete his final version centuries later. Either way, this does not of itself discredit the techniques described in *Lingshu* 51, but it does challenge their assumed antiquity.

So we have here for the first time clear indicators that moxa can both tonify **and** disperse dependent upon discrete techniques. The most basic conclusion we can draw from this section of text is that, subject to the desired effect, minor adjustments in technique may be necessary and even critical to the outcome of the treatment.

Attempts to clarify this subject by looking through the other available classic acumoxa texts serve unfortunately only to confirm that information on the subject still remains a little unclear, because of the problems in clarifying the authenticity of particular chapters as much as from the self-evident complexities and contradictions in the texts themselves. These inconsistencies almost certainly derive from their multiple authorships from probable differing traditions, being gathered beneath an illusory umbrella of a homogenous medicine which may never have actually existed.

The idea of justifying the rationale or authenticity for our treatment methods from the earliest texts available, however, has been a captivating and pervasive one for acumoxa practitioners across the centuries. If we are inclined to attempt this, we can actually do so with more confidence by searching the pages of the *Jia Yi Jing*, the "Systematic Classic of Acupuncture and Moxibustion", written by Huangfu Mi in the third century AD. Huangfu wrote this huge and influential work in an attempt to distil and rationalise for himself and his contemporaries the available (already distorted) material he was encountering in his own lifetime. Huangfu explicitly stated his source material to have been his contemporary versions of the *Suwen*, the *Zhen Jing* (the "Needle Classic" which has generally been accepted as being the *Lingshu*), and the *Ming Tang* (which was subsequently lost). Indeed it is actually on the basis of surviving authentic versions of his work that parts of the current received versions of the *Lingshu*, for instance, have had to be based because of the corruption of the text through the centuries.

In Part 1 the Roots we have already identified that the *Jia Yi Jing* generally tended to ignore moxibustion in favour of needling, but in Huangfu's Book Four, Chapter 1 (on Pulses) there may be some further clues as to contemporary understandings of moxa and its mechanisms which may have been prevalent at Huangfu's time. What is more, we can reasonably assume such understandings to have been derived from contemporary versions of the three classics referred to above. This particular passage (on Pulses) pretty much reflects *Lingshu* 48.

"Tightness" (緊 *jin*) in the pulse, we learn in this section, requires needling followed by moxibustion. The overall meaning from this sentence is far from completely clear, since neither the applicable technique for either treatment modality nor the locations for it are identified. But, more importantly, how should we actually interpret this tightness in the pulse? "Tight" pulses are referred to in the *Lingshu*, and they reflect cold. We just might suggest that this implies initial dispersion with the needle to disperse the blood (possibly even involving bloodletting) followed by supplementation with moxa to supplement or tonify the cold – and this would be in some accordance with the idea expressed in *Suwen* 28.

Interestingly, a somewhat similar approach to bloodletting exists in modern Japanese acumoxa teachings. When micro-bloodletting is used, for example, in order to promote circulation in an area which is clearly stagnated, a technique involving micro-bleeding and cupping is advocated to remove the stagnant blood. After this is completed, it is a common practice to apply warming moxa directly over the point or area which has been punctured.

But we are researching in the *Jia Yi Jing* specifically in relation to pulse types and the associated application of moxa. With a "sinking" pulse type we are confronted with a little more clarity in the text – such a pulse is stated as requiring treatment **exclusively** by moxibustion because of "blood binding in the vessels, which causes static blood and cold blood". This idea clearly echoes the similar endorsement to use moxibustion with a "sinking and depressed" (or a "sagging" 陷下) pulse in *Lingshu* 48 which suggests this was the possible source for this passage, although in the current versions of the *Lingshu* there is no mention of either blood binding or static cold.

Extrapolating from this, since it is clear elsewhere that the pulse should naturally be more sinking in the winter season, we might further assume that we have here a clear endorsement to use moxa at this time of year, particularly if there are appropriate indications from the pulse, and that this treatment would potentially free up the sluggish cold blood. If the pulse is found sinking at any other season, it might suggest even more generous moxa treatment to rectify what might be seen as a clearer pathological condition. It has to be said, however, that this remains wide open to interpretation.

Elsewhere in *Lingshu 48*, a "sagging" pulse is given a similar endorsement – again to treat with "moxibustion only" but "particularly at the brooks and rapids points".

Unfortunately, as with the *Suwen*, we encounter nothing in the Systematic Classic which tells us exactly *how* moxa was being applied. The section in Book 8 on Cold and Heat diseases indicates moxa at both hard points ("the place that feels hard like sinew above the clavicle") and at points in depressions, most interestingly at the back *shu* points "that have been found to be depressed." In terms of current thinking on these types of palpatory findings at acupoints, we can categorise the first type of point as being a sign either of an excess or chronic stagnation, and the second as a sign of a chronic deficiency, but again we can be far from certain on the matter.

We have to start somewhere, however, so in an effort to force some increased clarity into the business, let us assume initially that we might want to apply moxa to disperse an excess. Firstly, the moxa might be less refined, since we will intend it to burn hotter and slower. There is a suggestion from *Lingshu 51* that the cone might also be larger (we can hardly "propagate" the fire of a tiny cone to any major degree after all). The moxa might also be more tightly packed, so that it burns more slowly with a denser heat. It **could** be blown on (if the practitioner is feeling brave), and should almost certainly be burnt down fairly close to the skin, or even to the skin surface. This concentrates the heat on the point and should also increase the perception of temperature accordingly. Obviously, dependent on the size of cone, some degree of care will be needed to avoid blistering, and the cone will need to be smartly extinguished or lifted off as the full effect of the heat is felt.

If we are attempting to make total sense of these passages from earlier times, however, we have to accept that blisters quite probably were being caused deliberately. Today, this just might be acceptable with much smaller cones, but it will most definitely present problems for the western practitioner-patient relationship with cones any larger than the size of a grain of rice and should not therefore be contemplated.

Intentionally blistering suppurative moxa is known as *danokyu* in Japan, designed to create ulcerations with the additional application of an irritating herbs, and is still occasionally used there. Oddly enough it is said to be relaxing for the patient who often reportedly becomes quite sleepy, despite the fact that a large cone is burnt right down to the skin. Dr Yoshio Manaka occasionally used it with difficult cases, but he injected lidocaine before burning the point[116], so whether this treatment really is as relaxing as is sometimes claimed is up for debate. The practitioner applies very firm pressure with his fingertips around the cone as the heat hits, and this is said to distract the patient from the intensity of the heat. Such treatments are more "one-offs" than regular treatment, however, and are also beyond any sort of code of safe practice which exists in the West so they need not take up much of our attention.

Examples of what might be seen as a basic dispersive approach might be in the application of moxa on excess *xi*-cleft or other reactive points when there is acute symptomatology related to the channel, or at Du14 to break a fever, or even perhaps in treating excess points on a channel affected by herpes zoster. In the first case, fewer cones might be used; in the others perhaps twenty or more.

Interestingly, in the modern era, some Japanese authorities suggest using more points with fewer cones as a rule of thumb if dispersing. However correct such a general principle may be, if a patient has a clearly excess constitution and an excess condition, it seems reasonable to suggest that dispersive moxa with many cones might be useful, otherwise the technique should perhaps be approached with caution and only few cones used.

---

[116] Stephen Birch – private communication.

In fact, most of our patients and their chronic complaints fall into more deficient types, so the rationale in *Lingshu*-style tonifying moxa treatment seems altogether of more interest for us. In this case the moxa should be refined, more aged (generally meaning more gold or yellow in colour rather than green) and should be loosely formed so that it will burn relatively fast but with less intensity at a lower temperature. The clear implication from *Lingshu 51* is that the cone should be smaller – because "in a moment it will go out by itself". Large cones never go out "in a moment". This idea was corroborated by Sun Simiao in his "Thousand Ducat Formulas" a few centuries later[117]. For tonification fewer cones should generally be used on judiciously selected fewer points.

The late Sung Baek, a modern Korean proponent of moxibustion, was quite clear that the smaller the cone, the better will be its tonifying effect, the largest possible cone for this effect to occur being rice-grain sized. He hypothesised that this is because the effect from the moxa application works in a proportionate way to the amount of energy of the heat released. He theorised that an acupuncture point cannot handle the absorption of too much energy at any single point at once without releasing some of its own, meaning that more heat results in a release of energy, whilst less heat results in its absorption.

This is an intriguing idea, adding strength to the idea that dosage is perhaps **the** principle factor in determining tonification or dispersion, and particularly also that the individual constitution and state of the patient must be considered in this respect. For tonification, Baek also rather poetically endorsed placing the cone lightly on the skin "as if it was floating on the point[118]." Again the idea here is of the loosest possible moxa covering the tiniest of areas of the skin.

Moxa can also be cowled whilst burning to attenuate the heat. If using rice-grain size or smaller, this can be done by forming a cowl over the cone with the fingers. This reduces the flow of oxygen to the nap which will visibly reduce its burning power, and the cone can even be extinguished under this control before it completes burning if deemed preferable[119]. This technique might sound tricky, but actually it is not difficult to master, requiring only the first finger and thumb to work effectively.

A trade off occurs here between temperature (which is thus reduced) and burning time (which becomes extended as the burning slows). Bearing in mind Sung

---

[117] Because of the problems with establishing the authenticity of particular chapters of the *Lingshu*, it remains a distinct possibility that the writings of Sun Simiao in the Tang dynasty may actually ironically predate this part of the *Lingshu*, even though the classic is reputedly of the Han.

[118] Sung Baek 1990 "Classical Moxibustion Skills in Contemporary Clinical Practice" (Blue Poppy Press) p 5

[119] Stephen Birch – various teaching seminars 2001-3.

Baek's idea of the overall amount of heat being the determining factor for absorption of energy or its release, it seems quite reasonable to suggest that controlled cowling is most likely to create supplementation.

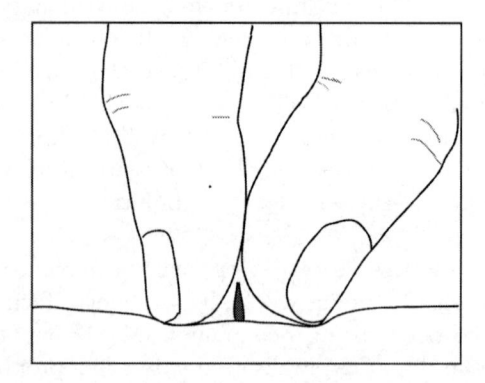

The one caveat to this technique is that, if one suddenly switches from cowling to extinguishing because of heat build up (which is a tempting action if the patient suddenly reports feeling heat), this can result in a sudden **increase** in oxygen as the cowl is released and the finger comes down on the cone to put it out, resulting in a corresponding sudden increase in heat. This might largely negate everything that went before and will increase the final heat for the patient and possibly alter the treatment's effect. If the patient perceives that the heat is building up too much whilst cowling is being performed, it is far preferable to close the cowl completely than to lift it off or snuff it out.

It should be added at this point that the terms of tonification and dispersion might best be viewed as loosely as possible. It is quite reasonable to suggest that they mean significantly different things to an acupuncturist or a herbalist, so it is equally reasonable to suggest that the same may be said for the practice of moxibustion.

For tonification purposes there are two methods available which might be prefereable to just letting it go out – particularly if we are working with a new or sensitive patient. We can either cowl the cone to purposefully and ultimately extinguish it by starving it of oxygen in a controlled fashion so that the patient only just feels the heat, or snuff it out quite early (or lift it off). Such approaches are particularly advisable for the first cone at each point,. It is certainly the best approach to use if one is absolutely intent on avoiding blisters [120]. Either technique, however, (with or without cowling) is "tonifying" by design, and can be selected according to the patient's relative condition, as well as an assessment of the condition of the point itself at which the moxa is to be applied.

---

[120] Edward Obaidey calls this type of approach "soft-*kyu*" – North American Journal of Oriental Medicine. 14;3:10.

In somewhat similar fashion, Masakazu Ikeda, a modern Japanese authority, suggests that, when tonifying, moxa cones should be burnt one on top of the other. This is to soften the effect of the heat in contrast with dispersive techniques whereby each cone should be removed after every application and a new cone placed directly on the same point on the skin. My own crude experimentation with cones burnt on softwood suggested in fact that burning on top of the pre-burnt ash of previous cones does not actually reduce the charring effect on a timber surface. This would in turn imply that the consequent heat trauma at the skin from either technique may be much the same, although the overall result of burning on existing ash on the softwood did curiously seem to slightly widen the area which was charred. More importantly, however, the subjective perception of patients quite clearly supports Ikeda's idea – since patients feel a softer heat when cone is burnt on cone.

Junji Mizutani, another modern Japanese authority, in fact hypothesises that repeated direct moxa on a single point, with the fresh cone placed on top of the flattened ash of the previous cones, means that the carbon is repeatedly re-burnt, creating a beam of far infra-red radiation penetrating deep into the body tissue[121]. (This idea concurs to some degree with some of Edward Obaidey's ideas concerning the use of a tube which we will examine later in this section, since it clearly presupposes an enhanced therapeutic effect from the deeper penetration of heat directly into the underlying tissue.) Mizutani quotes Sorei Yanagiya who is reputed to have burnt a multiple series of cones in this fashion on a watermelon, and then to have dissected the watermelon directly through the point of combustion to reveal a line right through the fruit from skin to skin. Yanagiya, incidentally, was a rather fascinating character from the early part of the twentieth century who changed his given name to the first two word of the *Suwen (So)* and of the *Lingshu (Rei)* as an act of witness to his total commitment to his rallying cry of "Back to the Classics!". He was clearly not one to ever do things by halves. We might allow our imagination free rein and envisage him using a razor sharp sword to slice the melon in half in appropriate samurai style.

This particular reported effect, however, seems at face value to challenge Ikeda's assertion that the combustive effect is attenuated when cone is burnt on cone, and seems more to echo Obaidey's ideas about increasing the penetration of heat with tubes which we will also come to shortly. I have to record, however, that I have tried repeating Yanagiya's experiment more modestly with twenty cones on an apple, and have failed dismally in remotely replicating his reported effect. A small kitchen knife was my sorry substitute for the razor sharp samurai sword used by Yanagiya in my own fantasy. Lorraine Wilcox reports that she has attempted the

---

[121] Junji Mizutani 2005 "Practical Moxibustion Therapy" (North American Journal of Oriental Medicine)

same experiment but far more authentically – burning three hundred cones on the skin of a water melon but with similar lack of effect[122].

Modern research into the relevant temperatures reached and retained both at the surface and beneath the surface of the skin further enriches the opinions of these modern day masters. A rather unpleasant *in vivo* study of temperature changes both at skin level and in the subcutaneous and muscle layers of mice up to three weeks after the application of three (sizeable) cones of moxa suggest that the maximum temperatures serially **diminish** at skin level whilst they clearly **increase** sequentially in the deeper layers beneath the skin. The explanation derived from these findings was that the temperature reduction at skin level occurs because of the accumulating barriers of tar and ash at the skin, whilst the latter deeper increase in temperature occurs from the accumulation of heat from repeated applications.

What was also interesting, however, was the conclusion that the retention of heat lasted longer in the deeper layers[123]. A similar experiment compared the effects of "multiple" cones versus single cones. Not unsurprisingly, the maximum increases in temperatures with the single applications related to the relative sizes of the cones, but with "multiple" applications (up to six) there were significant differences which were seen as being as much dependent on the number of cones as the size of cones themselves: the time that the tissue stayed above 40° C was proportionally related to the number of cones as well as the weight[124]. We will examine the possible mechanisms of these accumulations of heat in much more depth in Part 4 the Branches where we will also uncover theories about the possible secondary triggers from chemical absorption.

Amongst the clinically useful conclusions we can draw from all of this is that it is indeed advantageous to burn repeated tiny moxa cones on top of the ash of previous cones since it promotes both deeper penetration of heat and a corresponding increased accumulation of temperature whilst potentially minimising sensation at the skin level. It also endorses the practice of careful cowling of the first cone to attenuate the heat as well as the usefulness of a rhythmical application of the subsequent cones to maximise the cumulative warming effects at the deeper levels, a technique which is well worth practising if we hope to both become more proficient and efficient at the same time.

---

[122] Private communication.

[123] Suagat et al 1988 "A Study on Temperature-Changes *in vivo* with Moxibustion" Journal of Japan Society of Acupuncture and Moxibustion; 38(3): 326-329.

[124] Aizawa et al 1985 "Effect of moxibustion on skin tissue. Changes of skin temperature during moxibustion" Journal of Japan Society of Acupuncture and Moxibustion; 35(2):105-110.

The Business of Tubes

The use of tubes appears to be a particular Japanese innovation. It involves the use of hollow bamboo tubes placed over the mugwort after it has been lit. Isaburo Fukaya, late in his career as a famous moxa specialist in the twentieth century, advocated bamboo tubes of varying sizes for this.

Fukaya's "standard" bamboo tube had an internal diameter of 15mm (5/8 of an inch) and a length of 120mm (almost 5 inches). Junji Mizutani, a current authoritative teacher of moxa technique in the West, commonly adopts this technique using a tube which is shorter in length (around 90mm) which he has adapted based on his own experiences. Other practitioners have developed the idea further, adapting tubes with vents or with apertures for observation. For the purpose of this review we will focus our attention, however, on the simple tube.

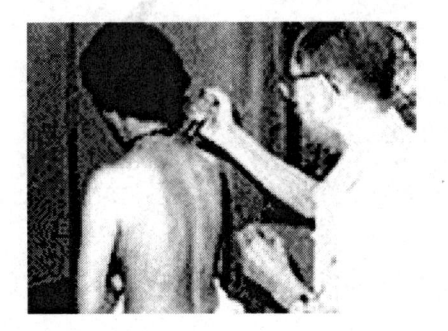

Fukaya using his tube

Relatively speaking, whatever the length, we can reasonably presume that the reduction of oxygen in the tube tends to some degree to diminish the intensity of the smoulder or to actually snuff out the cone of moxa completely as or before the heat touches the skin. Actually, careful observation of the way the moxa burns in a perspex tube leaves it far from clear that this is actually what happens.

Whilst Fukaya originated this particular technique, it is thanks to others that further discussions concerning its advantages and disadvantages can be best assessed. Whilst it seems quite possible that larger cones can be used in this way without causing pain or blistering because of the exhaustion of the oxygen within the tube, other modern practitioners have more developed ideas on the subject.

Edward Obaidey posits the slightly different view that, in general, the smaller the cone the smaller is the reactive and unwanted response of the defensive *wei qi* to the stimulation from the moxa. He sees this as an unwanted response which potentially prevents the deeper penetration of heat either to areas of induration or to the relatively deeper nutritive *ying qi*. This certainly adds an enriching extra dimension of "depth" to our understanding of the varying actions from differing techniques, although this does not necessarily mean that the factor of depth relates in any specific way to either tonification or dispersion.

It does, however, suggest a relationship between the depth of penetration of heat achieved and the idea of speed of burn – the faster the burn (as it is felt), the less time the defensive *wei qi* has to mobilise, which might in some way add to the treatment's effective tonifying potential. With the additional employment of the tube, Obaidey envisages that this defensive attenuating action of the *qi* at the skin's surface is effectively precluded, presumably by applying downward pressure on the tube which allows the heat to penetrate deeper still into the *yin* zones of the body. Exactly how this might occur, however, is a little unclear, particularly because it is evident that the cones burn slightly more slowly inside the tube, one effect quite possibly offsetting the other.

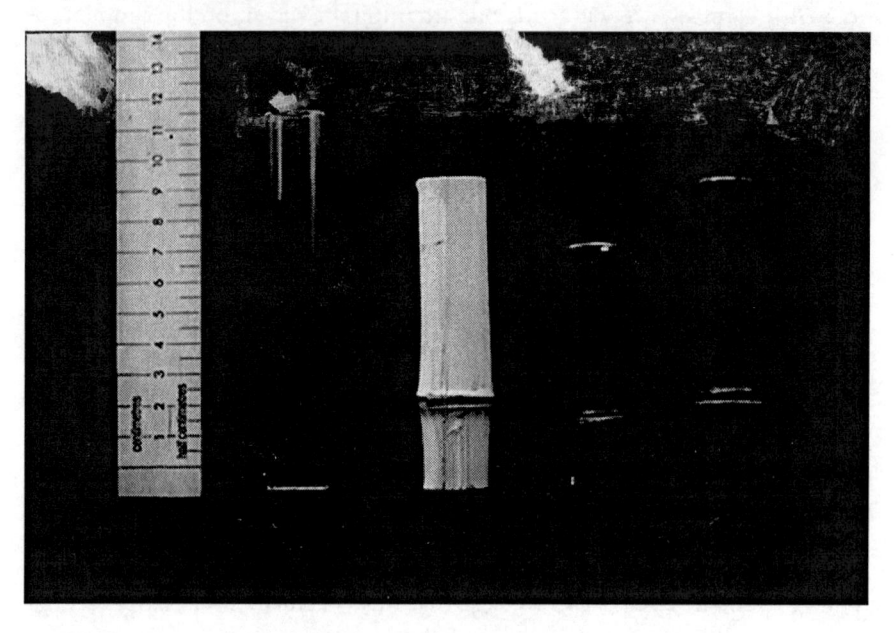

Tubes of varying size (bamboo and perspex)

One idea which is associable with Obaidey's hypothesis is a simple mechanical one: by pressing down with the tube, the superficial tissue in which he conceives the *wei qi* to liewill be compressed. Doing so would allow the heat and *yang qi* from the moxa simply to pass through it directly into the deeper *qi* levels of the body's fascia. This more mundane mechanical theory may be slightly more persuasive.

In fact, it may well be that this effect of allowing the heat from the moxa to reach deeper into the tissue is indeed more efficacious, but for slightly different reasons. By pressing the tube down into the skin as the moxa burns (and twisting the tube at the same time), there is clearly a sensorily distracting effect which reduces the degree of thermoception. This is a similar phenomenon to the pressing down of a guide tube into the skin at a super-sensitive site for needle insertion such as in the sole of the foot or the palm of the hand. But this very action of downward pressure more importantly also shortens the distance between the skin surface and the deeper tissue, meaning that the heat simply has relatively less distance through which to conduct itself to reach the blockage or stagnation, and to "melt" it, if this is what is intended.

Might this be equivalent to "tonifying" or "dispersing" as we understand the ideas? It is uncertain, but what is indisputable is the fact that this technique is very clearly effective for loosening tight areas in the deeper fascia or for melting indurations in muscle tissue which may be acting in some sense as trigger points for other problems.

Two further effects seem to emanate from the use of the tube. Firstly, the moxa does indeed tend to burn slightly more slowly, which is something which can be very clearly witnessed if a clear Perspex tube is used. The advantage of using clear tubes is that we can see what is happening inside with the moxa and the smoke, and it is actually quite intriguing as we will see.

This slower burn might allow time for more heat to build up in the burn, something which might be expected to cause more stress to the patient, but actually this seems not to happen since the patient's subjective thermoception is clearly reduced when using the tube. Less evidence of trauma on examination of the skin after the treatment similarly suggests that the peak temperature at the skin is slightly reduced since any visible signs are minimal.

One could argue that this slowing-down of the burn contrasts directly with the dispersive "blown" moxa technique which correspondingly apparently speeds up the burn, and that this also therefore might render this practice as being more tonifying. A slower burn, furthermore, does not necessarily support the idea of the reduction of the defensive effect of the *wei qi* at the skin surface allowing deeper penetration of the heat unless substantial pressure is applied on the tube, if only because the slower combustion would seemingly actually allow the *wei qi* a longer time in which to mobilise its defence.

A second effect, however, is much more interesting, and can be clearly seen through a clear tube. Clear perspex tubing of various diameters is commercially available and can be cut to lengths to suit different applications based on experimentation. It is interesting to experiment with small clear tubesof around 15mm internal diameter, which can be placed over the moxa and sealed by the practitioner's thumb to restrict the oxygen available for the burn.

What can be observed is that the smoke from the moxa, after rising from the cone, swirls back downwards and then actually accumulates around the smouldering cone. This fills the bottom twenty millimetres of the tube with smoke which then lingers over the skin around the cone with no inclination to rise up inside the tube in any type of chimney effect. What this would suggest is that any chemicals in the smoke itself could potentially be better absorbed at the burn site both during and immediately after combustion – certainly more than if the moxa is burnt in "open" combustion without the tube. The potential additional effect which might arise from this single factor would be extremely difficult to unravel from the complexities of the overall composite process, but if there is any significance in the treatment from the chemical constituents of the burnt herb itself and of its smoke (rather than from the simple temperature at the skin surface) then this practice may well serve to maximise them. Certainly some research from Japan has seriously suggested that the chemical components of moxa are important to the overall effect[125].

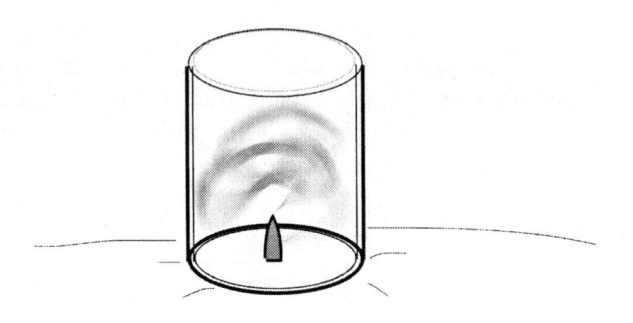

Smoke swirling around the moxa cone in a sealed tube

Heat Perception Moxa (*chinetsukyu*) Technique

Moxa use in Japan involves cones of varying sizes. Traditionally they have been identified in termns of bean, seed or grain sizes. The *chinetsukyu* heat perceprtion technique can technically use cones of any size, but more normally involve the use of cones of bean size or or larger.

A versatile and possibly much simpler way of tonifying (and dispersing) with moxa uses larger *chinetsukyu* cones. This is the sort of size of cone that is often taught for use on Ren8 with salt moxa, about 20mm across at its base (a veritable Asama Volcano of a moxa cone), but *chinetsukyu* cones do not have to be this large. The trick in this particular instance is to lift off the cone just when (or even just before) the patient feels any warmth.

As far as Japan is concerned (where smaller cones have been more the norm) this method, particularly using larger cones, can be traced to Keiri Inoue, one of the

---

[125] Aizawa S, Menjo Y, Tohya K, Nakanishi H, Toda S 2003 "Present Research on Moxibustion" Journal of Japanese Society of Acupuncture and Moxibustion; 53(5): 601-613. Japanese.

founding members of the Meridian Therapy (*Keiraku Chiryo*) movement in Japan in the earlier part of the twentieth century[126]. Inoue himself used this technique generally with larger cones and applied it more dispersively, and today Ikeda uses it exclusively so[127], allowing the cone to get quite hot.

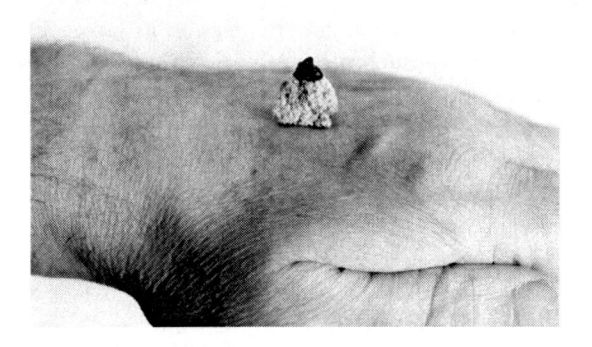

Larger cone chinetsukyu "heat perception" moxa cone

The Toyohari Association of Tokyo has adapted this application so that it is primarily a tonifying technique, however. The association was founded by Kodo Fukushima, a blind practitioner who regularly directed the use of this technique in his clinic to support his acupuncture root treatment. Given the general delicacy of Toyohari needle techniques, this adaptation of a surface protocol into an even more subtle one, one that is more clearly intended to tonify the patient's *qi* and is dependent upon careful employment of technique, may not be so surprising. With this particular method the large cone is invariably applied to a palpably deficient point and is removed as soon as the patient feels any warmth – and sometimes even before it is felt at all (prompted by careful monitoring of changes in the patient's pulse). This technique leads to clear tonifying effects which are observable both at the pulse and at the site of the moxa application where the palpatory "lustre" at the point can also be observed to improve.

In contrast, when applying the *chinetsukyu* technique in order to disperse, the cone is allowed to get very much hotter before it is removed.

The application of this technique is flexible. It can be applied to tonify a treatment point, to tonify an area, to target a symptom, or simply to disperse. Inoue's original general treatment principle was: "For replete conditions, apply one (hot) cone per point, and for vacuity, apply five warm cones", but in Toyohari often

---

[126] Kodo Fukushima 1991 – "Meridian Therapy Part 1". Toyohari Medical Association.

[127] The Society of Traditional Japanese Medicine 2003 "Traditional Japanese Acupuncture" (Complementary Medicine Press).

only two cones are used for tonification. Two warm cones will, for instance, more often than not rebalance an Akabane imbalance when applied to the back *shu* point of the organ associated with the respective channel on the deficient side, suggesting a pervasive whole body effect from this technique[128].

It will be noted that the traditional choices of odd numbers of cones for tonification and even numbers for dispersion based on numerological associations with *yin* and *yang* (or with even numbers of cones for females and odd ones for males) are treated with more general circumspection in Japan. Different grades of moxa, however, are accorded much more attention than elsewhere. Coarser grades of moxa are used to induce a more dispersive effect on the basis of an understanding that less refined moxa burns hotter. In such a case the moxa is burnt (and possibly blown upon) so that clear heat reaches the skin[129].

Using smaller cones of aduki bean size or similar and lifting them when the patient reports feeling the heat is a technique which was mentioned in Part 1 the Roots as being used widely in the UK. It is debatable in fact as to whether this technique is actually technically either "direct" or "indirect" but it certainly comes under the banner of "heat perception moxa". This particular technique has been accurately named "snatch moxa" by Peter Eckman[130].

The cones used in the "snatch" technique are about 8mm across at the base, and are definitely not allowed to burn to the skin, since the effect of the heat would be too much, but are swiftly snatched off the skin as the patient feels the heat. This avoids the risks of blistering which are inherent in more direct techniques, an issue about which there will be more wariness in a culture in which the therapy is unfamiliar. Eckman, who has researched the early influences on acupuncture in the West in the twentieth century, states that this particular "snatch" technique arose in Europe through the teaching of Jacques Lavier, a French sinologist and acupuncturist who greatly influenced the early development of acupuncture in Europe in the twentieth century.

Lavier's primary influences were Taiwanese, but Junji Mizutani, a Japanese moxa specialist who lives and practises in Canada, describes an almost identical method in Japan known as the "health promotion moxa of Sayama". It originates from

---

[128] It is worth noting that generally Chinese theories associate the back *shu* points very definitely to their associated organs; in contrast, Japanese approaches adopt a looser understanding, accepting that they also affect the associated channels and Akabane's ideas accord with this principle. See the section on the Akabane left-right Channel Balancing Method later in this section.

[129] The Society of Traditional Japanese Medicine 2003 "Traditional Japanese Acupuncture" (Complementary Medicine Press)

[130] Peter Eckman 1996 "In the Footsteps of the Yellow Emperor" (Cypress Books)

Osaka[131], and is a method which uses cones the size of aduki beans – much the same size as those used with the snatch technique[132]. Its leading proponent is Sukeharu Fukunishi. Mizutani categorises the technique as somewhere between direct and indirect (which adequately explains some of the confusions in terminology often encountered at acupuncture school) but he concludes that "it seems to give results like direct moxibustion." This idea is examined in more detail in Part 4 the Branches where the research on temperatures at the skin surface during moxa treatment is discussed in much more detail.

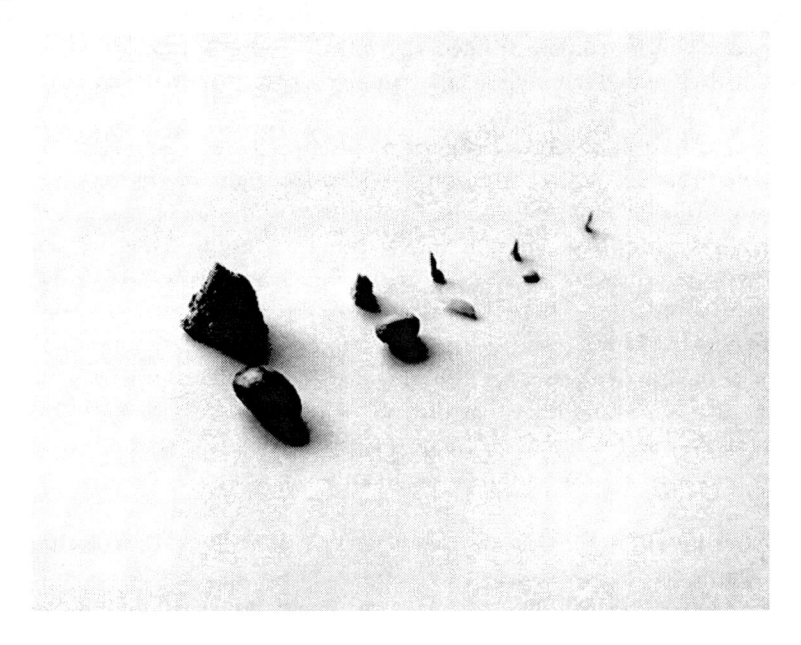

Cones of moxa of varying sizes:
Borlotti bean; aduki bean; rice grain; sesame seed; thread size

One differentiation concerning these two approaches (larger cones *chinetsukyu*-style, and small cones *toonetsukyu*-style) should be appreciated: the *toonetsukyu* rice-grain size small cone treatment can best be understood to be treating more chronic conditions by affecting the stagnated blood and disease which is manifesting at the blood or deeper level, often treating resistant chronic conditions which are less likely to respond quickly; the *chinetsukyu* larger cone can be best understood to be treating the patient more at the *qi* level, with changes being perceptible immediately the *qi* moves. When we revisit direct moxa techniques in connection with research data later, this differentiation may appear even more important than it might initially appear.

---

[131] It is evident that different traditions of direct moxa use have survived in different areas of Japan, and a strong tradition survives in the Osaka area.

[132] Junji Mizutani 2005 "Practical Moxibustion Therapy" (North American Journal of Oriental Medicine) p15.

Some subtle treatment strategies can be developed and employed by a more advanced practitioner. In the recently developed Toyohari tradition of Japanese acupuncture, sophisticated *ho-chu-no-shaho* ("tonification within dispersion") needling techniques are taught to both tonify underlying deficiency and disperse pathogenic *qi* simultaneously. These are seen to be particularly useful for addressing deficiency type diseases of the modern era. This approach is frequently used on a single channel, or even at a single point; arguably the same approach can be adapted by using moxa but require accurate pulse taking for them to be applied effectively. Using the principle "tonify first and drain second", a *chinetsukyu*-tonifying cone can initially be applied at a clearly depressed point in order to fill the point with *qi*, essentially filling the palpable depression, and possibly also the channel itself. In effect, this might also offer better access to pathogenic *qi* by floating it to the surface, and allowing it to be more easily dispersed. In order to do this, small (but hot) *okyu* can next be burnt on tight points on the channel. These can initially be carefully cowled to further promote the tonification effect from the *chinetskyu* heat-perception moxa, but then (as the warmth is felt) the cowling could be removed and the flat of the finger brought down smartly on the cone. The motion of the finger coming down on to the cone to extinguish it effectively fans the burning moxa for a second, instantaneously increasing its heat just at the moment of thermoception and just before the moment of the heat's extinction. If this technique is repeated, all ash should be removed each time a cone is burnt so that the effect of the heat is felt repetitively right at the surface of the skin, with minimal penetration of the heat to the deeper layers.

In a single channel the same point might well be used but different strategies of point selection can as easily or more effectively be applied. Simple choices of tonification and dispersion points might be used; but *yuan* source points (for tonification) and *luo* points (for dispersion) might well be better chosen capitalising on the "host/guest" principles and the idea that the *luo* channels are generally the most superficial zone of the whole channel and therefore may offer the most easily accessible locations at which this dispersion effect might be best achieved. Often the best combination is determined by careful palpation and a comparison of the relative reactions at the points concerned.

For self-treatment such techniques come into their own in terms of possibilities. One of the problems when one wishes to treat oneself using anything more complex than the most basic of needle techniques is that too often the points are in places that are difficult to needle. The advantage of using moxa is particularly relevant for points on the arms which are simply impossible to needle on oneself if the needle technique requires the use of both hands. Since one of the strengths of moxibustion is unquestionably that of home treatment, for the jobbing acupuncturist who wants to stay healthy, these slightly more abstruse techniques offer interesting possibilities for exploration.

Dr Yoshio Manaka, a famous modern proponent of acumoxa in Japan, made an astute suggestion for practitioners intending to extend their clinical abilities by developing original or innovative approaches. Firstly, he suggested, we should try such a technique out upon ouselves; secondly, we should try it out on a member of our family; and only then should we use it on one of our patients.

Direct and Indirect Techniques

We identified right from the very first page of this book that some confusions exist about what is or is not direct and indirect moxa.

As far as direct techniques are concerned, the issue seems fairly simple: the moxa is placed on the skin and burnt down to it – the only grey area arises if the cone is lifted off, particularly in relation to the moment in the process at which this happens.

With indirect techniques the issue is a little more confusing, however. Lorraine Wilcox identifies that the word most often translated from the Chinese as "indirect" is more literally "insulated", "isolated" or "separated". It therefore properly refers to the practice of placing moxa cones on an intermediary (or isolating) substance such as ginger or garlic. In this sense, the practices of burning moxa on the handles of needles or of using moxa sticks or poles are not strictly indirect at all but actually belong to a separate category again. For the purpose of this book, however, and in order not to unnecessarily confuse things, I have decided to take the liberty of designating all such practices as being "indirect" in the literal English sense of the word.

Indirect Moxa with the Moxa Pole with Tonification and Dispersion

When using a moxa stick, there exist quite simple general rules of thumb.

Dispersive action involves the application of the lit end of the moxa pole closer to the skin to elicit heat, often with a "sparrow-pecking" technique. This is when the pole is brought down for a short time close to the skin, then withdrawn for the skin to temporarily cool, then brought close to the skin again, repetitively. Some localised redness in the skin is desirable, but blistering should obviously be avoided.

Tonification techniques involve a far longer period of treatment, with the lit end kept farther from the skin eliciting a milder warming response, often with the pole being waved around in circles or figures of eight over wider areas. Signs of redness at the skin surface can be seen as an indication of potential overtreatment, so the pole should be withdrawn immediately if this is seen.

Indirect moxa on Intermediary Materials

As discussed above, the practice of burning moxa on specific materials is technically known as "isolating moxa". Since the mechanisms and effects almost certainly involve some level of synergy between the constituents or properties of the material selected and the constituents and combustive energy of the moxa itself, the idea of "isolation" may seem something of a misnomer – in consequence of which I have used the term "intermediary materials" in its place since it occurs to me to better reflect what may actually be occurring with these intriguing combinations of materials.

Particular intermediary materials have been traditionally selected and used for different purposes.

Ginger is described as being able to particularly tonify *yang* deficiency, a kind of doubling of the *yang* effect capitalising on the properties of both the ginger and the moxa. Appropriate points might be ones which energetically are regarded as regulating the *yang* functions – Ren8, Ren4 or Ren6, or perhaps Du4.

It also has a reputation for inclusion in infertility treatments and for treatment of premature ejaculation. Unsurprisingly, it is also considered to disperse cold and warm the Spleen and Stomach, in which case middle *jiao* points might best be selected, particularly if the symptoms indicating its use were clearly digestive ones with signs of cold.

Dr Tian Conghuo considers that ginger moxibustion is particularly effective for dispersing cold which has penetrated deeply, through warming and supplementing the *yang*. He suggests five cones at any point per treatment, with ten daily treatments constituting a course of treatment. His experiences suggest that this is an effective method with some difficult–to-treat cases[133].

Garlic, in contrast, is recognised for its medicinal, antibacterial and antiviral properties, and is therefore suitable for treating (cautiously) over local infections, or ulcers (in their early stages) or boils. It is reputed to relieve localised swelling and pain and to cool heat. It is also assumed to improve blood circulation. It is sometimes used in paste form at Ki1. It has been historically indicated for treatment on tuberculous lymph nodes (formerly described as scrofula). Centuries ago when syphilis first broke out in China, Wang Ji (1463-1539) was also known to cauterise syphilitic lesions with garlic. Moxa on garlic has also been endorsed for insect and reptile bites, replacing the slice every two or three cones using up to fifty cones of moxa.

---

[133] "Point Applications and Herbal Moxibustion – Tian Conghuo's Experience" in "Essentials of Contemporary Acupuncturists' Clinical Experiences" 1989 (Foreign Langauages Press, Beijing) pp 90-93

One unusual application of garlic moxibustion is the "long-snake" technique. This is a technique used during hot summer days for chronic, deficient or cold conditions affecting the Du channel, notably *bi*-syndromes, asthma, and even chronic digestive symptoms. The entire channel from Du14 down to Du2 is used. The patient lies face down and some garlic juice is sparingly applied. Following this, some *"Banshe"* powder is distributed along the spine[134]. Next, mashed garlic is applied in a band about 2 inches (50mm) wide and half an inch (12mm) in thickness. After this, moxa is carefully arranged over the garlic in the shape of a snake. This is then lit at the top, the middle and the bottom and allowed to burn out, and then repeated one or two times. Blisters, unsurprisingly, are to be expected, and these are carefully pierced on the third day (if they haven't already discharged their contents somewhat messily already). Amazingly, this protocol comes, not from centuries ago, but from the late twentieth century, from the clinical experiences of Dr Luo Shirong. Amongst other cases, he quotes its use in curing a patient of severe rheumatoid arthritis in the joints of all four limbs[135]. It is not clear what the underlying principles behind this treatment might have been, but it is nevertheless claimed to be effective.

Aconite as an intermediary material for indirect moxa is variously described as being formed by mixing *fuzi* (*radix aconite carmichaeli praeparatae* – perhaps the hottest herb used in Chinese medicine) with rice wine, or by using aconite "cakes" of thin slices of dried aconite with a further intermediate layer of gauze to protect the skin. Utilising the extreme heat properties of the aconite, this technique is understood to warm the *yang* in a similar but stronger fashion than with ginger and is particularly indicated for impotence and infertility.

It is important to note, however, that aconite is controversial in that it is highly poisonous when taken internally. In East Asian medicine it is known as the "emperor herb" but it is also known in another less healthy field of endeavour as the "queen of poisons". It **can** be absorbed through the skin, although with the processed herb this is highly unlikely. Nevertheless the use of gauze is imperative as a preventative measure for the patient's safety. "Pure" unprocessed aconite is best avoided, and the processed herb *fuzi* (which is steam processed with ginger) is recommended. The active herb is taken from the root, and it is definitely **not** advisable to use home grown monkshood root as a creative alternative to the prepared herb if this is difficult to obtain, since its toxicity will be completely unknown. Frankly the practice is probably best avoided by the more cautious practitioner, but it is widely regarded as being perfectly safe and highly effective if *fuzi* and gauze are used (but do wash hands carefully after handling or a numbness or mild tingling may result if you lick your foingers!). The raw herb unfortunately has been banned in many western countries, although this ban relates to its

---

[134] It is unfortunately impossible to identify exactly what this is.

[135] "Essentials of Contemporary Chinese Acupuncturists Clinical Experiences" 1989 (Foreign Langauages Press, Beijing) pp357-360

internal use and not for an external one, but as a result *fuzi* may currently be difficult to purchase.

Traces of aconite, incidentally, were reported as having been found in early post-mortem tests on the corpse of Bob Woolmer, the English cricket coach who died mysteriously during the cricket World Cup in the West Indies in 2007, just hours after the Pakistani team, which he coached, was unexpectedly ousted from the competition by Ireland. Initially he was strongly suspected of having been poisoned, and many still believe this to have been the case –particularly as aconite has been used as a poison for centuries in the Himalayan regions.

Also, in the UK in 2009, the so called 'Curry Killer' Lakhvir Kaur Singhpoisoned her lover with a curry dish laced with aconite: she was sentenced to life imprisonment with a minimum term of 23 years for the murder.

Salt is generally used for moxa application at Ren8. Salt conducts heat efficiently, and, of course, salt also has a traditional association with the *qi* of the Kidney. It might therefore reasonably be surmised that the "design" of this protocol is to use the salt to allow the *yang* warmth of the moxa to penetrate directly to, or resonate with, the Kidney. It is also commonly used at Ren8 to treat diarrhoea, and this effect may result from stimulating the Kidney's function of controlling water. Used in this way, it might also be indicated for symptoms of uncontrolled sweating. Ginger and salt are sometimes even combined together at this point, with a slice of ginger placed over the navel already brim-filled with sodium chloride. We examine this point in more detail later in this section.

Of the other materials less frequently referred to, **tangerine peel** is said to help "release to the exterior" and free the lungs in the case of a common cold, and so might be used at Du14 or Bl12 for increased efficacy. **Miso**, which is a messy material for moxa use, is supposedly good for both Stomach and Spleen, as well as having been used in the past for the treatment of sores. Finally, **loquat leaf** supposedly boosts the immune system by cleansing the blood, and is reported as having been used in Japan in cancer treatment.

One interesting technique which is both traditional and re-invented for the modern age is **moxa on ceramic**. This is a Japanese tradition, and is used in Buddhist ceremonies. Moxa is burnt on a ceramic bowl which is effectively warmed by it, and the ceramic is placed over specific areas of the body – the lower abdomen, the lower back or more often the head. The treatment (using a shallow bowl the size of a dinner plate) is known in Japan as *horoku kyu*. It is done ceremonially on older people in North-Eastern Japan on the 20th day of the first month, being believed to ward off dementia and is known as the *yaitozome* or the "moxa beginning".

There may in fact be some science to support this tradition. We will look at the potential effect of specific wavelengths of Infrared Radiation (and FIR) in Part 4 the Branches, particularly in respect of moxa on ginger, aconite or garlic. It is also known, however, that ceramic porcelain when heated to 400 degrees centigrade emits similar wavelengths which are known to have beneficial and stimulating effects on living cells.

Indirect Moxa-on-the-Needle-Head technique

Indirect techniques cannot be left without discussing the "moxa-on-the-needle-head" technique in which moxa is placed on the handle of the acupuncture needle and burnt. Sometimes this is described as the "warm-needle technique" or as the "periodiodically heated needle technique". It may have originated with Sun Simiao: "A great method is to settle the needle, then apply moxibustion to it[136]."

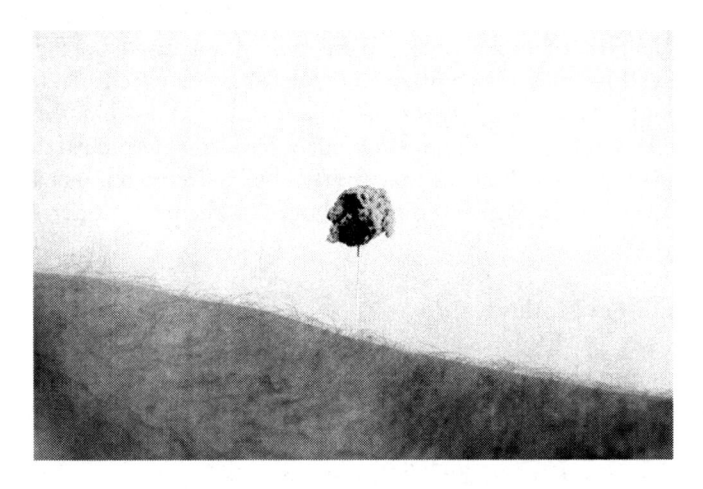

Moxa-on-the-Needle-Head technique.
The moxa should always be lit from the bottom.

It is often used to loosen tight tissue, and is particularly effective in cases of back pain as well as with knee problems. A question which arises is one that is fundamental to acupuncturists: is this technique tonifying or dispersive? As an answer this may seem like a cop out, but it seems likely that it is both: the technique seems to promote *qi* circulation and clearly warms, but also appears to clear stagnation at the same time.

In fact, it actually seems quite probable that its actions are three-fold: firstly, the tip and shaft of the needle stimulate the point and the surrounding tissue in the usual ways; secondly, the burning moxa creates a radiant effect (the patient invariably feels this as a pleasurable sensation and often describes as like lying on a beach in the sunshine); and the third is the effect of the heat passing directly down the shaft of the needle itself which dissipates beneath the point at which the shaft

---

[136] Lorraine Wilcox 2008 "Moxibustion, the Power of Mugwort Fire" (Blue Poppy Press)

has penetrated the skin where the heat passes into the local tissue. A heat gradient exists in the shaft from the skin level down to the needle tip itself where the remaining heat will finally dissipate. Curiously, the patient does *not* feel this particular heat in the shaft itself at all, which is without doubt just as well, because the shaft becomes extremely hot. The temperature reached at the actual tip of the needle is dependent on the quantity of moxa burnt at the handle (as well as on how long this takes), and the depth of insertion beneath the skin surface. Both vary enormously between practitioners.

Some sources suggest protecting the skin surface in case the moxa ball falls off the needle handle on to the skin. Such a precaution will almost certainly attenuate some of the effect of the radiant heat and seems best not to be adopted as a technique. Two simple alternative approaches effectively minimise any risk. Firstly, short lengths of moxa pole can be cut up and used (in fact proprietary short pre-pierced lengths are commercially available for exactly this purpose), or alternatively better "clumping" types of moxa can be used – like the "wakakusa" grades available from Japan. The latter also have the particular advantage of emitting far less harsh smoke than that emitted by less refined moxa which is used in moxa poles, something which is a major boon for the practitioner.

One other Indirect Method

One last wonderful more modern indirect moxa technique that is worth recording is moxibustion with "walnut shell spectacles". A curious set of spectacles are employed for this purpose in which the lenses comprise half-walnut shells which have been previously immersed in chrysanthemum water. Cones of moxa are then lit on top of the shells. Claims of effectiveness are made for conjunctivitis, styes, keratitis, myopia, cataract and optic atrophy. The walnut is said to relate to the Kidney channel, and the chrysanthemum to the Liver[137].

An unusual twist has been applied to this technique with the use of snail shells in lieu of the walnut shells. The idea of the snail shell treatment may have evolved from an earlier technique in which the inside of the shell, after having five small holes drilled in it, was rather unpleasantly filled with chicken manure. A moxa stick was then held over the shell – a treatment said to resolve toxins, disperse swellings and check pain[138].

---

[137] Li Zhiming's Clinical Experience "Essentials of Contemporary Chinese Acupuncturists Clinical Experiences" 1989 (Foreign Langauages Press, Beijing) pp 215-216

[138] Lorraine Wilcox 2008 "Moxibustion, the Power of Mugwort Fire" (Blue Poppy Press) p21

"Stick-on" Proprietary Moxa

Some innovative commercial products have been produced to exploit moxa techniques for more popular applications. They are generally known as "platform moxa" or *dai kyu* in Japan, and are more popularly known as "stick-ons" in the West. These can be particularly useful for home use, and also for children and sensitive or anxious patients.

Generally these products are designed to be used by the general public rather than the practitioner, although there is absolutely no reason why they should be avoided by the latter. Their effectiveness should not be underestimated.

Many commercial varieties of indirect stick-on moxas exist. These are easy to use and lack the inescapable fiddliness of preparing cones. They also offer uniform heat, and much less risk of accident. They come in a variety of forms, and with differing strengths in terms of heat. Most consist of a small rolled cylinder of moxa mounted on a sticky base.

Some of the cylinders themselves are made from smokeless material. With some the warming moxa heat slowly builds to a moment of more acute heat, and then recedes gradually. In others the heat is much milder. Holes in the base may allow both heat and smoke to circulate directly on the point. Small stick-on heat shields may also be applied to protect the skin from the heat if considered necessary.

One useful type consists of a small cardboard tube which is filled with moxa. The bottom of the tube is sticky and is adhered to the skin after the moxa within the tube has been pushed upwards to protrude from the top of the tube so that the underside of the moxa will be well clear of the skin. This creates a void within the tube within which the moxa smoke can also circulate.

Some more sophisticated "*Sennenkyu*" versions even employ bases made with miso, ginger or garlic. These latter three types are termed "harder" in terms of their warming properties.

A useful application for stick-ons will be found later in a discussion on Korean Hand Therapy (*Koryo Sooji Chim*). Proprietary stick-on moxas are specifically manufactured in Korea for use on the hand including ones mounted on small ceramic discs.

Personally, I like to use the small tubular stick-ons with smaller children, such as the Neo brand which is manufactured by the Yamasho Company in Japan, and I find them extremely effective. As important as their effectiveness is the fact that children cope with the treatment quite easily, whilst moxa hand-rolled moxa cones can easily create unhelpful anxieties for them even when the cones are rolled to thread size.

Towards the end of Appendix 1, some treatment protocols can be found which have been adapted from a list published by Sennekyu, one of the manufacturers of these products. The original list is meant for members of the public, but they offer a very useful source of points for a variety of conditions nevertheless, not only for use with these stick-on products, but also with moxa generally.

Since one of the core ideas of small cone moxa is that it should be done every day, these stick-on moxas offer a safe option for patients to do exactly this at home having been appropriately instructed by their practitioner.

Undifferentiated Moxa Treatment

Moxa specialists in Japan are separately licensed from acupuncturists and tend to be more pragmatic in approach, a little less attached perhaps to channel or excess/deficiency *yin/yang* theory than many acupuncturist colleagues. Their approach is typically both pragmatic and methodical: systematically palpate the body, locate reactivity, moxa and check the response. Some aspects of these approaches may have been heavily influenced by Japanese massage *anma* and *shiatsu* therapy.

Typical reactivity generally consists of tightness, pressure pain and/or indurations in the tissue. It is on this basis that the lists of treatment points and also the extra moxa points would appear to have evolved. Protocols for an enormous variety of conditions have been developed (often giving options of several points with a final selection being made from palpatory findings) and some of these are included in the Appendix.

The word invariably used to describe the techniques from almost any source on the subject is that these techniques can be "effective" – and more often than not this is prefixed by the word "very", "clinically" or even (in bold type) "**extremely**". These words are self-evidently not used lightly, and are supported by some of the research effects which are listed later. A common qualification to this, however, is a stipulation that the treatment should be repeated regularly for the total effect to be maximised.

Generally, as already mentioned, the concepts of excess and deficiency are largely ignored by those who simply practise moxibustion as specialists. As acupuncturists, of course, we have a kind of fundamental hard-wiring which makes it difficult for us not to try and make sense of symptomatic or palpatory findings in these terms, and then treat accordingly. With moxa, this approach may or may not be so useful.Since the points indicated are only used if there is some local abnormal reactivity at the points, any changes in reactivity give further guidance to the treatment. Abnormal reactivity might include pressure pain, tightness in the underlying tissue or indurations in the musculature.

There is a traditional Japanese "rule-of-thumb" guide to this type of application which may or may not prove helpful. The basic rule of thumb is: "If heat is felt, apply until the heat cannot be felt; if heat cannot be felt, apply until it can be felt". This is almost certainly an echo of Zhang Jiebin in his "Complete Works" in which he quoted: "When moxibustion is applied but is not painful, stop when the moxibustion becomes painful ... the effects reach good flesh, so there is pain. When moxibustion is applied and is painful, stop when the moxibustion is no longer painful." This particular historical adage, however, relates specifically to treatment over sores and ulcers, and it is worth considering whether this might be the limit of its application. Certainly the application of heat where it cannot be felt until it can be felt is a dangerously uncertain treatment principle, and one to be approached with caution if it is applied at all.

It is quite possible, actually, that the cumulative effects of direct moxa, particularly the serological ones which raise the host immune response, are at least partly dependent upon a relationship between the total number of cones being applied to the body and the general state of the patient. They need not necessarily be so dependent upon the number of cones per point. Although point selection is clearly important and in many cases is fundamental to effect, there may be other more general factors at work, something we will explore more deeply in Part 4 the Stems.

It is the critical nature of the total number of cones, regularly and repetitively applied, which appears to create the clearest effects with intractable or chronic conditions, and which most clearly relate to the references of the methods of effectiveness alluded to above. With states of general constitutional deficiency, the starting total may need to be very small, with the specific design of the treatment strategy being to slowly build up the dosage as the patient improves. This type of cumulative dosage effect can thus be seen, at least in some sense, to be a tonifying one. In Japan this is sometimes simply referred to as *mibyo-chi* or the activation of the body's self healing abilities and is seen as a vital part of moxa treatment.

It will be recalled that the word for "cone" in Chinese is *zhuang* or "reinforcement". In Japanese it is *sō* (壮). Similarly to the Chinese, this is a counting word, and basically means a "vibrancy" or "energy input".

Doctor Yoshio Manaka, who was not only a proponent of cumulative small cone moxa but also conducted some research into its effects, was renowned as a specialist and expert in treating difficult conditions. It is difficult not to take appropriate note, therefore, when he stipulated quite clearly that the judicious use of moxa is an essential treatment resource when other treatments are failing.

A paper published in Dutch by Dr Doortje van der Kamp on the Internet [139] suggests that the empirical treatment points on the trunk when indicated in the

---

[139] http://www.acupunctuur.com/scripties/vanderkamp.html#6 accessed 24/2/2010.

Japanese literature for specific complaints may actually be unrelated to the channel system. Her paper addressed the possible segmental nerve connections between the locations of these points, and the nerves supplied to the viscera and organs involved with the pathology. Her conclusions (which are in English although the rest of the paper is in Dutch) suggest at least more than a random connection: "Japanese moxibustion method is compared with the segmental innervations of the body. The dermatomes, myotomes and sclerotomes in which the points are located are then compared ... with the viscerotomes of the organs ... when you compare the points with the viscerotomes, a quite high percentage of correlation is found, especially with points that are located on the trunk." This research suggests that other complementary actions may be active in this type of treatment other than those discussed in the traditional literature, and therefore that some traditional concepts and approaches might even be waived in their use.

It is beyond dispute that a massive amount of systematic investigation deserves to be done if we are to more fully understand and more efficiently apply moxa today.

Moxa-only Treatment Protocols from China

Lorraine Wilcox, who is as an eminent English-speaking expert on the subject, has identified a shortlist of points which in China were traditionally reserved for moxa only. These were: the unnumbered "Four Flowers" *Sihua;* Bl43 *Gaohuang shu*; M-BW-24 *Yaoyan*; M-UE-45 *Zhoujian*; "Ride the Bamboo Horse" *Qihumaxue*; and M-CA-23 "Triangle Moxibustion" *Sanjiaojiu*.

Some of these points will be discussed in more detail in a later section, but, of the remainder, the following may prove of interest if only in the way that they provide a picture of how moxa may have been used in the past.

Zhoujian (Elbow Tip) is indicated in cases of intestinal abscesses, and nodules in the neck, axilla and inguinal regions.

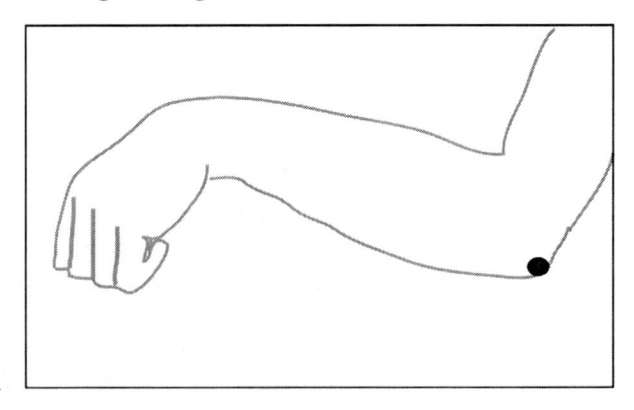

Location of Zhoujian

Sanjiaojiu utilises three points (Ren8 and two points located by constructing an equilateral triangle with the apex at the umbilicus – each of the three sides equal in length to the patient's smile). In the TCM literature this is now indicated primarily for chronic diarrhoea. Yoshio Manaka listed this as one of his favourite point combinations for sterility.

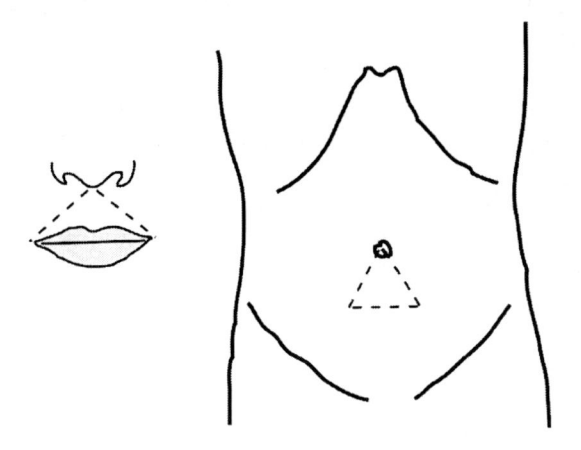

How to locate the two lower sanjiaojiu points

Qihumaxu, "Ride the Bamboo Horse" is as much a protocol as a treatment point but it would be difficult to restore it into the treatment formulary of the modern Western practitioner for reasons which will quickly become clear. It is such a wonderfully convoluted protocol, however, with such an evocative name that it simply begs inclusion, and has been meticulously described for us by Wilcox. A strip of bamboo is cut to length to match the distance from the centre of the elbow to the tip of the middle finger. The patient is then asked to remove all of his or her clothes and then to sit astride a stout bamboo carrying pole which is lifted off the ground so that the patient's legs no longer reach the ground, but so that the patient remains stable. The bamboo measuring strip is then used with one end abutting on to the top surface of the pole at the point where the patient's coccyx rests and with the strip aligned directly up the line of the spine. Where the top of the strip falls on the spine becomes a central marking point. Two points are marked, each one *cun* bilateral to this. Thirty-five cones are next applied suppuratively on these points with the patient still sitting on the pole.

This protocol is indicated for abscesses, malign sores and eruptions on the back as well as for breast abscesses. It was further proposed that, since the Heart vessel is said to flow through this point, any stagnant Heart fire will flow freely following this treatment and the associated toxins will scatter in response to this treatment.

It is postulated that the points themselves may correspond to Bl17, but the simultaneous stimulation or blocking off at the base of the spine seems to be as much a part of the treatment as the application of the moxa itself at any particular point. There exists an implicit idea of a secondary effect of the accumulated *qi* from the moxa treatment being released up through the coccyx to rush deep into the body at the moment that the patient "dismounts" (still naked, of course) from the bamboo horse at the end of the treatment[140].

More modestly, and certainly of more use to us, Wilcox also lists *Baihui* Du20 as being effective with moxa for raising *qi*, and conversely *Yong Quan* Ki1 for drawing fire down from above.

The following more extensive list comes from the comprehensive research in the traditional Chinese source literature by Deadman, Al-Khavaji and Baker. The specific original sources for each point can generally be found against each point listing in their extraordinarily comprehensive "Manual of Acupuncture". Neither the method of moxibustion application, nor the amount recommended is generally identified, so we must use our own discretion if we want to use these points in treatment.

> LI3 – toothache (lower jaw)
> LI10 – toothache (upper jaw)
> St29 – needle & moxa; warms the lower *jiao*
> St45 – draws fire down; insomnia
> Sp1 – stops bleeding especially in the lower *jiao*
> Sp17 – 200-300 cones to "secure life" in Spleen type disease
> SI16 – 50 cones for loss of speech and hemiplegia
> Bl12 – for attacks of wind cold
> Bl13 – chronic asthma or winter coughs ("intense moxa" in the summer)
> Bl17 & Bl19 – taxation consumption disorder (tuberculosis) – see section on the "Four Flowers"
> Bl32 (and the other 6 *liao* points) – difficult urination or defecation
> Bl67 – breech presentation and delayed labour
> Ki2 – sweating, coldness of feet and legs, cold diarrhoea, impotence
> GB36 – rabies (also with moxa treatment at the site of the bite)
> Liv11 – infertility
> Ren4 – longevity
> Ren6 – resuscitation of *yang*, profound deficiency
> Ren9 – oedema
> Du20 – prolapse of uterus or vagina, chronic deficiency disease, incessant diarrhoea
> Du23 – nasal disorders but caution against excessive use

A modern source also advocates Du14 *Dazhui* (dispersed with moxa) for an outbreak of herpes zoster (a clear heat condition) with daily treatment – using a moxa stick for the elderly and direct moxa for the younger[141].

---

[140] Lorraine Wilcox 2008 "Moxibustion, the Power of Mugwort Fire" (Blue Poppy Press) p83 From Zhang Jiebin – LJTY: 10-1-7.

The most frequently mentioned indications for moxa treatment in modern TCM literature, incidentally, generally appear to be for gastro-intestinal disorders, asthma, organ prolapse, bi-syndromes and herpes zoster.

There are certainly more moxa treatments in the canon of TCM, but this list is clearly not a very long one in comparison to the points listed elsewhere for needling, or indeed compared to the Japanese lists referred to above. Both incorporate hundreds of points for as many conditions. The wider picture which emerges from this is that moxa is viewed today quite differently in different countries, and the canon of acumoxa is very much still evolving. The diversity of practice we are so lucky to enjoy today should be cherished for this very reason, with exchange and debate between different "styles" to be encouraged and enjoyed for the benefit of the therapy iun the future.

Longevity and Moxibustion

No investigation into the subject of moxibustion could be deemed anywhere near complete without mention of the traditional associations of prolonged moxa use to promote longevity. In these days of conflicting claims for health enhancement, it is wise to treat what follows with healthy circumspection, but nevertheless there seems to be an investigable fire smouldering behind the smoke of anecdotal evidence.

The earliest proponent of moxa for longevity appears to have been Sun Simiao, who in the seventh century advocated that people should regularly apply moxa to prevent illness. He was himself in relatively poor health when younger, and yet was documented to have lived to the ripe age of 101, surviving seemingly as a testament to his own advice.

Several centuries later, Dou Cai, in the *Bian Que Xinshu* (his herb-and-moxa text of 1289), relates the story of Wang Chao, an infantry man living in the Song Dynasty who deserted from the army and became a bandit. At the age of ninety, he was still tyrannising local villages and kidnapping their women. Finally, however, he was arrested by government troops. The judge was baffled by Wang's brilliant, energetic, and youthfully chubby face and the fact that he was standing in front of him at the age of ninety accused of having his way with as many as ten of his kidnap victims in a single day.

The judge asked Wang to explain himself. "Every year, at the onset of autumn and the change of season, I treat myself with moxa," Wang replied, saying that each year between summer and autumn, he burnt more than 1,000 cones of moxa at *guan yuan* (Ren4). He claimed that it was this that had led to his insatiable appetite

---

[141] Li Huailin 1992 "34 cases of herpes zoster treated by moxibustion at *dazhui* (GV-14)" (Journal of Traditional Chinese Medicine)

for women, and was also the reason that he committed these crimes. "Even now, I have a patch below my navel which feels warm like fire," he said[142].

His creative plea for mitigation failed and he was still executed, but the executioner was said to have observed that, although the rest of Wang's body cooled as expected, the warmth in his abdomen remained after death. He was so puzzled by this that he supposedly cut open Wang's belly and found something hard within it that resembled a precious stone.

It is a fanciful tale, but an even more extreme (and doubtless equally exaggerated) tale on this subject comes from Japan. A farmer called Manpei, in the Edo period, was reported as living to the very ripe old age of 243. When questioned by the authorities, he reported that he had no secret to disclose other than burning moxa on St36 every day, just as his forefathers had done. His wife reputedly lived to 242, and his son to 196, his daughter-in-law to 193. He claimed that he had a grandson who was 151 with a younger wife aged 138. It clearly was something of a healthy family obsession.

Much more recently, however, another more authentic and reliable Japanese advocate appears in the longevity stakes. Dr Shimetaro Hara (1883-1991) was a more modern proponent for regular moxa treatment on St36.

He lived to the ripe old age of 108, for the last months of his life holding the cherished official title of "oldest male in Japan", and was also for some years almost certainly the oldest practising physician and scientist in the world[143]. Early on in his career in Japan in the 1920s and 1930s he was eminent as an important contributor to research into the effects of moxibustion. His story and the length of his life would suggest that any concerns of exhausting *jing* essence from frequent small-cone moxibustion are almost certainly ill-founded[144].

A complementary approach advocated for longevity is the "eight day method", a slightly less rigorous regime whereby moxa is burnt on St36 on the first eight days of each lunar month in the days immediately after the new moon. In the case of a woman, its beginning can be logically adapted to coincide with the end of menstruation rather than the cycle of the moon, although there is no reference to such an idea in any of the source literature.

---

[142] Liu Zheng-cai 2003."Health-Preserving, Life-Prolonging Moxibustion"- Acupuncture Today; Vol. 04, Issue 12

[143] http://www.grg.org/Adams/JapaneseCent.htm accessed 14/1/2009.

[144] Dr Hara investigated moxa over a working life of at least 60 years. The last paper I have found to which he was a contributor was published in 1981 when he was ninety-eight (the first in 1929 when he was forty-six). Not many researchers - if any - in the history of science have enjoyed a working lifespan of this magnitude.

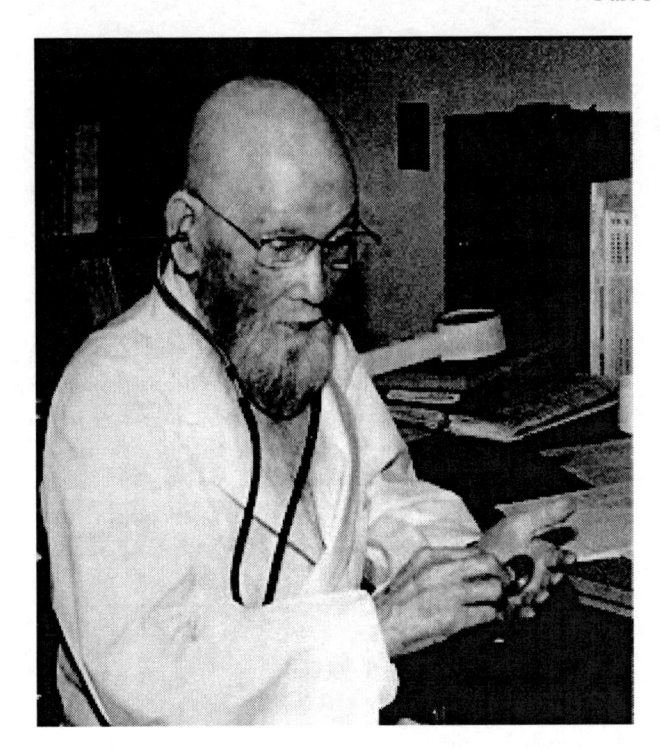

Doctor Shimetaro Hara

Other points have been similarly advocated in China for longevity. A classic example is a combination of Ren6, Ren4, Sp17 and Ren12, with the supporting theory behind its use being moxa's ability to support original *yang*. Dou Cai slid one of the most the most disarming lines in the literature of traditional East Asian medicine into his *Bian Que Xinshu* classic – that, although one may not obtain old age using these points, one can still maintain a lifespan of a hundred years.

Lorraine Wilcox writes on this same topic: "Nourishing life (養生 *yang sheng*) is a technical term that means promoting good health and long life in the absence of disease". Usually, nourishing life treatments are not begun before a person is 30 years of age. The intensity of the treatment is furthermore often recommended to increase with the person's age[145].

Wilcox describes how, from the age of forty, moxa can be applied in the spring to Ren6, and in the autumn to Ren4. She quotes *Suwen* 2 as describing how the sage nourishes *yang* in the spring and *yin* in the autumn, and that this protocol accords with this principle. Whilst the original texts may imply that a huge number of cones should be applied, it is not explicitly stated that this should be carried out in a single session. Wilcox suggests more sensibly dividing the total number by as

---

[145] For more information:
http://www.facebook.com/album.php?aid=108309&id=127985768455

many as ten separate applications on a daily basis from around January 30th to February 8th and August 2nd to 12th, either with small cones or with moxa on ginger. She does suggest, however, as many as 30 grain-sized cones a day.

A similar tradition existed in Japan for older people in the spring, incidentally, but in this case the second day of the second lunar month after the new year was identified as the most favourable (known as *futsuka kyu* or *futsuka yaito*). This would place the treatment most often in March or April.

Liu Jie-Sheng, a contemporary Chinese acupuncturist, endorses Dou Cai's opinion that moxa does not just support original *yang*, but it can also help to restore it. He encourages applying date-sized moxa cones on ginger at Ren6 for five days at the beginning of spring and at Du4 for five days at the beginning of autumn each year. He suggest that in these ten days one can use up to 300 cones, implying that he recommends 30 cones each day but with only five days' treatment in each season, with exactly half the total number of cones applied using Wilcox's methodology.

Moxa and Home Treatment

In considering the above we should keep in mind that moxa has been used in East Asia as a folk-therapy for many centuries. During the Southern and Northern Dynasties of the fifth century, Chen Yanzhi wrote the "Short Sketches of Formulas", a text which was subsequently lost but which was extensively quoted in later Japanese texts. He described moxibustion in terms which exactly suggest its suitability for folk-therapy and lay practice: "Even the ordinary person can apply moxibustion ... if a teacher has not explained the text [the *Neijing*] you can [simply] apply moxibustion according to diagrams and explanatory texts. However, in the uncultivated places without diagrams or anyone to explain the texts, you can [still] expel disease from a site by applying moxibustion."

Yet again we have evidence here of the lack of both training and skill needed to effectively apply moxa if only a few simple guidelines are adhered to, with little requirement for literacy and none for scholarship. Evidence for this idea appears frequently in the descriptions of the point locations in some of the moxa treatment texts which are clearly written in terms which describe how to locate the treatment points as simply as possible. No *cun* measurements for anatomical locations, no complex channel pathways – simple waxed string was frequently used, tied off to lengths standardised by measuring from simple landmarks on the patient's own body (the width of the patient's mouth, for instance) and then multiplied or divided as measurements using other equally obvious physiological landmarks[146]. This tradition of moxa's application for home use obviously has no

---

[146] As will be seen in the Appendix, this method was revived in the twentieth century by Isaburo Fukaya.

correlate in the West, something which presents a problem for many western practitioners, since, even if we advocate its use for our patients at home, its potential may well be culturally misunderstood by both themselves and their relatives.

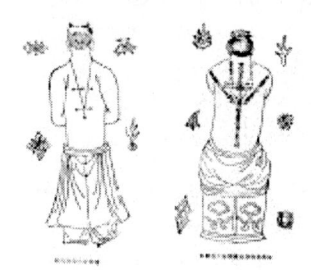

Early Chinese moxa point location drawing showing the use of string measurement

The relevance for its use as home therapy remains strong to this day, however, despite the population now being generally literate, simply because, as long as the points are appropriately and reasonably accurately located, it really does not matter who carries out the application. This relevance especially relates to daily treatment which is seen to create powerful cumulative curative effects and also to moxa's long-standing traditional reputation as a preventative therapy.

What is clear from Hara's writing, for instance, is his conviction that the effects are slow and cumulative. "A fluff of dust can accumulate to create a mountain," he wrote, "the important thing is not to hurry, keep calm and quiet and build a strong body…[147]".

Home moxa can definitely amplify the effects of our acumoxa practice-based treatment, and can also allow our patients to improve more easily and quickly. It may also do something else which may be as important: Kodo Fukushima perceptively pointed out that it "responsibilises" patients – something which results in our patients taking more active care and responsibility for their own overall well-being rather than becoming dependant upon their practitioner – which should surely be the goal of every responsible therapist. The venerable Dr Hara went even further – he suggested that moxa could put doctors out of business.

Both of these twentieth century Japanese sources obliquely reflect the earlier observation of Zhang Jiebin in China back in the Ming Dynasty: "In each and

---

[147] Dr Shimetaro Hara 1933 "Moxibustion Therapy effective for all Diseases" (Old Japanese) out of print.

every disease, apply three cones of moxibustion to *Sanli* every day. *Qi* will descend and the disease will stop[148]."

Stomach 36, Bladder 43, Ren 8, the Four Flowers, Suffering Gate, Sp17 and Ren4.

Specific points do seem to be especially suited to moxa treatment, and they deserve some discussion as a result.

We have already touched on **St36** *Zusanli*. Sun Simiao advocated it as a point for moxa which has a healthy down-bearing effect on the *qi*. As early as the *Suwen*, potential problems were identified from counter-flow effects arising from moxa treatment, particularly when symptoms indicated a "surplus above" situation or when they demanded a treatment using a large number of moxa cones on the upper back or chest. The additional effect of the input of *yang qi* into the upper body from the moxa was then to be treated with caution. In such cases it was warned that "when the patient is cauterised he will turn mute" (*Suwen* 40). To counter exactly such an extreme effect, moxa at St36 is frequently endorsed in later texts.

Wang Tao extrapolated this idea in his endorsement of this point for its anti-ageing effects – "Whenever people over the age of 30 do not apply moxa to *Zusanli*, qi is allowed to ascend, dimming their eyes. *Sanli* is used to descend qi[149]."

Since the *Huang Di Mingtang Jiujing* of the twelfth century, moxibustion at St36 has been regarded as being able to ward off wind-stroke. Zhang Gao, a physician and medical historian of the Song Dynasty also in the twelfth century wrote: "to be sound [of body], *San Li* should always be wet." The implication from this is that in his opinion the point should be to a greater or lesser extent rendered suppurative from regular direct blistering moxa treatment throughout the year[150].

It can hardly be considered controversial to suggest that this point, above any other, could lay claim to be **the** point for moxa treatment for any illness.

Dr Shimetaro Hara in his book "Moxibustion, a Treatment for a Hundred Diseases", which was published in Japan in 1933, advocated the burning of small half rice grain sized cones of moxa on this point on each leg on a daily basis.

---

[148] Lorraine Wilcox 2008 "Moxibustion, the Power of Mugwort Fire" (Blue Poppy Press) p54 From Zhang Jiebin's LJTY: 4-27-4.

[149] Lorraine Wilcox 2008 "Moxibustion, the Power of Mugwort Fire" (Blue Poppy Press) p30

[150] Honora Lee Wolfe 2005 "Moxibustion for longevity and health preservation" (Townsend Letter for Doctors and Patients)

"This is so simple, and almost too facile that it feels like a lie," he wrote. He advocated its use "at home, travelling, on the train and everywhere."

While moxa smoke, let alone moxa treatment, on a train is likely to create some unwelcome attention these days even in Japan, he seems to have been totally serious when writing this in the 1930s. Hara founded the "Great Japan Health Alliance" intending that hospitals should become "covered in cobwebs" as the population became healthier as a result. His language is delicious, although what happened to this organisation which consisted at one stage of at least 10,000 members is now uncertain. A catastrophic war intervened, first in Manchuria and then globally, finally ending in two horrific attempts at replicating Armageddon at Hiroshima and Nagasaki in 1945. Attitudes to moxa may have changed significantly within only a few years, however, an idea that can be supported by the fact that General MacArthur's occupational authority attempted to outlaw moxibustion soon after the Japanese surrender because of a misconception of its association with torture. These attempts failed as a result of public outcry, but moxa use has been increasingly neglected as a major part of Japan's traditional heritage ever since.

One of the oft-quoted attributes about moxa and this St36 point relate to the "three miles" in its name. It was said at acupuncture school that traditionally this point was moxa-ed by Chinese soldiers in order to be able to march an extra three miles (*li*) a day. While this seems a little fanciful there may be some truth to it. I used moxa on this point on a friend about to run the London Marathon in 1999 who at the time was 45 years old. He proceeded to run a better time than he had done two years previously (when he was two years younger and had trained much harder). He still talks about it over ten years later.

A far more beautiful reference to the power of this point comes, however, in the travelogue of Matsuo Bashō, the famous Japanese poet and master of the *haiku*. The particular entry has in fact provided the inspiration for the title of this book. In the very first sentence of his classic "Narrow Passages in the Back Country" of 1689 he wrote enigmatically: "I have sewn a torn part of my undergarments. I have changed the strings of my hat. I have burnt moxa on my *Ashi-no-san-ri*[151]. My mind is now totally occupied with the moon over the Matsushima Islands." In less poetic words, we can say that he was preparing himself for a very uncertain journey of 1500 miles in wooden clogs, a dangerous journey that he had no great expectation of ever returning from, envisioning at the jouney's end a view of bay filled with hundreds of pine-clad islands – something which he considered to be the most beautiful sight in Japan and is still recognised today as one of its most

---

[151] "Leg Three Miles" in Japanese.

iconic images[152]. He wrote how the branches of the pine trees "are curved in exquisite lines, bent by the wind constantly blowing through them[153]."

There is an interesting resonance to this same "three mile" characteristic which exists in terms of the global folklore of the mugwort plant itself which was discussed in the last section. In one way or another mugwort seems to be able to ward off fatigue, whether it be for Roman soldiers, haiku masters, medieval travellers, Chinese armies, modern sportsmen and women or mountaineers at high altitude. Though the means of creating this effect clearly varies, it always involves mugwort, this wayside weed.

Dr Yoshiaki Ohmura, a cardiac specialist with specific interest in acumoxa and kinesiology, suggested more recently that using moxa at St36 may have a part to play in cancer treatment, particularly if combined with more localised treatment since it may affect the release of killer cells and facilitate positive activity in the lymph nodes[154]. Whilst no-one is claiming that it can actually be used as a direct treatment for cancer (although researchers have definitely looked at this possibility) it offers a powerful supportive treatment. Certainly it can be highly effective at warding off neutropenia which often prevents the proper administration or completion of a chemotherapy programme, something which can have critical effect on ultimate treatment outcome.

Incidentally, Ilsa Veith in her study of the *Neijing* referred to a record of moxa having been used with radiation victims in Japan after 1945 to counter the effects of radiation sickness and fever and also quoted the source for this claim. While little other evidence is available to confirm that this actually happened and no specific evidence exists that the St36 point would have been a point of choice in such instance of treatment, circumstantially it seems a very reasonable possibility[155].

Another account from Japan does exist, however, albeit utilising another treatment point. John Hersey, a journalist sent out by the New Yorker in 1946 to report on the after effects of the Hiroshima bomb, subsequently published his report which was simply entitled "Hiroshima", a report which shocked the

---

[152] Tragically, many of these pine trees have been decimated by the tsunami of 2011. Most of the islands, however, were almost miraculously preserved by the outer islands that took the brunt of the wave.

[153] Matzuo Bashō 1694 "The Narrow Road to the Deep North and other travel Sketches". (Penguin Classics) p116

[154] Quoted by Mizutani 2005 "Practical Moxibustion Therapy" (North American Journal of Oriental Medicine)

[155] Shey Y C 1957 "Acupuncture and moxibustion cure radiation sickness". New Medicine in China (pub. Hong Kong); 34: 12.

English speaking world. He described how he encountered a pastor who was suffering from radiation fever. The pastor had been taught by a Buddhist priest how to burn "twists" of moxa on his "wrist pulse" (we could assume Lu7 or Lu8 although it might more logically have been Pc6). Hersey recorded that it helped reduce the pastor's fever at each application. Elsewhere he discussed the different characteristics and types of radiation sickness. He described two key symptoms of "second stage" sickness from which the doctors whom he interviewed judged prognoses – these were fever and lowered white blood cell count. If fever remained steady and high, they considered a patient's chances of survival as being poor. The WBC count was almost always found to fall below four thousand, but if it fell as low as one thousand the chances of survival were considered slim. It appears likely that moxa might have helped with both of these signs at this stage of the pastor's sickness.

There also exists some more recent research from the Czech Republic concerning the use of moxa to strengthen the immune systems of patients affected by the radioactive fallout from the Chernobyl reactors[156]. Although this latter report includes both acupuncture and homeopuncture (the use of homeopathic tinctures being mixed with the patient's blood and injected at acupuncture points) as part of the overall therapy, there is a quite clear conclusion that home moxa therapy increased overall efficacy.

There are two quite separate but eerily thought-provoking further co-incidences connected with these reports of moxa's use after radioactive fall-out. In this instance, both relate to geographical names.

The first is in the name "Chornobyl", the Ukrainian name for what is now largely a ghost town following the disastrous explosion in the city's nuclear power plant in 1986. This town was actually named directly from the Ukrainian word for common mugwort (pelymek cornobyl). The name is a curious choice, since the city was established in wetlands near the confluences of four rivers a thousand years ago, and would have been an unlikely prime growing area for mugwort. Ukrainian folklore, however, suggested that mugwort could banish mischievous water nymphs known as "*rusalky*". In keeping with those ubiquitous esoteric suggestions of mugwort's ability to ward off evil spirits, suggestions which exist across the northern hemisphere, the name of the city may just be another consequence of mugwort's capacity to deter mosquitoes as was discussed in the last section.

The second co-incidence in terms of geographical names also involves a nuclear accident and also occurs in the name of its location – that of the almost

---

[156] L.Kravrechenko 2007 "Immunity deficiency caused by the Chernobyl disaster and its treatment"– International Council of Medical Acupuncture and Related Techniques (ICMART) Symposium (Cyprus)

catastrophic accident which occurred in the United States in 1979 at Three Mile Island. This name curiously transliterates exactly to the very *San Li* (Three Miles) in this acupoint's common name in Chinese. The reasons for the choice of the name in the U.S. appear to have been almost the same as well – a demarcation of distance from a landmark. In the case of the point's name this is three *cun* down-channel[157] from the underside of the patella, in the town's name it is three miles down-river from Middletown, Pennsylvania.

These co-incidental and quirky connections between the point's possible functions for treating radiation sickness, a local European name for mugwort with its intimate association with the site of the world's largest nuclear catastrophe, the name of the location of an almost catastrophic nuclear accident in the United States, and the actual name of the point most commonly associated with moxa treatment especially for boosting immune response must be worth, at the least, a quizzical raising of an eyebrow.

One last mention of the Leg Three Miles point concerns the fact that it is sometimes contra-indicated in the literature for children, and there seems to be a watershed age of thirty before which moxa should be used with caution and beyond which it can be used with profligacy. This contra-indication is clear in the literature from the Ming dynasty, and may well have echoed forward across the centuries from Wang Tao's endorsement of the point for the over-thirties from nearly a millennium earlier. Dr Hara, it should be said however, in more recent times, did not share this view – but did caution against using adult doses of moxa on younger children. He was, however, using much smaller cone sizes than was being used in Ming times, almost certainly also with much purer moxa. I have on occasion successfully and effectively used stick-on moxas on young children at this point.

Bladder 43 *Gaohuang shu* was first discussed by Sun Simiao – "There is nothing that *Gaohuang shu* does not treat." But it was left to Zhang Zhuo in 1289 to complete this claim in connection with moxibustion with the publication of the *Gaohuang shu Xue Jiu Fa* ("the method of Moxibustion at Bl43"), a small text specialising in treatment indications for moxa on this one point. Zhuo considered himself to have been cured of life threatening disease including malaria by having 300 cones burnt on these points[158], and he obviously wanted to tell the world about it.

Lorraine Wilcox offers a graphic translation of Zhuo's experience as a refugee and his subsequent illness which was treated with moxa on Bl43. "I, being from

---

[157] Sometimes this is interpreted as "three-finger-widths" beneath the patella.

[158] Deadman et al 1998 "A Manual of Acupuncture" (Journal of Chinese Medicine Publications)

Xuchang [a city in Henan,], suffered the disaster of the Jin barbarians, the disaster of worry, fatigue, and danger. I was hit by contraction of cold and summerheat, through this descending into the east [he was fleeing toward the east]. I arrived in Sibin [today in Shandong province] on a Ding Wei day of the eighth month [probably July of 1127], and contracted malaria. When I reached Qinchuan [in modern day Jiangsu], I was improperly treated by a doctor, so my *ying* declined and my *wei* was consumed. At the end of spring of the following year [1128], I still suffered swelling on the dorsum of my feet, abdominal distention, hasty breathing, inability to eat, uninhibited stool, heavy body, wilting feet, and I needed a cane to get up[159]." He tells a sorry story.

Zhuo, incidentally, isn't the only famous practitioner to endorse the life-saving potentials of moxa: in the modern era, Denmei Shudo credits repeated moxa treatments for his recovery separately from TB, pleuritis and peritonitis, in his case, from application of "Sawada-style" moxa which is reviewed in Appendix 1. Isaburo Fukaya similarly credited moxibustion for his recovery from TB as a student.

It should be mentioned that some cautions do exist for multiple moxa on this point on the upper back, since it may cause some counter-current *qi* effects, and moxa on Ren6 and Ren4 are advised to accompany it as a counter-measure to root the *qi*, or alternatively at St36 as described above.

Zhang Jiebin, during the Ming Dynasty, adds his own poetry to the consistent endorsements for this point: "Apply up to 100 cones each on the left and right *Gaohuang shu*. Some apply three or five hundred or even more up to 1,000 cones. It makes *qi* move down, gurgling like the descent of flowing water"[160].

The *Zhenjiu Ji Cheng* "Compilation of Acupuncture and Moxibustion" in 1874 lists moxa at this point (along with the Four Flowers, Bl17 & 19 – and *Huanmen* M-BW-6 see below) as treatment for "a hundred syndromes of deficiency taxation". This would reasonably include any condition which involves exhaustion, but which also includes what was then known in the West as consumption and is now known as tuberculosis.

This *Gaohuang shu* point was enigmatically called "Rich for the Vitals" in my own initial acupuncture training, and it was endorsed for chronic illness particularly with accompanying physical or emotional exhaustion. Moxa was particularly advocated on the point, usually prior to needling. *Gao* and *Huang* have been variously translated as referring to relatively impenetrable regions between the

---

[159]Lorraine Wilcox – private communication.

[160] Lorraine Wilcox 2008 "Moxibustion, the Power of Mugwort Fire" (Blue Poppy Press) p21. Zhang Jiebin LJTY: 7-1-35

diaphragm and the heart where illness can roost, secure from interference from medicines or acupuncture -in other words the very home of intractable disease.

Junji Mizutani endorses moxa at this point with the patient sitting with upper legs flexed into the chest, in such a way that she can hug her knees, allowing the intrascapular region to open so that this hiding place of intractable complaint can be revealed and appropriately accessed. This is exactly one of the positions which Zhuo himself prescribed and it can be seen in the famous Song Dynasty painting by Li Tang of a man having moxa burnt on his back.

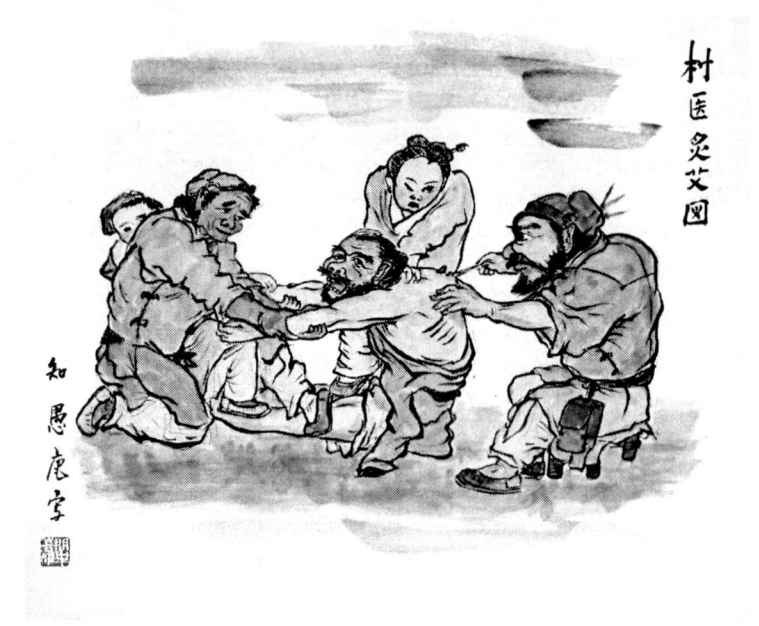

Li Tang's famous Song Dynasty painting – as recreated by Dr Yoshio Manaka[161]

The patient appears to be being supported by his friends during his treatment with two of them holding him down by his legs and pulling on his arms so that the intrascapular region will be most exposed, one of them looking pitifully at his friend's distress. A third holds his neck and seems barely able to watch the moxa being burnt. Close examination shows that one of this third supporter's eyes is shut tight, while the other open eye is staring at the site of the moxa burn. The practitioner, meanwhile, is intently focused on the work at hand. We can imagine that the patient could have been Zhuo himself! It is a wonderful picture, but the treatment hardly looks in any way pleasant.

---

[161] Reproduced by kind permission of Morinomiya University's Museum of Traditional Japanese Medicine.

Ren8 *Shenque* is another interesting point. The wider TCM and Japanese texts tend generally to assign it indications for treatment of diarrhoea while also suggesting it warms and rescues *yang*, something which seems broadly complementary to the accepted traditional actions of moxa. This *"yang*-warming" property seems a common attribute to all particularly moxa-friendly points. But again, my early acupuncture studies intimated something extra as well. We called it "Spirit Deficiency" rather than the conventional "Spirit Watchtower", and used it to nourish or calm the *shen*, especially with the patient in a state of collapse from depression. Most practitioners taught in this tradition will testify to its effects in this respect.

Zhang Jiebin talks of Ren8 as follows: "A lot of moxibustion is good. If three or five hundred cones of moxibustion are applied to it, not only will illness be cured, but it will also prolong life[162]."

In Japan it is listed by some sources as a point to use to counteract ill-effects from overtreatment from micro-bloodletting[163]. It is also indicated to reduce the risk of miscarriage both before conception and even in early pregnancy. Yoshio Manaka includes it as a favourite point for fertility issues, particularly when combined with the other two "triangle moxibustion" points (*sanjiaojiu*) as already discussed, found by constructing a triangle with the sides equal to the triangle formed by another one using the distances between the base of the nasal septum and the two St4 points on the face (the apex of the final triangle being Ren8).

The Four Flowers *Sihua***, (Bl17** *Geshu* **& 19** *Danshu*) are used with moxibustion in combination, traditionally for tonifying both *qi* and blood. They are also reputed to be effective for all types of respiratory diseases.

There is an alternative reference to the location of the "Four Flowers" originally dating from Wang Tao in the eighth century with a comprehensive later description found in Zhang Jiebin's "Illustrated Supplement to the Categorised Classic" published in 1624. In contrast to their normal description of lying "in parallel" as points on the Bladder channel in the locations of Bl17 & 19, according to both of these texts they lie in a diamond formation, centred on the spine. Their location is found by tying a loop of string around the neck, with a knot made at the level of Ren15 on the anterior abdomen at the tip of the xyphoid process. This "necklace" is then reversed to fall down the patient's back to become the focal centre of this alternative "Four Flowers" constellation. This focal point locates itself at the point where the knot comes to lie on the spine. The actual four points themselves are finally located by forming a cross with equal axes horizontally and

---

[162] Lorraine Wilcox 2005 "History of Preventative Moxibustion" – Journal of Chinese Medicine. From the *Leijing Tuyi* Categorised Classic, quoted from.

[163] Birch & Ida 1998 "Japanese Acupuncture, a Clinical Guide" (Paradigm Publications). The other points are Du14 with *chinetsukyu* technique, and Du 20 or St36 with thread-size moxa cones.

vertically from this focal point. The distance in each direction is half of the width of the patient's mouth.

My own interpretation is that these points may or may not lie either over intravertebral spaces or on the Bladder channels dependent upon patient anatomy, but they should be palpably reactive points for them to be clinically useful. The descriptions used for their location were almost certainly designed to facilitate their use in home treatment. Traditionally they were reputed to be effective for "all" respiratory diseases, but the symptoms Zhang uses to describe the indications for the use of these points once again points us towards an earlier treatment for tuberculosis. The treatment, however, is aggressive. He recommends the application of 7, 14, 21 or even up to 100 cones to each point, then stopping treatment at least until the sores either erupt or are about to heal, and repeating if needed because of limited recovery.

Zhang also adds another bilateral point into this combination – M-MB-6 *Huanmen* ("**Suffering Gate**"), sometimes assumed to be Bl15, although (with other "simplified" location methods using cut string) alternative locations emerge. Yang Jizhou, a contemporary of Zhang, advocates the number of moxa cones on these points as corresponding to the patient's age "plus one". The method of location may appear abstruse, but actually both Zhang Zhiebin and Yang Jizhou, in spite of describing two different location methods, both identify these points with Bl15. Zhang boldly claimed them to be "always effective". These points also reputedly originated (similarly to the "Four Flowers") a thousand years earlier with Wang Tao, but only received their name fifty years before Zhang wrote about them. Yang also named these points *Laoxue* (taxation point) on account of their application for treating consumption or TB. This sounds sufficient a reason in itself to substantiate the choice of "Suffering Gate" as an alternative name to "Heart *Shu* Point", but there may also be a Buddhist connotation in this nomenclature. Yang rationalised the use of moxa on this point because, since Bl15 *xinshu* is the back *shu* point of the Heart, it might have specific fundamental effects: "the Heart governs blood – that is why moxibustion is applied to it."

The number of *zhuang* indicated for these points perhaps also provides another pointer towards the significance of the name "the Four Flowers". There is a tradition that moxa "flowers" refer both to the blister formed by the treatment, and the resulting sore (an ironic euphemism if there ever was one). If this is the case, the implication is clear that, to elicit the sort of effects that Zhang is so clearly claiming for these points, there should be no holding back on the part of the practitioner, nor possibly on the size of cone, nor indeed of the endurance or suffering of the patient!

One further comment deserves a brief mention. Lorraine Wilcox invokes the spirit of hexagram 63 "Already Completed" of the *Yi Jing* in connection with this point combination.

With every line in its appropriate position, this is a hexagram of particular propitiousness. An anomaly is apparent, however. When the back is viewed with the cones placed on the *Sihua* and *Huanmen* points, only four lines of the hexagram are visible. Another two seem requisite to complete the image. There seem two possible ways to complete the hexagram: two lines above comprising Bl43 as the broken line at the top, with Du10 the next solid line; or alternatively and perhaps more promisingly two lines below comprising Du3 the solid line at the bottom, and *Pigen* (the bilateral extra point indicated for chronic disease in Li Ting's *Yi Xue Ru Men* of 1575) as the broken line above it.

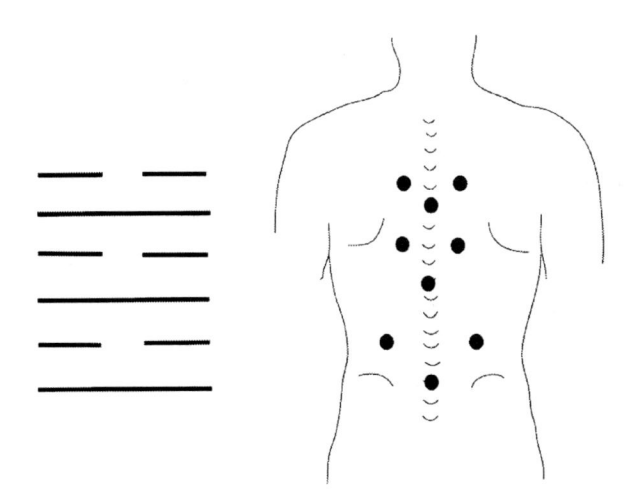

Indicative drawing of these points alongside Hexagram 63 (including Du3 and Pigen)

Today **Sp17** is known by the name *Shidou* or "Food Drain". According to Dou Cai in his *Bian Que Xinshu* (the moxa-only text of 1289), it was referred to by Bian Que as *Ming Guan* 命関, as "Gate of Life" or "Gate of Destiny". It seems to be an amalgamation of the names and perhaps the functions of the two powerful acumoxapoints Ming Men (Du4) and Guan Yuan (Ren4). Dou attributes to it the true post-natal energies of the Spleen, and promotes the point as being useful for literally any disease in which the Spleen might be implicated. Included in the list of diseases which might be involved in this syndrome are any chronic or acute digestive problems, problems with water metabolism, rheumatic heart disease, hepatitis and chest pain.

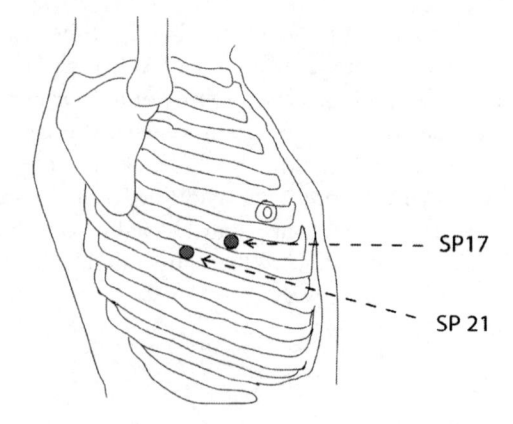

Location of Sp17 in relation to the more commonly used point Sp21

The location of the point is not widely taught since it is almost totally ignored in all other acumoxa literature and is not a point which is widely used in general acupuncture, but it is worth noting that the quantities of cones advocated by Dou Cai for use on it are immense, invariably between one hundred and three hundred *zhuang*. One can assume from this that it was being used by him to treat more acute, intractable or desperate conditions than most of us are normally faced with, and perhaps therefore that its use should be approached with discrimination. Nevertheless, the importance he ascribed to this point with specific reference to moxibustion suggests it is hardly a point which should be ignored.

One small twist can be added to enrich this point's possible application: dependent upon which side of the body the problem is on, the point can be used unilaterally. A clear Spleen related problem would involve the left side, as might a condition with a cardiac implication; a condition with a clear Liver connection would imply moxa on the right side. Palpation might be the best way of establishing the more likely side from which to create the best response, and clear tenderness on either side would indicate that the point might be particularly effective.

Returning to our modern clinical realities, however, this point may have appeal in the treatment of the chronically ill with much smaller dosages. Cancer patients, or those undergoing chemotherapy, might well benefit from small cone daily moxa at this point, using as few as three cones each side, although in the case of breast cancer, moxa anywhere near the site of the cancer necessitates special caution if not absolute contra-indication.

Ren4 *Guan Yuan* is another point which was endorsed for moxa by Dou Cai – he probably endorsed it more than any other. There may have been complex reasons for this – it is traditionally a crossing point on the Ren channel for the Spleen, Liver and Kidney channels as well as the *mu* point of the Small Intestine. Dou Cai invokes it (again commonly recommending two or three hundred cones) in just about any condition which potentially threatens life. If Sp17 tonifies the post-natal *qi* of the Spleen, it is not difficult to conjecture that this point must complement this action by tonifying the pre-natal *yuan qi* of the Kidneys. As such, this point may be likely to have a beneficial effect on any condition in which there is a suggestion of chronic deficiency with implications of Kidney involvement, although (again) much smaller doses would better suit the modern patient. The particular power of this point is its potential to pass on its supplementation to any other channel via the *qi* of the Kidneys.

Dou Cai even advocated its use as the best way to treat paralysis, increasing his prescription in such an event to as many as five hundred cones.

For health maintenance and longevity, the number of cones he suggested was somewhat more modest, the number of cones keeping pace with the patient's age: for patients in their 30's moxa on this point is encouraged thirty-five times every three years (about once a month); in their 50's, one hundred times every two years (about once a week), and in their 60's, three hundred times annually (practically daily). His logic was simple. He wrote: "When people reach their later years, *yang qi* is debilitated. That is why their hands and feet are not warm, the lower origin is vacuous and worn out, and movement is difficult[164]."

Much more recently, Dr Wang Fengyi endorses heavy moxibustion at this point. He considers it to be the storehouse of the essence for men and of blood for women. He describes a case of impotence cured by three treatments of moxa at this point using 150 cones each time, and another case of paralysis of the lower limbs complicated by incontinence which was cured with three moxa treatments of one hundred cones each. His endorsements make it quite clear that the multi-cone approach has survived to the present day[165].

The Possible Nature of these "Moxa" points.

So what should we actually be looking for, if we are considering applying moxa to a point? Or conversely, what might characterise a point which might give us pause and suggest that we might use moxa rather than a needle? Do we just accept the texts (whichever ones we assign the most influence over our treatment) and simply use them as a text book – or do we allow our sense of intuitive creativity some free rein, guided perhaps by the intelligence of palpatory findings? Probably it is a foolish practitioner who exclusively does either one or the other.

---

[164] Lorraine Wilcox 2008 "Moxibustion, the Power of Mugwort Fire" (Blue Poppy Press) p31

[165] "Heavy Moxibustion at *GuanYuan* (Ren4) – Wang Fengyi's Experience" in "Essentials of Contemporary Acupuncturists' Clinical Experiences" 1989 (Foreign Languages Press, Beijing)

By now the perceptive reader, having noted some of the recommended numbers of cones applicable for use on certain points on the body, may well have indentified a fundamental discrepancy in the underlying approaches to moxibustion. This discrepancy is particularly puzzling because these points are invariably indicated for conditions of extreme deficiency. If large numbers of cones are being recommended at such points under such circumstances when a general rule suggests that smaller numbers of cones create more tonifying effects and larger quantities dispersive ones, something contradictory seems to be occurring.

One reasonable explanation would refer us back again to Sung Baek and his idea that moxa could either result in an absorption of *yang qi* or a release of it dependent upon the relative dosage at any specific point. We might reasonably suspect that these are points with special properties that might enable them to soak up a lot more of the *yang* energy from the moxa without it overflowing into dispersive effects, or at least that they might at least act in this way in response to certain extreme physical conditions.

It might also be the case that the localised tissue damage from multi-cone treatments, triggers long-term potent biological effects which are completely different to the more traditional theories so far described.

There certainly seems to be an interesting contrast between the prescribed use of these points and the described application of moxa for health and longevity. In the latter case, the secret is described as being a slow cumulative effect possibly over many months, using small quantities of small cones with the specific intention of creating cumulative effects. In the former, the approach is diametrically different – massive quantities of apparently larger cones are prescribed with the clear intention of creating blistering "flowers", after which some form of cure of the disease is to be expected. The reason may be as much to do with the nature of extreme conditions of disease that must have quite regularly confronted earlier physicians – ones that demanded desperate measures which included these extreme amounts of moxa.

We encounter many references to moxa's use in life-threatening primary care situations in the older texts. These date right back to the seminal texts, and survive right through to the twentieth century. Acu-moxa practitioners of previous times would have been regularly faced with medical scenarios which are way beyond our own experiences in our cosy treatment rooms where we often find ourselves treating the (relatively) healthy and wealthy. Nevertheless such reports from the past still provide context and illumination for us, if only in terms of the extent of their contrast to our own day-to-day treatments.

Thankfully, the debate remains theoretical in the modern age, since the idea of using massive numbers of cones is clearly beyond the realms of anything which could be considered "safe practice" today. Even direct techniques with small cones must be approached with caution.

One primary contradiction in these texts persists, however. Clearly, in many instances, the intention is to create blistering effects at these points, sometimes added to by the application of preparations of herbs to the moxa sores for the purpose of prolonged suppuration. Without these effects, some of the authors quoted above considered their treatment incomplete. What contradicts this approach, however, is the core idea of moxa being "warming", something which was also clearly identified in the literature. A gulf of difference in terms of subjective perception of heat exists in the modern human between something which might be described as "warming" and something which is hot enough to blister the skin. We will take this discussion in a fresh direction in Part 4 the Stems when we discuss dosage. Meanwhile we should look at the ideas behind "warming moxibustion".

Warming Moxibustion

Aside from the aggressive techniques which permeate the older moxa literature, another term is often encountered – that of "warming moxibustion". It seems impossible that moxibustion which can be experienced as being "warm" can possibly be the same in approach or intention as that which causes the blistering "flowers", even allowing for the legendary long-suffering endurance of the Chinese.

Just how could these massive doses possibly be described as warming? One possible explanation is that, when used as a "warming" technique, intermediary substances such as ginger, garlic or aconite were used. Unfortunately, however, if this was indeed the case, it is not explicit in the literature. "Doctors who favour warm supplementation" writes Lorraine Wilcox "tend to use more cones". By "more" in this case we are talking of up to a thousand. A thousand cones of the size considered beneficial in China, if burnt to the skin, will create something more akin to a third degree burn than a blister, so the technique being advocated clearly must require a different approach.

Discounting the endemic contradictions frequently encountered in anything more than a superficial study of East Asian medicine, we seem at first glance to have a serious discrepancy at play here. But there is a simple explanation. Warm supplementation does not in fact specifically relate to moxibustion. It is one of the seven schools of Chinese medicine with its focus being on keeping *yang* strong. The concept of warming supplementation originated with Dou Cai in the twelfth century, but formally developed as a school during the Ming dynasty, particularly developed by Zhang Jiebin. In essence, warm supplementation is an idea formulated by a school of herbal medicine but its advocates often favoured the use of moxa (and not much in the way of acupuncture).

The idea of warming supplementation revolves around the concept of the primacy of *yang qi* in the restoration of health. Interestingly, whenever Zhang specified the use of grain-sized cones, he also generally prescribed smaller numbers of cones. When he prescribed larger numbers of cones, no size is mentioned but in every case, he advocated the standard collection of moxa-friendly points described previously. In fact, he too was actually far from reluctant to suggesting a hundred or more cones to some of these points, but when it comes down to moxa at other points he seems to have taken a far more cautious approach. Rather than encourage profligate application of moxa at these other locations, particularly on the arms, legs and head, however dire the condition, his applications became far more conservative both in size of cone and in numbers used.

It seems possible that the methods he was prescribing for these secondary points on the extremities might be very much more in line with the techniques described in Japan to this day – small cones and limited dosage. It also seems quite possible that the "warming supplementation" of which he was such an authority is very much more connected to the principle moxa points he relied on – all of those usual favourites which we have already identified. In truth it is difficult to really know what to make of all of this, particularly as his approach is not as closely linked to blistering methods as are other moxa masters, but if we are to interpret them at all in ways which we can adapt to usage today, we must, as ever, be cautious.

Perhaps the simplest and most practical interpretation involves equating Zhang's "warming" with Fukaya's "soft heat". Whether this involves the careful cowling of small cones, or the semi-direct "snatch" techniques using bean-sized cones, or indeed using larger Inoue-style *chinetsukyu* supplementing techniques, we should bear in mind that we would be using larger numbers of cones in ways which would not necessarily be the same or even similar to those which stimulate resuscitative response as described above. In such instances of "warming", however, we can still proceed with the idea that we are supplementing the *yang* by adding warmth.

Whether we have to use such large numbers of cones ultimately remains a matter for further debate. As western practitioners, we can at least hope that we can get away with much less and yet retain some of the power of the original treatment. The evidence from Japan would certainly support this idea. Moxa cones at the right points at the right moment clearly can create effects with only a minimal amount of treatment – effects which can include fundamental changes in a patient's subjective perception of cold inside his or her body. On this basis alone it seems that it may not be so necessary to use hundreds of cones.

Some practitioners may feel it important to adhere to these larger numbers of cones, however. It would be certainly be advisable for them to consider resorting to the "snatch moxa" technique describes earlier. The risks of blistering (and overtreatment) can then be absolutely minimised.

Moxa and the Divergent Channels

This section contains a personal and idiosyncratic approach to moxibustion theory and practice which, to my knowledge, has not been explored previously – certainly not in the English literature.

It may serve best first to briefly describe the origins of Divergent Channel theory, and afterwards explore the implications of this theory in terms of moxibustion. The Divergent Channels are described in only one chapter of one of the seminal acumoxa classics – in *Lingshu* 11. We have to assume from this that they represented a singular tradition which somehow became incorporated within the whole. To complicate or frustrate things further, unfortunately, their descriptions are unhelpfully sketchy, and most frustratingly, their clinical applications are not described at all. We can conjecture that they were at best used by only a small minority of contemporary acupuncturists, and were far from comprehensively understood, but that there was a potent enough reputation concerning their use for them to have been included in the needle classic. Such factors have merely served to whet the appetite of acumoxa theorists through the centuries, particularly because of one specific aspect of their use – what are described in this chapter are channel pathways which are conceived to reach directly into the interior of the body to home in on particular internal organs.

It will be recalled that the diseases typical of those living in the cold of the north are those characteristic of cold in the *zang* organ – the *yin* organs of the interior – and that moxa was seen as being particularly applicable in order to disperse this cold. We have also already noted the possibilities raised by the text of *Lingshu* 73 which suggests that this interior territory may be particularly accessible via the *he* sea points. We are thus offered clear potential clinical viabilities arising out of these convergent themes, and with this text in chapter 11 of the *Lingshu* we are presented with a unique treatment model which has particular interest for moxibustion practice.

In this eleventh chapter, each of the twelve main "regular" channels, which had been meticulously and topographically described for the first time in the *Neijing* corpus in the previous chapter, are ascribed a divergent channel of their own.

Generally, slightly different principles apply to the divergent channels either of the arm or the leg. Irrespective of the direction of flow of the main channel, the divergent channels of the leg separate at particular locations on the lower limbs, and each one then "homes" in on or "enters" its associated organ and also disperses within its *yin/yang* paired organ. Each then also flows through the Heart itself.

In slight contrast, the divergent channels of the arms, after diverging from their main channels on the upper limbs, then "home" in on or "enter" their respective associated organs whilst also flowing through the throat.

In the cases of the *yang* channels generally, they then resurface to rejoin their main regular channel somewhere near or on the head. In all the cases of the *yin* channels they resurface at the same places as their paired *yang* divergent channel resurface, in effect joining up with their respectively paired yang channels. The direction in every case is caudal regardless of channel flow in the main channel.

With respect to moxibustion, these individual points of divergence can be logically suggested as being of particular interest since they can be interpreted as providing particularly potent surface locations from which to access the interior from the exterior – something which has great implication for the practice of moxa if we intend to pass warmth into the interior to disperse the cold.

The challenges of *Lingshu* 11 are somewhat complicated, unfortunately, by the inconsistencies in the descriptions of these points of divergence or at least in the difficulties in definitively interpreting their descriptions. This problem has dogged commentators throughout the centuries with many differing general interpretations having been posited for these divergent locations – from the *jing* points, to the *yuan* points, to the *he*-sea points. Such interpretations represent wide and challengeable assumptions in every instance simply because they are at such variance with each other.

The latter theory (that the channels diverge at the *he* sea points) certainly makes most sense in terms of heterogeneity with other chapters of the early acumoxa classics, since traditionally it is understood that it is at these points that the flow of each channel is seen as deepening, and in some sense the *qi* flowing within them becomes less accessible for general whole body regulation. Certainly it is widely accepted that the overall vacuity or deficiency of the channel can best be influenced by treatment distal to these particular points, but the *he* sea points are traditionally also regarded as being good locations from which diseases of the organs themselves can be best treated with acupuncture, particularly in the case of the *yang* channels.

In theory at least, therefore, we can surmise that an effective way of influencing deep cold within the body with moxa, particularly if it relates to a specific organ, might be at this last point before the channel runs relatively deeper (or at the point of divergence, or, as is described in *Lingshu* 11, at the divergent channel's "confluence hole" if it is the same thing).

The problem then becomes just a matter of agreeing whether this might be the case.

These various interpretations have generally suffered from a constant flaw – they attempt to force consistency into the locations, something which is missing from the original text. If we consider the original text to be the most reliable reference point, the logical thing, of course, is to review it. From the text of Chapter 11, the points listed below can be considered as prime candidates for accessing the interior via a divergent channel.

Point of Divergence	Interior organs accessed
Bl40	the anus, the **bladder** and the kidneys
Ki10	the kidneys, the **daimai** and tongue
GB29	both gallbladder and liver
Liv 3	the liver
St30	**stomach**, spleen, pharynx and nose.
Sp12	spleen, throat and root of the tongue.
SI10	small intestine
Ht1	**heart**
Pc2	the chest and **triple burner**
LI15	large intestine and **lungs**
Lu2	lungs

(The entries denoted in bold are those particular organs or vessels described in the text as being "homed" on by the divergent channels, and therefore of potential particular clinical significance.)

Disappointingly, it will be quickly realised that only a couple of these points are actually *he* sea points.

No point, it will be noted, is listed for accessing the divergent Triple Burner channel. Two reasons exist for this: one, that the point of divergence is oddly listed as being Du20 – a discrepancy which has simply posed too many problems for interpreters over the centuries; the second is that the pathway of the Triple Burner divergent channel does not actually reflect the general pathways of the other divergent channels of the arms as described above, basically completely doing its own thing[166]. On this basis it would seem wisest simply to keep treatment options reduced to eleven of these divergent channels, particularly since the Triple Burner itself is said to be accessed in the interior by the Pericardium divergent channel anyway.

The key targets for treatment with moxa would thus refine themselves to be:

Cold in the bladder	Bl40
Cold in the Kidney	Bl40 or Ki10
Cold in the Daimai	Ki10
Cold in the Stomach or Spleen	St30, Sp12, St36 or Sp9

---

[166] Those interested in this topic will benefit from reviewing the fascinating study by Charles Chace and Miki Shima 2001 "The Divergent Channels – Deeper Pathways of the Web" (Blue Poppy Press)

I have personally found that using this approach is occasionally a clinically efficient strategy when other approaches are not working, particularly so for increasing warmth in the lower or middle *jiao*. One way that this can be optimised is to tonify or supplement the respective channel first to improve the flow of *qi* in the channel before the moxa is applied. So, for instance, is there is cold in the middle *jiao*, and there is a clear Spleen deficiency, then Sp3 might be tonified with a needle, and then Sp9 has moxa applied with better effect as a result.

Moxa and the Muscle Meridians or Channel Sinews

These channels, the *jing jin*, are first described in *Lingshu* 13. They have been relatively ignored by most commentators down the centuries and are certainly not addressed to any great degree in standard curricula of acupuncture schools or colleges in the West.

The description for their treatment in the original text involves the use of the *fan zhen* or "fire needle" (or more accurately the "blazing hot" needle) – a thick needle that is heated to red heat and then inserted swiftly into the muscle channel and then immediately removed, often five or six times across an area. This, of itself, may help explain why they are so widely ignored in modern acupuncture.

This treatment, however, was cleverly adapted by Dr Manaka in the twentieth century. Dr Manaka himself was not averse to using the "fire needle" technique itself, but was happier teaching how its use could be substituted using the instant heat of direct moxa.

In respect of the Muscle Meridians he similarly employed both fire needle and direct moxa in two distinct ways – in simple "channel stretching with release" techniques, and in channel stretching in conjunction with *sotai*. In both cases the application of heat is used to amplify a release of tension which is deliberately induced to correct a restriction of movement and/or structural imbalance – in other words as a treatment which can reasonably be described as principally musculo-skeletal. This description, however, might be to under-sell the treatment, since Manaka was convinced that structural imbalances (or "biases" as he termed them) had direct impact on chronic and organic disease and even on the functions of the internal organs themselves.

It is beyond the scope of this book to comprehensively describe these techniques. The best that can be achieved is a brief description and to direct the inquisitive reader to the relevant text on Manaka's defining work "Chasing the Dragon's Tail" – or better still the practitioner should learn the techniques properly in a workshop.

Channel stretching involves stretching specific channels identified for treatment from a simple range of movement tests. Having established the relevant channel for treatment, the practitioner then palpates the likely moxa points for pressure pain reactivity and then places a small grain-sized moxa cone on the most reactive point that is identified. The patient is asked to breathe in and then immediately to extend the relevant limb in a specific way which is intended to stretch the constricted channel sinew, whilst slowly breathing out with the limb still extended as directed. While the patient breathes out, the practitioner lights the moxa cone and allows it to burn down. The intention is that the patient should complete the exhalation, and then count aloud from one to three with the help of the practitioner whilst the lungs are still empty with the limb still in extension. At this last moment (on the count of three) Manaka would normally rapidly insert and withdraw his fire needle, immediately asking the patient to totally relax the limb and resume breathing normally. The moxa practitioner, however, strives to carefully time the moxa so that the "hit" of heat coincides as closely as possible to the last moment of the count of three when the cone can be put out exactly as the patient is instructed to relax.

Immediate improvements of range of movement can often be achieved with this technique, but it will be immediately recognised that timing is critical, and the technique requires practice, dexterity, co-ordination and confidence on behalf of the practitioner.

Points are generally investigated and located around the shoulder and upper arm for arm channels, and upper leg and hip for leg channels. Understandably, its use is favoured for problems of the arm rather than the leg or foot as a result, and is most commonly applied for what Manaka described as "stagnation" in the Lung, Large Intestine, Triple Burner and Small Intestine channel sinews which he found to be typically involved in neck and shoulder stiffness. The best indications for this treatment are abnormal tension accompanied by restricted movement with accompanying pressure pain at the likely treatment points.

Typical optimal treatment points for neck and shoulder problems are:

Lung	Lu1, Lu3 or Lu4
Large Intestine	LI15, LI14 or LI11
Triple Burner	TB15, TB14 or TB9
Small Intestine	SI11, SI10 or SI9

Generally the moxa treatment consists of three cones on a single point (i.e. three repetitions of the extensions), but two or more channels might be used if they show similar reaction.

Moxa with *sotai* stretching can involve a more complex range of movement testing and subsequent treatment but with similar potential for immediate release. *Sotai* itself was a physical treatment technique in its own right and was developed by Dr Kaizo Hashimoto, principally to adjust left and right differences in the neck, torso and legs. The basic intentions behind the treatment are to restore such physical imbalances into a more balanced state. In order to do this *sotai* employs gentle physical movements (usually these movements are **towards** the most comfortable position and **away** from the discomfort or pain) combined with specific movements of the breath. To accentuate the effect from the *Sotai*, Manaka added both fire needle and small moxa cones.

Each movement is made slowly and gently towards a certain more comfortable neutral position at which point a slight amount of resistance is applied against this movement – right at the movement's end. Similar to the channel stretching described above, whilst this movement towards comfort is being made a cone of moxa is lit by the practitioner and the patient is simultaneously asked to slowly breathe out. Timing once again is key – the intention is that the exhalation should be completed at the same time as the movement is completed at which point the resistance against it is applied. Once again the rhythmic slow count of "one, two, three" is employed at this point with the lungs still empty, at the end of which the heat should hit, the cone snuffed out, and the patient instructed to "relax" as much as he or she possibly can and to resume breathing as normal. Typical treatment points might include Bl18 and Liv3, and sometimes Du10 or Du12.

Those readers interested in finding out more about *Sotai* itself are directed towards Dr Hashimoto's comprehensive text book "*Sotai*, Balance and Health through Natural Movement" which offers a comprehensive explanation of the techniques although there are only one or two references within it to the use of moxa. For simple *sotai* protocols combined with moxa treatment from which one can develop a more and flexible application of these techniques, one should review the section on the "Treatment of Channel Sinews with *Sotai* Exercises" in Manaka's "Dragon's Tail" pp 197-203.

Moxa and the Eight Extraordinary Vessels

A lot has been written about the Eight Extraordinary Vessels in English, much of which is less coherent than might be desirable, and which has definitely at times been subjected to creative interpretation rather than strict attention to original texts. The fact that some of these original texts themselves bear witness to the way that quite differing approaches developed across many centuries has hardly helped the matter.

For the past six centuries the dominant approach to utilising these vessels has been via their "master" and "coupled" points, but even with this approach differing views on how best to access them have developed. What follows is a further idiosyncratic interpretation, and, as with any such interpretation, judgement should be made by assessing both clinical usability and effectiveness.

The basis for this approach is adapted from the fascinating work of Dr Yoshio Manaka, who, in contrast to almost any other approach to their use in treatment, saw them as being particularly effective as the core of a root treatment. Most other approaches in the literature use them for their symptomatic effects. In our case, we will also review their effect on symptoms, particularly to treat pain, but will do this by borrowing some of Manaka's insights and ideas on the subject and look at how moxibustion can be used with this in mind.

The use of the various master-coupled points has consistently been intended to "open" one of these vessels with a view to increasing treatment effect as a result. Normally this is done with needles, generally using some sort of polarity effect or by weighting the stimulation of the needles in order that the patient's *qi* system might respond in specific or predictable ways. In the modern era, this is often done for a specific vessel by needling its master point on the left (for a male) with its coupled point on the right (or vice-versa for a female). The thinking which lies behind this is that, for a male, the dominant side is left (being as it is more yang) and for a female the dominant side is right (and *yin*). Whether this is really consistently the case is a matter for debate, and in any case may be significantly affected by symptomatology.

A common response to this dilemma in Japan in the last fifty years has been to look for other ways to weight or polarise the needles. Various solutions have been found, often referred to as "minus-plus" or "mp" treatment. Many different methods have been used including using different metals (gold-silver or copper-zinc typically), north-south magnets, or (specifically in Dr Manaka's case) his famous ion-pumping cords. In this way, both master and coupled points can be used in any combination in terms of sides of treatments, ipsilaterally, contralaterally, and (with the ion pumping cords) even bilaterally-contralaterally, in each case offering a clear polarity to the stimulation.

What Manaka's work revealed is that, rather than defining these vessels as eight distinctly individual ones, they can be practically divided into four groups of two, each pair being defined by their common points (in other words their master and coupled points and by specific symptomatologies). In this way the following groups emerge:

Ren/Yin Qiao Mai	Lu7 and Ki6
Du/Yang Qiao Mai	SI3 and Bl62
Chong/Yin Wei Mai	Pc6 and Sp4
Dai/Yang Wei Mai	TB5 and GB41

This idea arises directly from the writings on the subject from the Ming Dynasty. Manaka together with his innovatively inventive circle of collaborators in the Topological Acupuncture Society developed some creative ways of accessing these so-called extraordinary vessel pairings using polarising techniques which included using magnets and different metals applied to the skin surface. They also added several other clinically useful topological pairings to the four so far described, one of which is particularly useful for the approach about to be described.

The Moon over Matsushima

This "extra-extraordinary" vessel pairing is:

    Yang Ming pairing   LI4 and St43

In this way it will be seen that there are now confusingly **ten** extraordinary vessels, not eight! But as importantly, it will also be noticed that, in each case, one point is on the upper body and the other on the lower.

Whilst Manaka used these treatments primarily as the first step in his root treatment, other approaches have focused much more clearly on their usefulness for symptomatic effects, particularly focusing on the pathways of the particular channels on which these key points lie to identify their possible applicability. So, for instance, a problem on the medial aspect of the knee might be helped by using the Chong/Yin Wei pairing because of the pathway of the Spleen channel, and a problem of pain in the facial sinuses might be treated distally by the Yang Ming pairing for similar reasons. In each case, the treatment is understood to have its effect by opening up the area of the body either by freeing some stagnation of *qi* in the affected area or by improving the flow of *qi* into the area itself. This idea has been extensively explored already and it is not the intention to explore it any further except to look at its clinical usefulness to add to the possible effect of moxa in the treatment of pain.

It has been the experience of the author that the effect of local moxa for pain attenuation can be effectively improved by adding these distal points to open up the area whilst the moxa is locally applied. We are immediately confronted by two questions, however: how best to open up the vessels; and then how best to effect the local treatment.

Many readers will hold their own existing ideas about how best to open up these vessels, and it is not my intention to challenge them. I do, however, want to propose a simple method that might be worth trying which might prove clinically useful, and in so doing offer some simple rules of thumb based either on the experiences of master accomplished practitioners or on my own experiences.

Let us suggest a particular case. A thirty-five year old female presents with left side elbow pain. There may be many covert causative factors at work, but we will consider none of them simply because doing so will serve only to confuse the picture. What we need to decide first is which channels may be most affected (or might be having an effect) on the elbow. The patient complains of pain on moving her elbow, but careful palpation reveals a clear focus of pain on the LI channel just a little distal to LI11. We can thus be particularly alert to the likelihood that the LI channel is a clear contender for playing a part in the problem. So we then can palpate along the channel, and we might then find that there is also both tightness and tenderness on two or three points along the channel going up into the shoulder. And we might also confirm that there is clear tenderness at LI4, which is the treatment point for this extra vessel treatment. This would clinch it!

We can now reliably conclude that the LI channel is involved, and since the problem is on the left side, we can reasonably choose the left LI4 point at its most tender location as being the best "master" point to use. But if we are attached to convention, since the patient is female, we could compare this point's sensitivity with the same point on the right. It is unlikely, but it just might be the case that we find this point even tenderer. If so we would then have to decide to go with either the symptom or the tenderness. Either option may be effective, but my own choice would be to go with the symptom.

So we can now turn our attention to its coupled point, examining around St43. Should we choose the left point because the patient is female (and the coupled point is typically selected on the left for a female) – or should the the opposite right side be chosen because we have selected the left side for the master point, or should we simply choose the left side because that is the side of the problem? All are logical choices. Once again, we can simply resort to careful palpation of the point, and a final decision may be made based on palpatory findings. The patient's body is effectively leading us to our final clinical choice based on what we are finding.

Thus far we have selected the primary affected channel and then selected what we considered to be the optimal master and coupled points to "open" it to improve the *qi* circulation around the symptom. Now we have to decide how best to actually "open" the vessel. Most practitioners will use needles at this point. Standard acupuncture needles will probably be sufficient: the weighting has already been effectively created by the symptom as witnessed by the palpatory findings. But some practitioners may favour using different metals, ion pumping cords, or even a thicker needle at the master point. An effect can in fact be created merely by placing small discs of copper and zinc or ball-bearings of gold and silverplate over the palpated points – copper on LI4 (in this case) and zinc on St43. Such techniques have been developed to high degrees of sophistication by the research committee of the Toyohari Society in Japan, using sophisticated pulse feedback assess both accuracy of point location and efficacy of treatment.

Typically, polarising LI4 and St43 by whatever means is selected, the discomfort in the elbow may well be seen to reduce – almost immediately – but we may do even better if we bring in some moxa. Once more we can look at the tender points we found on the channel. We may find that they have moved a little, but wherever we find them we should burn three to five cones on the tenderest points. We may even choose to use the bamboo tube as as has been previously described. We could even use stick-on moxa cones if we have a very sensitive patient. What we should expect to see is a significant increase in the reduction of discomfort.

There are a couple of other aspects to this particular approach that are worth considering.

Firstly, there may well be more than one channel affected. In this case, for instance, it would be worth palpating the other key *yang* points on the arm – SI3 and TB5. If we find tenderness, we may suspect a secondary channel involvement, and to confirm the treatment's applicability we can cross check by palpating their respective coupled points – Bl62 or GB41 on both sides. As a result, we may chose to open up a second extraordinary vessel, and, if we do, we should do so before using the local moxa in order to allow its effect to be enhanced and maximised.

We might even decide to open the channel just with moxa itself. This approach was taught by Kodo Fukushima with patients in more acute pain. In such a case, small cones are burnt at the selected points, three cones on the arm point (in this case the master point on the channel affected by the symptom) followed by two cones on the coupled point, and this is repeated continuously until the patient reports a reduction in pain. Fukushima was reported in some instances to have used an **awful** lot of moxa cones before the patient finally reported relief, but this would much more typically be in cases of pain of internal or more organic origin. In principle, using moxa in this way is a perfectly valid treatment in that it adapts the same ideas as those used in the last six centuries to open up these vessels – it effectively weights the stimulation in favour of one of a pair of points to provide a clear energetic message to the patient's *qi* system. It can be argued that it may even be a **better** approach in that the effects may actually last longer than the needles – and furthermore the treatment could even be repeated at home by the patient or the patient's relative in lower dosage.

Moxa and the Akabane Balancing Protocol

In contrast to the preceding sections, Akabane's "heat-sensitivity meridian-balancing" protocol, whilst clinically interesting of itself, serves to cast an alternative and interesting light on the topic of warming meridians as opposed to warming the interior. It also offers us another interesting and often effective treatment approach. Furthermore, it also provides a potentially richer access to individual points which might be particularly responsive or "live" to moxa treatment but which might otherwise remain unconsidered or ignored.

Kobei Akabane (1895-1983) established his "theory" concerning heat sensitivity at the *jing*/well points in the early 1950s. He became fascinated by the possible pathological implications of a general lack of sensitivity to heat at these most distal channel points, and found that this imbalance could be easily restored with holistically beneficial knock-on effects.

Measuring the relative thermoception at these points constituted the primary part of his diagnosis. To do this Akabane used thick incense sticks or tapers. Initially he touched these rhythmically to the *jing* point, but the diagnostic method has evolved to rhythmically sweeping the tapers to and fro at a consistent height over the *jing* points of both toes and fingers from the comparative insensitivity of the nail-bed. He counted the strokes made with the tapers until his patient reported the sensation of heat from the taper at each particular *jing* point (both left and right), and he then tabulated and compared the results between each side for each channel. Between five and ten strokes was considered "normal", anything less than five represented relative excess, and anything more than ten indicating a deficiency. A sizeable relative difference on an individual channel between the left and right side constituted, for Akabane, an imbalance which required rectifying.

Akabane was specifically most interested in the amount of deviation between the two sides, and was not so much interested in the greatest relative excess or deficiency between specific meridians. This represents a fundamental difference between his approach and that of the *Keiraku Chiryo* (meridian therapy) practitioners with whom he was associating at the time in Japan. His treatment criterion was simple: to be treatable, the difference on any single channel should be at least twice the count of the opposite side.

The standard explanation for this diagnostic protocol is that the Akabane diagnosis measures the relative state of *qi* left and right in the individual channels. Accepting the theory that the thermoceptors kick in more quickly at the distal end of a channel which is more replete with *qi*, an interpretation of the relative "fullness" or "emptiness" of *qi* in a channel of any meridian could thus be seen as being easily and reliably diagnosable without resorting to far more challenging and challengeable naked-sense diagnostic techniques such as pulse-taking and abdominal diagnosis.

It is generally true that a relative imbalance identified by a higher count (i.e. a slower thermoception) may well indicate a deficiency of *qi* in the channel, which can be further confirmed by alternative means. It may, however, indicate other pathology on the channel pathway itself. It remains unclear, in fact, whether this general interpretation of relative assessment of *qi* is totally reliable or correct, since sometimes channels with very small scores (which indicate an excess) can be actually diagnosed by alternative methods as being very clearly deficient.

A more plausible explanation is that the amount of heat stimulation which any *jing* point can accept before eliciting a sensed response on the part of the patient more simply reflects the capacity of its particular channel to absorb heat. Simply put, once this capacity is met, the heat-sensing thermoceptor cells kick in and fire and the patient immediately feels the heat. Taken one step further, what this might mean is that this diagnostic technique indicates the relative state of heat and cold in any particular channel, particularly between left and right.

Akabane's actual treatment method was to immediately rectify this imbalance. His approach was quite simple and serves to shed further light on his idea. He simply treated the back *shu* points relating to the most deficiently imbalanced channels with the intention of rectifying the original scoring at the *jing* points. Initially, he was reported to have used intradermal needles (which he himself invented) using them on the deficient side, along with a quick insertion and withdrawal of a "thick" needle (1.5mm thick) on the excess side, but he refined his method to simply applying moxa to the vacuous side, and then needling the excess side only if required because the imbalance had failed to immediately completely resolve itself. Here we have yet another interesting echo of *Suwen* 28 that suggested that moxa is most suitable for supplementation whilst needling is useful for dispersion.

The fact that Akabane came to favour moxa for supplementing the deficient side may help us in our better understanding of moxibustion. In Japan in the seventeenth century Doctor Gonzan, it may be remembered, believed that the cause of illness was connected primarily to a defiency of *yuan qi* caused by cold. It seems that Akabane's method evolved to reflect this view. In fact, we can go so far as to argue that what the Akabane diagnostic method measures is not necessarily the relative left-right amounts of *qi* in the channels at all, but rather the relative left-right amounts of **cold** in the channels. This seems particularly probable given that the most effective method for measurable restoration of balance was found by experience to be the application of heat or warmth on the colder side. While it is tempting to equivocate heat with *qi*, we should be cautious in doing so, since the presence of heat, of course, can also be accompanied by an absence or deficiency of *qi*.

The moxibustion method used by Akabane involved the use of large cones of aged moxa, although it is unclear as to how hot he allowed these to get. As we have discussed, some modern Japanese theories about moxa, based on the classical literature, regard gentle warming with large cones as tonifying. Inoue, who developed the large cone *chinetsukyu* "heat perception" moxa technique, was a contemporary of Akabane, and it is improbable that ideas would not have been exchanged between them. In my own experience, the use of quite gentle warming with large cones on the deficient side is extremely effective in creating a clear response in the *jing* point readings. The application of only two or three cones on palpably deficient back *shu* points can generally create such an effect. Just by using this simple method, the readings at the *jing* points will in most cases improve immediately.

Akabane's belief was that left/right imbalances were central issues in all diseases, and, if attended to, the remaining pathologies would largely take care of themselves. In this sense he saw this re-balancing as a root treatment. From the perspective of moxa treatment, this is fascinating, because what it implies is that his diagnostic method reveals specific treatment points on the back which, with moxa treatment, may have clear whole-body effects with minimal intervention.

In previous sections we looked at a limited number of points which have been traditionally identified as being particularly "moxa-friendly". With Akabane's method of treatment, however, we immediately find ourselves equipped with more, whilst also being presented with a way of treating them which can be conceived as constituting fundamental root treatment and which can furthermore immediately be monitored for effect. These points can thus be seen as being ones which could be the most particularly "alive"[167] and therefore the most potentially responsive to warming with moxa and which may be the most appropriate to the patient exactly at the time when he or she is being diagnosed and treated.

If cold is, as Gonzan suggested in the seventeenth century, perhaps **the** major causative factor of disease, and if the Akabane method (as Doctor Manaka suggested) contains clear prognostic indicators for health and recovery[168], then the Akabane method provides us with a remarkably neat way of locating the most efficient and efficacious way of restoring heat or warmth where it may be most needed, and one, furthermore, which is both simple to diagnose and is remarkably reliable.

It should finally be mentioned that some minor variations to this general approach exist. Amongst others, super-fine direct moxa (*okyu*) has also been prescribed on the *jing* points on the deficient side for tonification, and the author has occasionally seen clear efficacy with this technique when the conventional back-*shu* point treatment has failed.

Moxa and *Koryo Sooji Chim* Hand Microsystem

Several acupuncture micro-treatment-systems have been developed in the last sixty years. One of the most interesting is the hand acupuncture system developed in Korea by Dr Tae-Woo Yoo, originally conceptualised whilst he was still an acupuncture student in the 1970s. What makes this system particularly interesting from the perspective of moxibustion is that the system's treatment methods can be applied at several levels, one using a simple reflexology-type system in which particular parts of the hand are deemed to reflect particular areas of the body, and others in which this idea is extrapolated to incorporate a full-blown meridian model complete with increasingly complex theories in terms of diagnosis and application of technique which can be adapted to treat more difficult cases. Probably for this very reason, this particular method of microsystem acupuncture

---

[167] In Japanese acumoxa there is a pervasive idea of *ikita tsubo* or "live points" – points which are reactive, and possibly not at the standard locations but which are particularly indicated for treatment.

[168] Manaka and Itaya drew some extraordinary conclusions about the capacity of their readings of meridian imbalances made via the Akabane method to offer accurate prognostications for response and recovery.

holds special appeal to acupuncturists – this and the rather persuasive fact that it can be a very effective and adaptable form of treatment.

One further advantage for us, of course, is that the hand can be accessed for judicious moxa treatment in a way that most other microsystems simply cannot.

Dr Yoo's Korean Hand Therapy (KHT) system includes moxa as a legitimate and important part of the total treatment repertoire. The method he advocates uses stick-on heat shields and small proprietary "KHT" smokeless or smokey stick-on moxa cones. As a rule, if a point is selected which turns out to be extremely sensitive to heat it should be avoided; a slow build-up of heat should be looked for with a clear sense of heat developing not just at the skin surface but in the tissue of the hand itself beneath the point.

A couple of clear advantages can be seen immediately. For patients with very limited mobility (in wheel chairs, or bed-ridden for instance) moxa can be used safely and effectively in a way which would otherwise be impossible. This is also the only way that a practitioner can possibly self-moxa his or her own back, through applying moxa to the areas which reflect the back on the dorsum of the hand – and since treatment for the back is such a key part of effective moxa treatment, this single fact should hold no small attraction for the practitioner who might need or want to treat himself in order to maintain his or her health.

It is not the intention to go into treatment techniques in any great detail since this is a subject in its own right, but some broad principles can be usefully outlined quite easily.

Firstly, several points can be identified for treatment and heat shields can be applied to all of them, but only half the number of actual cones need be used as points chosen: as a point become hot the cone can be lifted and switched to another point while the cone continues to burn. With moxa on the hand there need be no concern of the heat perception being hot rather than warm as long as it builds up slowly, but the cones should always be moved before they start to become uncomfortably hot. Both palmar and dorsal surfaces can be treated, although they should not both be treated at the same time. Generally, on the palmar surface, points which relate to the middle and lower *jiao* may benefit most from moxa, whilst, on the dorsal suface of the hand, points can be more liberally selected. Points can be quite simply selected by degrees of reactivity, established normally by application of a probe. Probes of variously sized rounded ends are usually rubbed across the surface of the hand looking for two principle findings – pressure pain response on the part of the patient and/or knotted or indurated tissue.

Clear warmth can often be felt on the reflexive area of the body after judicious moxibustion on the hand. For instance, moxa burnt on the hand on the area which is reflective of the left-hand lumbar region can quickly result in palpable warmth in the left sided lumbar region itself. This can even be tested using a thermographic camera. If moxa is burnt on the left hand on the area designated as the left side of the spine, then an image taken thermographically of the skin surface on the left side of the spine itself should almost immediately start to show itself to be warmer than the rest of the back.

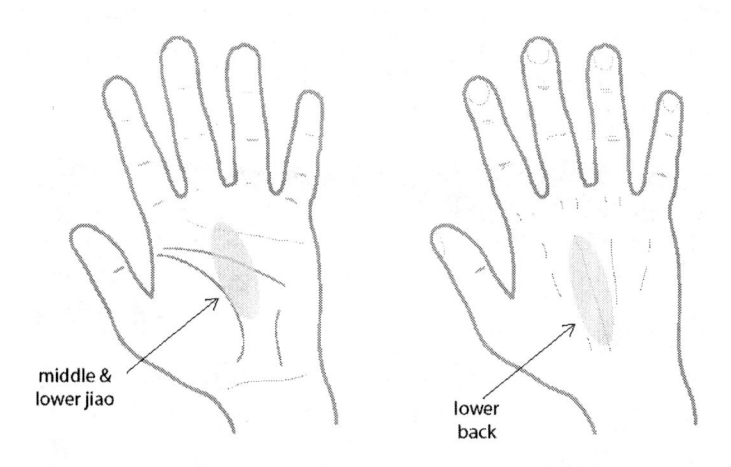

middle & lower jiao

lower back

Koryo Sooji Chim advocates simple popular protocol treatments using smokeless moxa on the palmar surface both for men and women. The system encourages self-treatment by anyone with minimal training, simply because it is seen as being effective and extremely safe.

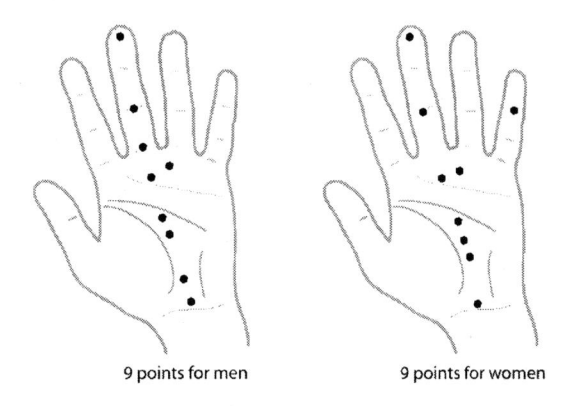

9 points for men

9 points for women

Classic protocol treatments for stick-on moxa on the palm of the hands

169

The Moon over Matsushima

Regular moxa can be applied using these protocols for simple health maintenance. The points used are A1, A3, A6, A8, A12, A16, A20 A30 & N18 for men, and A1, A4, A6, A8, A12, A20, A30 N18 & F6 for women[169].

A question naturally arises as to whether small cone direct moxa may be as effective, or even more effective, than the stick-on smokeless KHT proprietary versions which are commercially available but which are comparatively more expensive. In the case of hand moxa this does not seem necessarily to be the case. The key seems to be in the slow build-up of palpable heat which clearly contrasts to the quick hit of heat from small cone moxa.

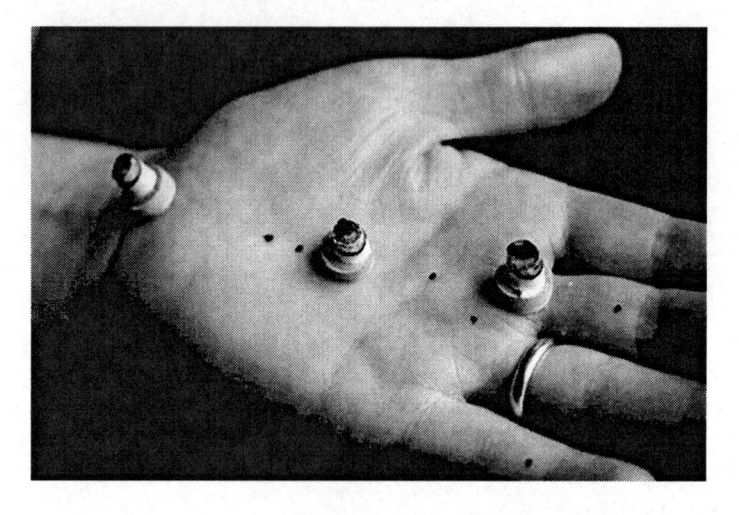

Stick-on moxa-on-ceramic being burnt on the protocol points on the palm

An interesting KHT application uses proprietary stick-on moxas which are mounted on small disks of ceramic. These utilise processed mugwort with a similar convenience to the smokeless stick-on cones but with a potential extra effect from the heated ceramic. The only draw back is some smoke, but this is quite limited.

One other way of controlling the heat if raw moxa is being used is to use small bamboo tubes of 10 or 12 mm internal diameter. With careful timing, the heat from the small cone can be softened quite effectively, since the smaller tube serves to extinguish the moxa faster than the standard size tubes of 15-16 mm diameter.

Point selection for any approach can actually be quite simple: painful or "gritty" points can be looked for on the line of the spine or just to the outside of it. These will often be found to be the same on each hand. Moxa can then be burnt directly over these points. The same approach can be utilised on points on the central

---

[169] These point numbers relate to the KHT numbering system, "A" points being on the Ren channel on the hand, "N" points on the Liver channel, and "F" points on the Spleen channel.

"Ren" line of the palmar surface. A little more care needs to be taken in applying moxa here because it is particularly sensitive to heat.

One drawback to the raw moxa method is that the skin on the palm particularly absorbs the oil from the moxa very quickly leaving small stains on the palm of the hand. If we assume that chemical absorption is as important with this technique as with body moxibustion, then this may be a good thing, but cosmetically it may well be seen to be an issue. If there is no intent in the treatment to invoke an immune response, however, (which with this treatment it probably would not be for reasons which we will review in Part 4) chemical absorption may well not, in any case, be relevant to this treatment at all.

If smokey moxa is preferred because it may seem to be more natural as a product, a neat modification to the technique is to use ginger as an intermediary material in a similar way to the descriptions earlier in this section. This is a particularly interesting option for points on the palmar surface in the zone that corresponds with the lower *jiao*. In this case a slice of ginger about 20mm by 9mm and 3mm thick can be prepared and placed on the palm. The ginger is then placed on the line of the *Ren* meridian on the palm, and individual "rolls" of moxa can then be placed along the ginger and lit.

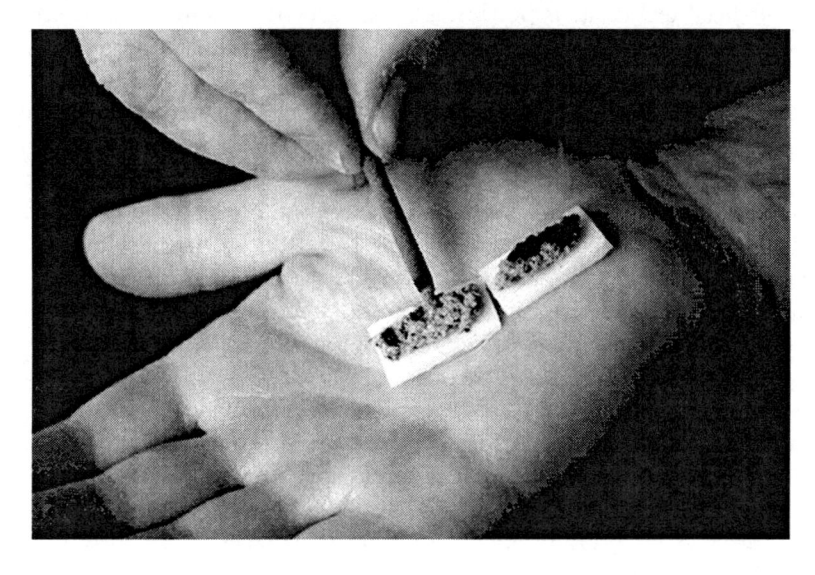

Moxa on ginger on the palm

The width of the moxa rolls should be a little less than the width of the ginger strip (say 7-8mm) and they can be burnt repetitively until clear warmth is felt through the ginger. As with the standard technique, the ginger should be pierced in several places to allow some of the smoke to penetrate to the skin below, and the ginger can be removed if the heat becomes excessive.

Another method is to adapt a *kyutoshin*-style technique for use on the hands using *hinaishin* intradermal needles rather than normal acupuncture needles. This is a technique that has been developed by Aaron Rubinstein of Austin, Texas, and he calls it *kyutohinaishin* or moxa-with-intradermal. The technique itself is designed for the treatment of blood stasis in the hands, feet and elbow, particularly utilising the transmission of heat down the shaft rather than the radiant heat itself. To my knowledge, Rubinstein does not adapt it to the microsystem in the particular way that is being suggested in this text, but the same principles for point selection would apply. Generally subcutaneous tissue which is dense or tight is targeted for treatment.

The intradermal needle was originally designed by Kobei Akabane to be inserted almost horizontally, literally between the skin layers; in this instance the needle should be inserted (with tweezers) more vertically. Rubinstein recommends between 30-35 degrees from horizontal, although it could be steeper as long as the moxa is secure.

The technique involves the use of small chunks of moxa wedged carefully in the loop or eyelet which forms the handle of the intradermal needle after the needle is inserted. The moxa is then lit and burnt in the same way that normal moxa-on–the-needle-head technique is performed. Generally the depth of insertion need be no more than 1-2mm. If a 7mm needle is used, this should leave 5mm of the shaft above the skin. As ever, a pair of tweezers should be on hand in case the heat produced becomes excessive, so that the needle can either be adjusted or removed. Rubinstein (who actually uses this technique for treating problems in the finger joints), endorses what he calls "chain moxas", repeating the moxa on the same needle 3-9 times. He likes to apply the second cone to the first (and so on) actually while the first cone is still burning to maximise the development of the heat in the shaft, since, with a small needle like an intradermal, the heat dissipates very quickly. Some practice on a banana and then on oneself is a very sensible start before using the technique since it is not an easy technique to master.

Rubinstein acknowledges that Dr Manaka along with his assistant Kazuko Itaya sometimes heated intradermals for specific purposes, but Rubinstein himself has developed this treatment in a slightly different and novel way[170].

The technique is best not attempted on palmar surfaces where insertion may be excessively painful, but could be used in creative ways on dorsal surfaces of the hand to treat areas of the back if access to the neck itself were difficult. As a useful way of treating neck tension, this type of treatment can be considered on the dorsal surfaces of the middle finger between the interphalangeal joints on reactive points. For lower back pain in a patient confined to a wheel chair the

---

[170] Aaron Rubinstein 2011 "Kyutohinaishin-Intradermal Needle Warming Technique (parts 1 & 2)" North American Journal of Oriental Medicine, Vol 17, Nos 50 & 52

treatment could be used on reactive points on the back of the hand, particularly on either side of the third metacarpal bone.

Another innovation using Dr Yoo's microsystem system involves adapting a much older treatment by using moxa on the hand. In Part 1 the Roots we discussed a treatment method used by Goto Gonzan in the seventeenth century in Japan, specifically his "Five Pole Moxibustion Method" which he felt could treat most diseases[171]. The locations were: the "upper pole" – at the spinous process of the first thoracic vertebrae, which, on the dorsal aspect of the hand would be just below the PIP (proximal inter-phalangeal joint) of the middle finger; at the "lower pole" at the coccyx (which is in the hollow just proximal to the base of the third metacarpal); at the "middle pole" (midway between the upper and lower poles which, on the hand, would be halfway between these two points); at the "left pole" 1.5 *cun* left of the middle pole point (which on the hand would be on one edge of the metacarpal); and at the "right pole" 1.5 *cun* right of the middle pole (which would be on the opposite edge of the metacarpal bone).

If Gonzan saw the disease as "opening on the surface", he would apply ninety moxa cones to the left and right poles. If he saw the disease as manifesting more as "pathogenic *qi* in the channels" he would use sixty cones on the upper pole, and also the same on points located 1 cun above the left and right poles. If he saw the disease as already having "penetrated the viscera", he would apply sixty cones on points 1.5 cun lateral to the upper pole and on both left and right middle poles. If he recognised the disease as simply being truly chronic and stagnated he would apply a staggering fifteen hundred cones on both left and right middle poles, and three hundred on the lower pole. In practice each treatment might involve a blended combination of two or more of these approaches.

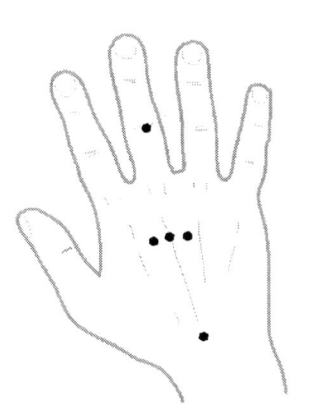

Five pole moxibustion method on the hand

---

[171] Tetsuya Fukishima 2010 "Goto Konzan's Theory of Qi Stagnation and Five Pole Moxa" North American Journal of Oriental Medicine, Vol 17, No 49

The Moon over Matsushima

The number of cones originally prescribed for these treatments are quite astonishing, but the basic ideas which lie behind the treatment can easily be adapted to moxa on the hand using the Korean model. The dosage can be proportionally weighted to the number of cones originally advocated by Gonzan, the treatment can be carried out on both hands, and, using the stick-on cones, can even be done daily by the patient for best effect. For a resistant chronic condition, for instance, it might be worth palpating these points on the dorsum of the hand, and if they appear reactive this would be a treatment that might prove effective. Ten cones of raw moxa could be applied to the left and right middle poles of the hand, and two on the lower pole. With stick-on cones, on the other hand, the focus of treatment would be on the middle poles, with less heat applied to the lower pole.

Incidentally, in cases of contracture of the hand, quite significant nodules can appear in the tendons in the palm of the hand. "Melting" these with repeated applications of moxa using a small bamboo tube can also be a very effective treatment.

Moxa and Needling Combined

Current codes of safe practice, if applied to the letter of the law, pretty much preclude the combination of the techniques of needling and any sort of direct or semi-direct moxibustion at the same point in the same treatment, although this has hardly always been the case. Irrespective of such codes, the ideas behind combining the techniques at a single point remain worthy of review if only in the hope that it casts clearer light on their wider application. In what Peter Eckman called "Leamington-Acupuncture"(or "LA") as developed by Jack Worsley, the procedure of applying moxa first followed by needling was actively encouraged, particularly on points like Bl43 *Gaohuang shu*. The idea was that the warmth of the moxa would activate the *qi* before the insertion of the needle. Pea-size moxa cones were used with a "snatch" technique to remove them as they became hot. This order of approach actually reflects the endorsements of Sun Simiao who also believed that moxa generally should be applied before acupuncture.

Other styles, both Chinese and Japanese, advocate the opposite order, their logic being, one surmises, that the needling facilitates the arrival of *qi* at the point, which can then be more easily warmed by the moxa. This practice to some degree reflects the use of the moxa stick around the needle if it is retained in place, or indeed the moxa-on-the-needle-head technique. Furthermore both Shudo and Mizutani [172] separately suggest that, if the insertion of a needle to relieve tenderness or reduce an induration is not effective, then direct moxa should follow. This would initially seem to be a step too far under the remit of modern

---

[172] Shudo Denmei 1990 "An Introduction to Meridian Therapy" (Eastland Press)

codes, but actually what is often found is that the locus of discomfort, or even the induration itself, can be found to have moved a little from the needled location, allowing direct moxa to follow, as long as it is deemed acceptable by the appropriate governing authority to palpate a point which has already been needled – something which may or may not be the case.

Clearly both approaches can be seen to have their individual rationales and advantages, but the arguments for-and-against are largely academic if one interprets such codes to the letter. The reality we face is that, if we want to use direct moxa in our practice we cannot easily combine it with needling at the same points[173] – pushing us towards focusing on just using moxa where we feel it might clearly be more effective than needling, something which may well ultimately be to our patients' benefit.

One method of combination which is sometimes used in Japan, however, is still acceptable: combining the *chishin* retained-needle technique (thin needles superficially inserted 1-2mm only) with half-rice size cones burnt just beyond the point of insertion. This technique is known as *kyu kon shin* or moxa-shaft needling. An alternative method is to use deeper needling with thicker needles, and to use a moxa stick to heat the needle shaft. The author personally has little experience using either technique, but knows of practitioners who use this over tight points on the back and report great effects quite similar to moxa-on-the-needle-head technique.

The above does not, of course, in any way preclude the probability that both moxa and needling may be effectively combined in a single treatment at different points and in different phases of the treatment. Some reflection on this and particularly the optimum order in which this may be applied is deserved since it may make treatment more efficient and outcome more effective.

Firstly, it may be advantageous to reconsider the traditional differentiations as to the effects on the *qi* from either method. A classic interpretation of acupuncture is that it balances and regulates the flow of *qi*. In subtle contrast, the action of moxibustion is said to actually add some *yang* to the body in the form of the warmth, and since *qi* is essentially *yang* in nature, then moxa may logically actually add some form of *qi* as well. (This would assume, of course, that the particular application of moxa is primarily not intended to be dispersive or releasing.)

We enter challenging areas of energetic metaphysics if we dare to ask just how effectively we might be able to add *qi* into the body with moxa since we would

---

[173] Under current UK guidelines, for instance, one would have to swab the point which has been treated with moxa before needling, something which, while possible, self-evidently would potentially counteract the warming effect of the moxa. If applying moxa after needling, the site of puncture would also require swabbing, effectively pre-cooling the point before the moxa is applied.

first have to agree on exactly what the stuff is. It is clearly an important issue: Dr Manaka, for instance, identified that, of the fifty thousand characters in the Suwen, for instance, roughly one in fifty is *qi*.

Over the ensuing centuries, it has been a term that has been used and interpreted in different ways. The scholar Manfred Porkert helpfully summed it up by suggesting that whenever Chinese thinkers were unwilling or unable to fix the quality of an energetic phenomenon, the character for *qi* inevitably flowed from the tips of their brushes[174].

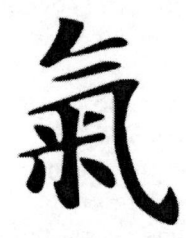

The consensus today, as far as traditional East Asian medicine is concerned, is that it remains a relatively indefinable and abstract non-substance and that we can do little more than do our best to attempt to understand it in relation to the complexities of acumoxa therapy in the best way we can.

Certainly it would be difficult to convincingly argue that we can **permanently** inject an influx of *qi* with moxibustion, but we could strongly suggest that we may be able to **temporarily** do so. Assuming this to be the case, it begs a logical question: is it better to add this *yang qi* before regulating the system, or vice versa? Or might it even be better to add some in the middle or towards the end of the treatment? There is no simple answer to this, only preferences and prejudices which for any practitioner are likely to change from time to time, dependent upon our sense of the state of the patient, of the flow of the treatment or from simple intuition. The decision is ultimately the practitioner's.

We could liken the situation to that of a motor car: is the servicing of a car or the tuning of its engine more effective because one has just filled the petrol tank? Frankly it is unlikely that it is. Mostly it just doesn't matter. It may, however, be a risky trip from the mechanic's ramp to the forecourt of the petrol station if the tank were still particularly empty just after the service. In such a case, the finest available krypton tuning of the engine would not make the slightest difference to the outcome of the journey.

If we extrapolate this analogy a little further, however, we can also observe that the act of filling the tank is performed many times more often than the act of servicing the engine. This offers food for thought, especially if we consider the idea of long term daily moxa treatment, or of home treatment for our patients between visits to the clinic. We also know that a good service can mean that our engine runs more efficiently with better fuel consumption, something which is important if the fuel is too expensive or in short supply. How far this analogy can be stretched is debatable, but the idea would certainly support the idea of home moxa treatment between acupuncture treatments.

---

[174] Manfred Porkert 1974"The Theoretical Foundations of Chinese Medicine: Systems of Correspondence"(MIT Press)

Two personal preferences do, however, seem worth mentioning.

Firstly, when I use moxa to rebalance "Akabane" *jing* point imbalances, I generally use this before any other regulation of the *qi* system. If, however, I am using direct moxa with the specific intention of fortifying the patient's constitution, I actually tend to do so <u>after</u> other *qi* regulating techniques. It is my experience that careful use of direct moxa, even if used symptomatically, does not upset a more balanced pulse – in fact it rather does the opposite, leaving the pulse stronger and more consolidated if done well.

My approach contains a basic contradiction, however. Generally my own preference in treatmentis to tonify **before** dispersing, something I have been personally taught as an idea which originates from the text of the *Nan Jing*[175]. Many modern acumoxa practitioners favour the opposite order, a practice which is an orthodox part of *Zhong Yi* TCM. My own rationale for the "tonify before deficiency" model is based on a perception of most of my patients as being fundamentally deficient (another concept founded on teachings I have received but which have also been endorsed for me by experience). "Tonifying first" seems a very sensible approach for such patients. Adopting the principle that one of the primary functions of moxibustion is to tonify whilst the mechnanism of needling is more regulatory, however, the concept of "moxa first, needle second" might seem to be a more plausible rule of thumb to adopt than the one I actually use, and is one which certainly would not jar with the use of the Akabane method as described at the start of the previous paragraph; it also would not jar with the teachings of Sun Simiao.

---

[175] Nan Jing chapter 69: "One should fill first, and drain afterwards".

The Moon over Matsushima

Part 4 – The Stems

> "DO NOT BELIEVE JUST BECAUSE WISE MEN SAY SO
> DO NOT BELIEVE JUST BECAUSE IT HAS ALWAYS BEEN THAT WAY
> DO NOT BELIEVE JUST BECAUSE OTHERS MAY BELIEVE SO
> EXAMINE AND EXPERIENCE YOURSELF"
>
> The Buddha[176]

The Actions of Moxibustion

Some of the actions and effects of moxa have already been touched upon in the previous sections although these have been generally couched in the terms of traditional East Asian medicine. In this section we will begin to try and unpack some of moxa's possible mechanisms by looking at them through two different lenses, one traditional, the other more biomedical and scientific.

In examining the issue of moxa's mechanisms this way, we face something of a challenge since using these two lenses together – the one traditional and holistic and the other reductive and scientific – tends not necessarily to help bring things into that sharp a focus. Looking through one lens without considering the same shape when seen through the other, however, will (in my opinion) leave our considerations of this therapy very much the poorer, because there is much to be learnt from each. We are children of the twenty-first century, like it or not, and we organically absorb and adapt to the current pervasive cultural conclusions about the nature of reality. As part of a deepening of life experience, we may choose to challenge such conclusions by embracing alternative older philosophical ideas, but in order to be heard at all in the wider world, we need to be able to talk in the language of its dominant paradigm. To put it mudanely, our treatments may well be enriched by embracing and exploring the laws of the five phases and the concept of qi, but we will make ourselves seem delusional if we ignore the laws of gravity in the process.

---

[176] The *Kalama Sutra*. This was a sermon given by the Buddha when he passed through the village of Kesaputta. The villagers there asked his advice concerning all of the many holy men passing through, wondering whose teachings they should best follow. He suggested that the words of the wise should indeed be heeded but should not to be taken on absolute trust. The Buddha included in this category words associated with tradition, with repeated hearing, words ascribed to a "teacher", to experts, to scriptures, deduced from suppositional reasoning, and (most challenging of all) from common sense.

The Moon over Matsushima

In order to use the scientific lens at all in a holistic sweep of the subject, however, we have to adopt strategies which are problematic if not downright risky. One is that we have no choice but to objectively review each and every claim made by any party; the other (which is far riskier) is that we have to attempt to conflate quite different paradigms. At best this can be a challenging experience – at worst a bewildering one. Adopting this strategy may also put off some readers who have enjoyed the book so far, particularly since the tone and approach of this section necessarily has to stand in contrast to the previous three parts. But, if we have any serious intentions for the future of this therapy, I personally think that it is worth taking a deep breath and accepting these risks.

It seems to make most sense to start this review by listing the most widely quoted actions of moxa that are stated in the standard current TCM literature. It should be borne in mind from the very start of this section, however, that some of the general properties attributed to moxa **anywhere** (in either the older or the newer literature) may not be moxa properties *per se* but may be only associable with moxa when applied at specific locations.

Moxa is generally said to –

- warm meridians and expel cold and damp

- induce the smooth flow of *qi* and blood and move stasis

- tonify *yang* and strengthen *yang* from collapse

- prevent disease and maintain health

Lorraine Wilcox adds several further effects which deserve listing, writing that moxa:

- warms and scatters cold evils
- warms the channels and frees the *luo* vessels
- disperses stasis and scatters "bindings"
- quickens the blood and stops pain
- eliminates dampness and scatters cold
- "up-bears" *yang* and lifts the fallen
- supplements the centre and boosts *qi*
- regulates and contains the *chong* and *ren* vessels
- repositions the foetus
- "down-bears" counterflow and descends *qi*
- calms the Liver and subdues *yang*
- dispels toxins and discharges heat
- prevents disease and safeguards health

She compiled this list from two modern Chinese books on moxibustion from the People's Republic of China, PRC - He's 2003 publication "Utensils and Methods of Moxibustion", and Liu's 1991 "Collected Essentials of Chinese Moxibustion". It can be reasonably assumed from this that deeper understandings of the actions of moxa currently exist in the PRC than those which prevail in the mainstream TCM literature in the English language. The fact that most of these ideas remain out of the global TCM info-stream suggests two things: firstly that moxa is not that widely embraced within orthodox TCM as a therapy which in any way "stands alone"; and secondly that it is not seen as being so globally exportable as acupuncture and herbs have proved to have been.

Whatever the truth may be, it is important for us to bear in mind that many if not almost all of the actions identified in the second list are point and/or technique specific, whilst those in the first list are more general and furthermore may be more generally related to indirect techniques.

In quite marked contrast, the majority of the modern literature on the subject emanating from Japan suggests that direct moxa exerts actions in ways that are much less traditional and more often than not couched in the language of bioscience. It is variously claimed that moxa:

- increases white blood cell count (WBC) dramatically (as much as twice its normal count with repeated use)
- maintains this raised WBC with regular treatment
- increases phagocytic activity of white blood cells
- increases blood glucose counts
- increases red blood cell count
- produces analgaesic effects
- creates anti-inflammatory effects by promoting blood coagulation and regenerating granulation tissues
- inhibits the spread of infection
- increases the capacity of the body to produce antibodies
- causes localised vasoconstriction accompanied by more widespread vasodilation
- increases calcium ions in the blood and decreases magnesium ions
- emits radiation at Far Infrared Frequency which is healthy to cells
- promotes alkalosis and suppresses acidosis
- expands peripheral circulation
- improves peristalsis
- decreases urolobin in the urine indicating improved liver function
- balances the autonomic nervous system, possibly promoting parasympathetic responses
- potentially creates thermo-electrical effects in the fascia and connective tissue
- promotes recovery from fatigue

- facilitates oxygen uptake
- reduces total cholesterol
- whilst bolstering immune response, does not exacerbate auto-immunity
- produces minute amounts of histotoxin (denatured protein) or creates immunohistochemical expressions of HSP (Heat Shock Proteins) and CGRP (Calcitonin Gene Related Peptides) which may stimulate blood changes[177].

We can wonder whether this set of claims in any way adds up to something similar to what is claimed in the traditional Chinese literature, or whether it is made simply with a different terminology basing itself on a different paradigm and means something essentially completely different[178]. Hopefully what follows will clarify the matter a little.

Some of the claims made in the Japanese list, it should be said, are at the very least challengeable, and some of them may even raise clinical concerns. In addition, as with the list from the PRC, it would be wrong to suggest that all, or even most, of these effects occur whenever or wherever moxa is applied to a human body independently of point selection or technique. Indeed many of these effects, if they can indeed repetitively be proven to occur under controlled conditions, will also certainly be dependent on technique, dosage and/or point specific treatment.

One thing is immediately clear – far more detailed information is required to render these claims properly valid. We have no alternative but to initially review them with some circumspection and to review some of the research on which some of these claims are made, although we will see in the course of doing this that there is some interesting evidence available which goes some way to strongly support some of them.

It is a shame that most of the "credited" explanatory research into the mechanisms and effects of acupuncture (rather than moxa) that is generally published and recognised in the English speaking world is focused on the pain perception response and particularly on potential responses in the brain, but remains frustratingly inadequate in terms of investigating the more holistic claims of traditional *jingluo* channel-based acumoxa. Moreover, such research is generally averse to embracing the idea of multiple mechanisms of effect because of further complicating research approaches which are hard enough already. In contrast to

---

[177] Manaka et al 1995 "Chasing the Dragon's Tail" (Paradigm Publications) Appendix 2; and Junji Mizutani 2005 "Practical Moxibustion Therapy" (North American Journal of Oriental Medicine)

[178] It is important that the reader should understand that the field of literature is being deliberately simplified: there has plenty of biomedical research into moxa in China and there is also plenty of Japanese literature on moxa which is firmly wedded to ideas from the traditional canon.

this, some of the available fruits of moxa research, however, seem to be strongly hinting at measurable whole-body effects, although much of this data is pretty much unknown outside of Japan. Neglecting it may well be to the broader detriment of the acumoxa profession. The overall picture that we will draw will also point very strongly towards multiple mechanisms. For moxa to have such a profound effect on the body as is about to be suggested, its application maywell create something of a cascade effect on wider body systems arising from the single initial stimulus from a moxa cone. Whether or not this cascade does occur, at the very least it is unlikely that the original stimulus works does not work through several synergistic mechanisms.

There is a wealth of research in Japanese, right up to the present day, which focuses on vertebrate immune response after moxibustion. A list of interesting papers which specifically relate to immune response forms an appendix to this book. Most have yet to be translated into English, but many have abstracts in English that are at least comparatively comprehensible.

The trail begins early in the last century. A revealing list of nearly fifty early research papers published in Japan from 1912-1940 is to be found in English in Manaka et al's "Chasing the Dragon's Tail" (in its Appendix 2). It was collated by Kazuo Itaya who collaborated with Dr Manaka for many years, and it documents quite clearly how continuous scientific research has been carried out in this field for a full century.

We can immediately draw a few conclusions. Firstly, there is an enormous corpus of moxa research which has for many reasons been largely ignored outside of East Asia, whilst literally **none** has been conducted on moxa in the West. Secondly, that this research may well support the idea that it is direct rather than indirect techniques which are most effective in creating whole-body self-regulatory effects, since these are what are primarily described in the research quoted above. And thirdly, that moxibustion research may yet prove to be more convincing than acupuncture research in terms of measurable whole body response if only because its methods of application contain fewer variables of technique particularly in terms of practitioner skill. Despite this, clear problems in moxa research do exist, and we will come back to the endemic problems faced by future researchers of moxibustion in the West in Part 5 the Leaves.

Moxibustion and White Blood Cell Count (WBC)

For large parts of what follows the author is indebted to the collaborative research of Jenny Craig. Much of the following work on temperature particularly is almost entirely hers, as are some of the more evolved ideas about receptor proteins. Some sections of text which are included in the following discussions were originally co-written with Jenny and published in various articles on the subject in acumoxa journals. Without her persistence and thorough research-mindedness, some of the most interesting parts of this consideration of immune response from moxibustion would have been completely missed.

Reports of rapid or prolonged increase in WBC heightening immune response are probably the most oft-quoted modern descriptions in the English speaking world endorsing the actions of direct moxa (and sometimes even of indirect moxa) although they are often quoted, unfortunately, from relative ignorance. A typical googled search for "moxa and immune response", for example, will regularly turn up something along the following lines on websites created by a wide range of practitioners who use moxa in quite different ways: "The white blood cell count begins to increase immediately after direct moxibustion, and reaches a peak 8 hours later. This peak is maintained for 24 hours. The number remains elevated for four or five days after treatment. The white blood cell count almost doubles with moxibustion, but when applied continuously for six weeks, the increase is sustained for up to even three months after moxibustion is discontinued". Sometimes such websites read word for word the same even though the moxa techniques described are different. Unfortunately vital information concerning the distinct methods used to elicit these effects in terms of technique, size and numbers of cones, and the points used are never properly identified. Sometimes as well (quite worryingly) this generic statement even accompanies a description of indirect moxa pole technique, something which is grossly mistaken, since this technique almost certainly cannot induce or reflect these particular effects and has little direct connection with the related WBC research.

Some fundamental questions need to be evaluated in the light of the available literature for a truer assessment to be made. Unfortunately the problem is exacerbated by the lack of detailed information in the English language. Generally, at least, a much better idea of specific dosage and method of application needs to be established before any clear conclusion can to be drawn.

The bulk of modern research on this subject emanates from Japan and is in Japanese, but it is fraught with contradiction at worst and lack of clarity at best. Since the 1920s, an observed response (that regular moxa treatment has beneficial effects on the human which suggest that it has a broad non-specific effect on the immune system or increases the phagocytic activity of the WBCs) has stimulated repeated research on the subject on both humans and animals. Unfortunately, with the benefit of modern understandings of human immunology, such an idea of non-specific immunological response will no longer suffice – and even the oft-quoted claim that "moxibustion increases White Blood Cell Count" can now be seen as being relatively meaningless in the light of more recent post-HIV/AIDS developments in understandings of immunology. These have significantly deepened understandings of the different actions of the various sub-types of white blood cells which make up the overall count, thus challenging the overall import of these more popular claims. Unless we know **which** white blood cells moxa may affect, we cannot today draw any truly useful conclusions as to how moxa might be best used today.

It is important to appreciate that many of these earlier findings, and much of the corpus of Japanese research (although not all of it), together with most of the intricacies and complexities of the recorded response from earlier papers were far from understood when they were first investigated in the way that they might be interpreted today.

This apparent dramatic rise in WBC, as quoted above and so widely quoted on the web, can actually be directly traced back to some earlier research from 1929, which was done using rice-grain sized cones on points on the backs of rabbits. It cannot, of course, be readily assumed that a similar response should be expected from a human subject, so the general exploitation of this study's results to endorse human moxa generally is unfortunately misleading and quite justifiably challengeable.

If we assume for a moment, for instance, that the immune response of a human might indeed be similar to that of a tiny mammal, how might we best evaluate the dosage used? If we were assessing pharmaceutical dosages we might adopt a simple linear approach, but extrapolating from the relative size of a mouse to a human, it becomes evident that quite large cones might be required to create a similar effect in a human. A 1mg cone on a 25g mouse, for instance, is going to be equivalent to a 3 gram cone on an average human, if one were to extrapolate weight for weight. That would make for a frighteningly large moxa cone which would be guaranteed to cause first degree burns if left to burn to the skin. If cone sizes were kept smaller, which would clearly be desirable for the human subject, it is possibly arguable that a similar dosage might be achieved by using a huge amount of cones, in which case we are reminded of Yang Jizhou's seventeenth century endorsement of the number of cones per point for his "guaranteed" effective treatment of chronic disease with moxa to be "the number of years of age plus one"[179]. But this can hardly be seen as a conclusive answer to the dosage anomaly.

To complicate this further, we also have to consider the fact that, while the body mass of small mammal and human subjects might be vastly different, the sizes of the dermal cells that the moxa may affect are actually the same, and if a temperature threshold is required for effect, this of itself may well be cone-size dependent, and bear no relationship at all to body mass.

Additionally, the general conclusion that "white blood cell counts rise" may not even of itself be that helpful. Might it be that peripheral circulation is increased by the moxa, mobilizing WBCs from storage in immune organs or from what is referred to as the "marginal pool" of immune cells into the peripheral circulating blood circulation, or is it that there is an increase in the "manufacture" of the WBCs themselves? What ratios of lymphocyte subsets and natural killer cells exist

---

[179] Yang Jizhou 1601 – "The Great Compendium of Acupuncture and Moxibustion" – (Chinese) as quoted by Lorraine Wilcox.

immediately after moxa application, and at varying times after it? Is it even fair to generally assume that a similar response exists in humans to that recorded with the rabbits in the research? How much do these readings vary dependent upon dosage, and are these variables also dependent upon point selection? One would certainly expect them to be, and we will review the available data as best we can to draw some tentative conclusions.

The findings from the research certainly do promote the idea that particular protocols might conceivably be designed to specifically address certain immune compromised conditions — treatments which might thus be especially and even invaluably applicable in more "bare-foot" or basic primary care applications.

But might even the general significance of raised WBC itself be fundamentally questionable? Certain drugs, such as lithium for instance, clearly also create increased levels of WBC as part of their general effect, but do nothing to enhance the immune system. So just raising WBC count may be of no significance at all, unless we can also simultaneously confirm accompanying therapeutically beneficial effects — something which reassuringly does indeed seem to be the case with moxibustion.

We might also wonder whether it is advisable for the human body to operate with raised levels of white or red blood cells for any length of time as is suggested might be the case with prolonged prophylactic or longevity-based treatment if we take the Japanese claims at face value. If the moxa stimulates the manufacture of WBCs, for instance, might it create a cumulative exhaustion of bone marrow from long term moxa treatment, equivalent in terms of traditional East Asian medicine, perhaps, to a pernicious exhaustion of *jing* essence? Or might the recorded co-agulatory effects pose serious risks of cardio-vascular events for certain patients if platelet levels remain raised for lengths of time? Such suggestions clearly conflict with the longevity treatments which we reviewed in the last section, which were surely based on empirical observations, so there may be no cause for concern. But such questions are justified nevertheless.

Perhaps more importantly, are the immunological and anti-pathogenic actions of moxa as effective against viruses as they may be on pathogenic bacteria, or might some techniques even be modulated particularly for anti-viral applications? These questions deserve clearer answers than currently exist. It is undeniable that the mechanisms of moxibustion are far from fully demonstrated or understood.

To make better sense of this all, particularly in terms of today's biomedicine, we have to carefully pick over the evidence from the research available to us, and then try to reframe our understandings in the light of what we find.

There are some limited sources of information in English available to us which offer useful starting blocks and might even prove really useful as signposts to avenues for further exploration. We need to return to the oft-quoted 1929 research – in which Dr Shimetaro Hara applied seven "rice grain sized" cones of refined and aged moxa to ten points on both rabbits and humans. He duly reported in the Fukuoka University Medical Journal that WBC counts peaked eight hours after treatment and remained high for three days. Hara, who survived until the age of 108 to become the oldest official living male in Japan in 1991 when he died, remained a life-long proponent of moxa therapy for general health maintenance. He also published papers on the effects of moxa on Red Blood Cell RBC count, as well as conducting some controlled research, which is still compelling to this day, concerning the recovery tendencies of guinea pigs infected with TB in a controlled environment, groups of which were treated with moxa using varying regimes.

Five years later another researcher, Shoichi Tamura, similarly investigated the WBC response to moxa, but this time used four differing weights of moxa. He applied different doses – of 0.17, 0.5, 0.75 and 1.0 mg per kilogram body weight – and reviewed the response with each dose. It should be noted that this approach (regulating cone size relative to body weight) differs from Hara's approach which used the same cone size (approx. 1mg) for both human and rabbit. The points Tamura used unfortunately also remain unclear, as do the number of cones used. The lowest weight he used (0.17mg per kg) produced no response at all under the conditions he employed. With the largest dose a rapid response was noted, and with the two intermediate doses a more gradual increase took place over one to three days. Dosage, therefore, seemed to Tamura to have a possible important linear role to play in overall effect. But using his relative cone-size-to-body-weight principles, in an average man of 75kg, cone sizes of between 32-50 mg might be needed for a gradual response, and a quite frightening 65mg cone would be required for a more acute situation if one were to extrapolate the weight.

A half-rice grain sized cone weighs approximately 1mg, so a cone fifty or sixty times this size would hardly seem a safe direct moxibustion technique.

Many papers, currently still only available in Japanese, may yet throw more light on this subject since these two seminal papers, whilst both reporting increased WBC counts, appear to do so according to important differences in principles: Hara's various papers depend upon moxa cones of approximately 1mg for effect based on attenuation of temperature for histological effect; Tamura's research depends upon extrapolated weights of moxa for their effects which are far in excess of what Hara was using.

It is surprising but characteristic of general claims made on behalf of moxibustion's effect on immune response that little attention is paid to possible different response at different acupoints. There may be fundamental differences of approach which might help explain this apparent deficiency. Many of the more biomedical researchers may not have been so attached to explanations of body changes based on the channel system. Doctor Hara himself, whilst publicly endorsing St36 as a major treatment point and not being in any way dismissive of moxapoints based on channel theory, was nevertheless not a huge advocate of the *jingluo* channel system. Nevertheless, he used quite specific points and, in fact, his approach echoed loudly back across the centuries to the same tune of the simplified approaches of the old Chinese moxa texts – approaches which had as much to do with facilitating simple treatment protocols with limited points which could themselves be easily located by an untrained and even illiterate patient group. To some degree, his basic point selections still support the idea that specific points on the body might create specific effects.

The variation in the selection and use of points used in different research protocols, of course, has been a hindrance to efforts to draw any unifying conclusions about moxibustion's mechanisms, and this may well be precisely because of exactly such point specific effects. One earlier paper quite clearly supports the idea that different points can create different measurable effects – "Changes in Content of Blood Serum through Moxibustion on Acupoint Equivalents" published in 1983[180]. Moxa was applied at either Liv14 or Sp15. Whilst relatively huge doses were apparently applied (on mice), something which immediately makes the results questionable in terms of their extrapolation to human treatment protocols, it was clear that quite different changes in blood serum were observed with identical applications of moxa at these two different points.

Before we further examine some of the ideas suggested by the available research, however, we need first to step back and review the human immune response through our two discrete lenses – the one of traditional East Asian medicine and the other modern orthodox medicine. We must also summarise a more modern understanding of immunology than was available to either Hara or Tamura when they were conducting their early research.

Wei qi and the Immune System

As the concept of the *wei qi* is far from being a universally defined one, it invites both whimsical re-invention and blatant mis-construction, and so it is to be approached at best with care and caution. But, in spite of these potential pitfalls, it is a subject that is just too tempting to ignore if we wish to consider the possible effects of moxa on the immune system in the light of traditional acumoxa theory.

We can start by discussing exactly what this *wei qi* (*eki* in Japanese) might or might not be. It is most often translated as the "defensive" *qi*. Broadly, it can best be defined as a discrete type of *qi* which flows outside the *jingluo* channels (as opposed to the *ying qi*, for instance, which is generally defined as the *qi* which

---

[180]Sakamoto et al. 1988 Journal of the Japan Society of Acupuncture and Moxibustion; 38(3):320-325

flows within them). Beyond this, things become increasingly less clear, perhaps like the character of the *wei qi* itself.

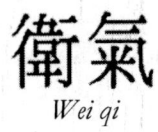

衛氣
Wei qi

The character for *wei* is generally accepted as "defense" or "guards" as opposed to *ying* which is often translated as "army camps" or "barracks"[181].

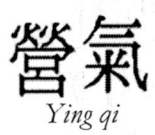

營氣
Ying qi

We can reasonably consider it to be the most *yang* of the variously described types of *qi* which circulate throughout the body. It is described in differing terms – as acting like the walls of a house, as being prone to sinking into the interior when affected by cold, as decreasing around a new moon, as being "fast and smooth" or "fierce and nimble" and flowing between the skin and muscles or running towards the slackened areas, and being associated with sweating. Its "abnormality" in one instance has been rather grandly defined as the "mother of all diseases"[182]. Its origins within the body are subject to differences of opinion from the earliest of times – some sources hold that it emanates from the upper *jiao*, and some conversely that it comes from the lower. Some suggest that the key to supporting the function of the *wei qi* is actually in supporting the middle *jiao*.

It is frequently asserted that it is principally a type of *qi* which gravitates to the body surfaces, but its distribution within the body can quite reasonably also be assumed to be literally anywhere outside of the channels. As such it holds an intimate association with the *jin* fluids which are anywhere and everywhere as well.

---

[181] Paul Unschuld refers to *ying qi* as "camp qi", a term which is perhaps open to misinterpretation despite being probably more accurate. I have translated it as "barrack *qi*" which is how Volker Scheid refers to it. The clinically useful perception that *wei qi* is distributed throughout the body rather than on the surface and superficial fascia, as is often popularly assumed to be the case, is also Scheid's.

[182] Zhang Zhicong commenting on *Lingshu* 59 which discussed *wei qi* when it is "out of its usual order" in his *Huangdi Lingshu Jing Ji Shu* of 1670. In it he stated "I have not dared to impose my ideas on it in a single word" – but the work was immediately criticised by Wang An, another contemporary scholar, who suggested otherwise: "they may have applied their own ideas to fathom the sages" he wrote – something we may all be guilty of! It may be that this idea of the *wei qi* being the mother of all diseases is a prime example of this scholastic crime; it is a compelling idea, nevertheless, particularly for the modern era.

A pervasive tradition survives that says that it circulates in some way which is complementary to the *ying qi*, one circulating in the day, the other supposedly at night.

Does all this actually matter? In some sense, most surely it does, but in the wider scheme of clinical acumoxa we can wonder exactly how much. It seems at the very least quite reasonable to suggest that what may be being presented to us across the centuries is fundamentally a working concept – a concept which forms part of a larger theoretical model of human health which is implicit and fundamental to the traditional practice of acumoxa. As such it may have been as much an intuitive idea (like *qi* circulation itself) as it was either a theoretical or clinically practical one: and it might just be that, even if *wei qi* does not actually exist at all in the way that it is described, its conception is a metaphysical necessity to complete the traditional East Asian theory of human health and disease.

The larger explanatory model of human health and disease as described in traditional East Asian medicine at its core depends upon the interplay between three fundamentally different forces: *xie qi* (the evil or pathogenic invader), *wei qi* (the skirmishing defending soldier), and *zheng, zhen, jing,* or *ying qi* (comprising the remainder of the armed forces in terms of ordinance, communication, supply and support, billeted in the barracks and encampments, as well as in the depots and palaces or *zangfu*).

The generalised axis of conflict being presented in this paradigm of health and disease centres on the balance between the relative strength and opportunity of the enemy (a term often implying external invasion but which can as easily include endogenous and pernicious "enemies within") and the overall strength, mobility, response, adaptability and intelligence of the host army. Conceptually, this idea allows us to flexibly and creatively tell the story of disease in the language of traditional East Asian medicine in ways which are still immediately understandable to our patients today. This is not to denigrate it: almost all explanations of human health and disease tell such stories even today. Such explanations almost invariably reflect and borrow language from the dominant technologies of the day: in ancient China the *jing luo* theories reflect the vital management of the river systems, for instance; in the first waves of modern medicine, in the 19th and 20th centuries, the idea of "man as machine" dominated, and to a degree it still dominates medical thought. More recently newer ideas have emerged, however – of neural pathways acting like complex networks of tele-communication, or of the brain being like a super computer, each superimposing new ideas in the light of emerging technologies. All of them are explanatory stories which both enrich and limit our understandings of the workings of the human body since none of them can possibly tell us the whole story. The fact that this particular Chinese story survives to remain quite real when explained to a patient in the twenty-first century suggests that, as an explanatory model, it still has strikingly healthy working legs. We can surmise that this story of disease would have been equally understandable to patients living two thousand years ago with vastly different ideas of what might constitute human health. The basic principles of both offensive and defensive warfare, of course, are much the same today as they were two thousand years ago.

What is quite irresistible, however, is the possibility that this relatively less developed explanatory model of disease might still be used to interpret some of the more complex understandings of modern immunology as they exist for us today, and the original story can be extended to become an even richer one, very much one for our times.

In terms of external invasion, using one of the classic models of the development of illness, the *wei qi* comprises the first line of mobilised defence at the frontier. There is a clear hierarchy of progression of disease which appears repeatedly in the *Suwen* to support this idea. This theory described the initial penetration of the external *xie qi* through the skin into the superficial *luo* channels, next into the regular channels, then penetrating further into the deeper blood levels that are so prone to stagnation and finally into the interior itself where it can lodge in the *zangfu* and become ever more difficult to shift.

This model of systematic penetration by an external agent of disease, of course, really only applies to external and infectious disease for which acumoxa has much less application today than it had in the past. Clearly this was not always the case, since acumoxa was widely used in the past as a primary treatment for fever and seasonal or epidemic disease. Nevertheless, this same model can still be imaginatively employed to deepen our understandings of human illness, but it may be far too simplistic to stick with the idea that *wei qi* just provides the first and outermost defence at the body's frontier zones – and it might even do the model a disservice.

A deeper appreciation of what *wei qi* might just be can be gained by bearing in mind that this same *wei qi* can be seen to add the "living" *yang* component to all of the body's blood and fluids (resonant of the western concepts of "vitalism" in fact). As such it simply **must** have access to the deepest parts of the body where it may also play just as important a role in terms of defence or response. Infection in early East Asian medical theory was clearly conceived of as a real phenomenon, although it was hardly described in the way it is today. One early idea, for instance, described invisible "worms" being the principle carriers of infectious disease, something which would stretch credibility a little today, even if they might be argued to resemble bacilli or parasites. But since one of the traditional descriptors for consumption (TB), for instance, was "passing from door to door disease", it is quite clear that some diseases were identified as carrying some higher index of what we would today describe as infectivity than others. And we can bear in mind that moxa was favoured as a treatment for just such a disease.

The descriptions of the endogenous causes of disease in traditional literature offer us another slightly evasive target to aim at, possibly reflecting as much the predominant philosophical or political views of each age as those of any particular author or clinician. It is a subject all of its own. In the modern western versions of the traditional East Asian medical literature, endogenous causes of disease relate primarily, of course, to the role of the emotions, something which, in our New Age of psycho-spirituality and ideas of "BodyMindSpirit", is difficult to dispute. In addition to this, however, we find within the traditional canon another layer of etiology – the so-called miscellaneous causes of disease which include overwork, diet and lifestyle, again ideas which are far from controversial to us today. In fact we can unfortunately add to this list so that it includes the iatrogenic effects of modern medicine, and the pernicious effects of pollution from a variety of sources.

From a bioscientific perspective, however, we are confronted with fundamentally more complex understandings of disease today given as it is understood at cellular and humoral levels – understandings which now serve to blur such definitions as exogenous or endogenous causes of disease. Endogenous antigens, for instance, are created by exogenous viruses clandestinely replicating within host cells deep in the interior, but first they will have had to evade detection by the roving defence force by sneaking past the frontier posts in tiny undetected sorties, or at least to have survived its defensive response to its initial intrusion. Some endogenous disease is also understood to be the result of the demonstrable decay or corruption within the host cells themselves, the control of which is seen as a fundamental and implicit role of the immune system. Both instances make for difficulty in treatment.

It is fairly common today, of course, for the attentions of acumoxa practitioners to be drawn to exactly such covert intractable conditions. In many such cases the biomedical etiology is often largely unknown or not fully understood, or is of such complexity that treatment and even diagnosis is rendered difficult for any form of medicine. An exogenous disease can be further complicated by an endogenous response to the allopathic drugs used for orthodox medical treatment. Often such conditions involve causative factors which may be provoked by psychological predispositions by insidious environmental influences, or sometimes simply by nutritional ones. Even in terms of such complex levels or stages of internal disorder we can find that the *wei qi* model can still enrich our understandings, since, not only does the *wei qi* seemingly seamlessly operate on the exterior levels, but it patrols the interior zones as well.

More significantly, in certain cases the *wei qi* can quite easily be seen to become the problem itself.

Out of its own frustrations or lack of discipline it can clearly be conceived of as sometimes creating unwarranted or undesirable responses of its own. To resort to the military metaphor, no nation would want an army or defence force which is anything but ruthlessly focused and lethal when called upon to defend the realm. If this same force should be let loose deep in the peaceful provinces without good discipline and direction, however, these self-same aggressive qualities can become extremely disturbing to the peace of the realm. With such lack of good discipline or indeed of basic supportive supplies, in fact, the effects can quite simply become catastrophic.

On account of his very "fierce and nimble" nature, the archetypal universal soldier has always had a propensity to become a problem whenever his natural aggressive qualities are not required, particularly so if they are not being appropriately channelled or restrained. Rigorous discipline and demanding training is part and parcel of the regular regime of any model army. So it might be in exactly this sense that we can best understand Zhang Zhicong's classic idea that abnormalities of the *wei qi* can constitute the mother of all diseases.

Similarities between Traditional and Modern Understandings

The similarities (equally militaristic in nature) between the traditional East Asian model of defensive *qi* and the modern immunological ones will probably already have been noted and are actually quite striking. This "fierce and nimble" nature resonates strongly with the very modern nomenclature of Natural Killer Cells, for instance – in fact the one description seems to complement the definition of the other, adding a richness that edifies rather than depletes an integrated understanding of the aetiology of disease.

One of the simplest and most understandable modern descriptions of the immune system written for a lay readership by a scientist exactly summarises these very similarities:

"The business of the immune system is to defend the body against foreign intruders, and it does so with a huge onslaught of cells and whole cascades of different molecular weapons. The complexity, and diversity, of the mobilisation is overwhelming: whole tribes and subtribes of cells assemble at the site of infection, each with its own form of weaponry, resembling one of the ramshackle armies in *the Chronicles of Narnia*. Some of these warrior cells toss a bucket of toxins at the invader and then move on; others are there to nourish their comrades with chemical spritzers. The body's lead warriors, the macrophages, close in on their prey and envelop it in their own "flesh" and digest it…they are large, mobile, amoeba-like creatures capable of living for months or years. When the battle is over, they pass the information about the intruder to other cells, which will produce antibodies to speed up the body's defences in the next encounter. They will also eat not only the vanquished intruders but even their own dead comrades-in-arms[183]."

---

[183] From Barbara Ehrenreich 2010 "Smile or Die" (Granta Books) – a book which offers a sharp and captivating critique of the modern obsession with positive thinking. Ehrenreich has a PhD in micro-biology, incidentally.

To offer a better insight into the relative "presence" of this force at any time in the human body, we can consider the total mass of leukocytes or White Blood Cells (which can simplistically be described as the prime constituent members of this roving army) circulating around the realm of the average adult human at any one time. Its gross mass is roughly equivalent to that of the liver or the brain. The "*wei qi*" portion of each and every one of us therefore (if we elect to see it in this light) can be seen to be the size of either one of our two largest internal organs. Most of the time, of course, the majority of these cells are quietly patrolling the peripheral blood or are strategically posted out in the wider lymphatic system ready for immediate mobilisation if required (within some of the very *jin* fluids of traditional East Asian merdicine we referred to above).

Modern understandings of the immune system condense into two principle levels of operation and response: the "acquired" or "adaptive", and the "innate" or "non-specific". We can still observe how the language and imagery, however, remain strikingly appropriate to the traditional East Asian theory of defence: overall the immunity, whether of a human being or a primitive plant, can be generally described as something which is defensive to its host and which endeavours generally to recognise, kill and dispose of pathogens and tumours as well as dead cellular matter. The levels of complexities in terms of the various components of this defence force, however, have developed in complexity as the living entity has become more and more evolved.

The "acquired" processes have continuously adapted over millennia to recognise, respond to and remember more insidious pathogens ever more efficiently, thus providing better protection at potential future encounters. (In terms of the *wei qi* model, one could hypothesise that this could represent a more highly trained, mobile, intelligence-led and adaptable defence force responding to the cunning mutating tactics of the anticipated invader, but the same can equally be said to describe the workings of the immune system).

The "innate" immune system, in contrast to the "acquired" part, is universally recognised as being one which is more primitive in nature and of much older evolutionary stock. In general terms, its processes are less sophisticated, and its responses to any type of assault are correspondingly clumsier and in many circumstancesless effective. The pervasive militarist analogy still applies however to this part of the system: the use of a less-trained and less well-equipped foot soldier is one that is almost universal in the modern defence strategies of most sovereign nations. We can associate this with the reserve force which is called up in support of the regular, more specialised and more technically equipped army.

The similarities as well as the subtle dissimilarities between the two models (ancient and modern) provide much food for thought. The principle differences lie in the fact that the actions of one system can be observed under a microscope and are massively complex, whilst the actions of the other remain tantalisingly more confined within the realms of theory and metaphysical philosophy and are accordingly much less defined. Nevertheless, since the latter are so captivatingly simple they are open to more creative adaption and application. The question for us is whether, within this simplicity, there exist opportunities for clinical usefulness with moxibustion today.

Reviewing the early literature, however, we may find ourself initially perplexed since there are no acupoints indicated specifically to tonify or supplement either the *wei qi* or the *zheng qi*[184], which might seem something of an omission given the extraordinary scope of the theoretical idea behind each of them.

It is curious that these implicit intuitive understandings of the body's defence seem to remain so frustratingly in the conceptual realms of theory and philosophy rather than in the realm of immediate clinical application.

At best, the original theories of traditional acupuncture see the therapy as combating the invader or the endogenous evil by regulating the channels along which the *qi* flows, adjusting excess and deficiency, dispersing pathogenic *qi* and promoting free-flow, as well as by balancing *yin* and *yang*. Anything else, as acutely observed by Bunkei Ono[185], one of the founders of the movement of Japanese meridian-based acupuncture in the twentieth century, is not really traditional acupuncture at all, but is rather some kind of stimulation therapy or simple piercing treatment.

It should be born in mind that, when *yin* and *yang* are appropriately balanced, it is traditionally understood that the pathogenic *xie qi* finds it much harder to gain access. This is a key fundamental axiom behind the idea of disease prevention in acumoxa theory. The same is true if the channels are relatively balanced in relation to one another and are free-flowing. It can thus be reasonably argued that the actions of acupuncture can support the *wei qi* in its defensive capacities in exactly this way – as a result of the act of regulatory balancing. As such it can also be argued that these actions help promote and provoke the very first more external preventative resistance to invasion (literally at the borders themselves) and that they may thus effectively prevent the actual access of the pathogenic *qi*. It might equally be argued that acupuncture may facilitate the actions of the *wei qi* at deeper more endogenous levels by suppressing endogenous pathogenic activity. As a way of explaining why one member of a family, for instance, might contract an infectious disease whilst another escapes it, such ruminations are captivating; but

---

[184] More modern interpretations of point function would suggest otherwise - Bl12 might be considered as a point which supplements the *wei qi*, and St36 both the *zheng qi* and *wei qi* but there is nothing written about this in the classic seminal texts.

[185] Bunkei Ono was an influential practitioner of *Keiraku Chiryo*, a five-phase based style of meridian therapy developed in Japan in the twentieth century. He may have had an indirectly profound influence on acupuncture in the West as well since it is suggested that he may be one of the "masters" who taught Jack (J.R.) Worsley parts of his particular approach to acupuncture.

this idea frustratingly remains a mere theoretical rumination unless we can apply treatment grounded upon it to demonstrably improve our clinical effectiveness.

Both the nourishing and the protective forms of *qi*, whether inside or outside of the channels, can, of course, be acceptably recognised as being largely produced by digestive and respiratory processes, so, theoretically at least, we can add that anything which might support and promote either function could also be interpreted as supplementing host defence. In this sense it can also be reasonably suggested that there may be various indirect means of tonifying both processes in ways which will fortify the host, whether the invader is at the gate or covertly subverting the state from within.

But we are discussing moxibustion, and it is specifically with this treatment method in mind that we can look further for grounds for speculation on this topic – particularly in view of the Japanese research which so strongly connects direct moxa with immune response.

Firstly, we can consider that it is popularly recognised that moxa "puts in" *yang/qi* in a way that acupuncture cannot. This idea can be traced right back to acumoxa's seminal texts. In the context of immune response and *wei qi*, however, it can be suggested that (using the pervasive militarist model of health and disease) the defensive army might thus be rendered stronger or reinforced as a result of moxa treatment. This suggestion is made somewhat more convincing by recognising the repeated endorsements of the *cumulative* effects of moxibustion. Moxa is not necessarily normally considered within the Japanese tradition as either a one-off or once-a-week treatment modality – it is best used as a daily treatment done over as much as a year from which, dependent upon the starting place, maximum effect might be gained. No-one, it seems, should expect to revitalise an army overnight.

Secondly, we have previously looked at particular points (in Part 3 the Branches) which have, over centuries, been particularly identified as being responsive to moxa therapy. The list bears repeating: St36, Bl43, Ren4, the Four Flowers, Ren8 and Sp17. It seems at the least a reasonable possibility that this list includes points from which the *wei qi*, the *zheng qi* and indeed the immune system might best be supplemented or, perhaps even more importantly, can be better regulated.

Moxibustion and Tuberculosis

Tuberculosis is an opportunist invasive infectious bacterial disease, one of the oldest diseases to afflict mankind, and frighteningly is still the second most lethal infectious disease affecting humanity today [186]. An astonishing one-third of

---

[186] It is quite arguable that it remains the most lethal being as so many of those infected by HIV actually die of tuberculosis. In Africa, for instance, TB is recognised as the defining illness for HIV/AIDS.

mankind is estimated to be latently infected with this disease – in other words over two billion people. It is opportunistic in that, under normal circumstances, only 10% of those actually infected by the bacillus go on to develop full-blown potentially fatal infectious disease. The 90% majority of those infected manage to disable this infection to a state of latency most probably with the strength of their own immune system[187]. We can thus construe that, in every instance of infection which remains latent, the invader will have somehow slipped past the border guards, but will have beensubsequently walled in by the interior defence force, effectively becoming (in modern anti-terrorist parlance) something similar to a "sleeper cell". In effect, Homeland Intelligence is unable to eradicate it completely but manages to control it by boxing it into a tiny area in the lungs and then somewhat hopefully sealing it off. It is generally only when the host immune system becomes in some way compromised or distracted that TB becomes an active and lethal disease by breaking out of its confinement – in other words, only when the internal host "defence" is distracted, deficient or depleted (often after having being exhausted by battling another illness or simply because of poor diet).

Today TB is treated using aggressive antibiotics, classified as "first" and "second" line dependent upon their effectiveness and degree of toxicity. These drugs clearly serve to attack the pathogen from the outside of the host, having destructive effect not only on the bacterium itself, but also more generally on other host immune cells as well. If we return to our traditional model of disease, we can suggest that these drugs assume both defensive and offensive roles in relation to the pathogen, taking control from the host force like some kind of imported mercenary army. In reality, whilst this may be effective in knocking back the disease into a non-infectious state, it also causes more than a certain amount of collateral damage in the process and simultaneously confuses, demotivates and further weakens the existing host defence force. Given the lethal nature of the disease this can be seen as an acceptable effect, of course, if the outcome ultimately saves lives, particularly if no other treatment is available.

In the past, however, these drugs were not available, but moxa was reportedly widely used in East Asia for well over a millennium as an effective treatment for tuberculosis, at least effective enough to knock it back into latency. Whilst it is currently impossible to be definitive, the treatment appears to have effectively bolstered and promoted the defensive and offensive functioning of the host defence system just when it was being effectively overrun. Such an interpretation very strongly supports the idea that the judicious use of moxa in some way reinforces the *wei qi* and/or the immune system, depending upon one's preferred explanatory model.

---

[187] This figure is unfortunately misleading in that it fails to identify just what a dreadful disease this can be. The estimated global death toll from TB in the 19th and 20th centuries was a staggering 1 BILLION people. The second of these centuries, of course, included fifty years during which effective drugs had already been developed.

The Moon over Matsushima

Two questions arise – how exactly might it do this, and could moxa withstand a rigorous scientific investigation concerning its effects on patients suffering from this disease? If it could, it could well tell us a lot about moxa's clinical usefulness in supporting the functionality of the *wei qi*.

The points used to treat TB with moxa have varied across the centuries, which must give us further clues – perhaps of individual points' effectiveness, or even that, with moxa, sometimes the actual points may not be as critical as we might wish them to be; we may even conclude that that different dosages or approaches at differing points produce different or complementary effects.

Older Chinese sources tend to include the following points, most of which we have already reviewed in Part 3:

- Bl43 – *Gao huang shu*
- Lumbar eyes – *Yao yan*
- Four Flowers – *Si hua* – Bl17 & 19
- Bl15 – *Huan men* or *Lao xue*
- "Three cun behind the breast" – possibly Sp17

The techniques used were aggressive and often suppurative, involving single treatments using many cones and almost always involved blistering and scarring.

More recent Japanese sources (from the treatments of Sawada) list the following indicated points for pulmonary TB:

- Du12, Bl13, Bl12, Bl11
- Bl17, Bl15, Du10, Du9
- Lu6, Lu5, LI11
- Ren12
- St36

Japanese techniques used relatively tiny cones, only a few at each point, applied on a daily basis with minimal scarring.

Both approaches claimed efficacy, but apart from Bl17 and Bl15 they have no points at all in common. They both, however, appear to have exerted some similar form of stimulatory effect on the host immune system if they were indeed as effective as was claimed. We will look at these possible differences a little further on. With both approaches, however, something implicitly *strengthening* seems to be happening to the host, and we can perhaps now tentatively suggest that what is being strengthened in traditional terminology is the *wei qi*.

In so doing so, we can recall the Chinese counting word *zhuang* which is translated as "cones" but more literally means "reinforcements" and the Japanese equivalent *sō which* means "vitalisations".

Auto-immune Disorder

Before we can be entirely satisfied with such an idea, however, we must confront another common spectre of immune disorder – one which we are far more likely to encounter in our treatment rooms than tuberculosis. Let us consider a situation in which it is actually the immune system itself which is in disorder: that it is still functional – but that it is acting inappropriately. "That which is wild, defensive and rushes harmoniously is qi, if the movement is reckless and rushing it is fire", Zhang Jiebin wrote in Ming times. Re-writing this sentence and substituting the words "healthy immune response" in place of "*qi*", and "auto-immune response" in place of "fire" would perhaps make some sense to an immunologist interested in auto-immunity today. The key words are "harmoniously" and "reckless" respectively. Zhang notably, however, was not in this instance differentiating this particular *qi* into *wei* or *ying* sub-types, and there may be some significance in this: we can logically surmise, using the military analogies described above, that a strongly ordered "barracks" full of *yingqi* would automatically make for a more orderly and controlled extra-meridial roving *wei qi*. We could go so far as to suggest that this "harmony" might most critically be in the relative dynamic relationship between these two distinct forces, suggesting that such a disharmony between the two might equally easily unbalance the whole fighting force.

This may seem a simplistic interpretation of an auto-immune disorder, and it probably is, but such interpretations can usefully lie at the heart of modern explanatory models of immunity. We might go so far as to surmise that a term like "immunological friendly fire" paints a much clearer picture for a modern lay person trying to understand auto-immune disease than a term like "T and B cell discordance".

Further logical questions immediately confront us, however. If such a scenario exists, how does one regulate the *wei qi* without emasculating its very nature, and/or how does one fortify the *ying* back at the barracks to counterbalance the imbalance without sacrificing the flexibility of the roving *wei qi*? Even more importantly, might we inappropriately over-reinforce one type, and in so doing create the expectation among the defence force that this particular type of *qi* should be doing the job of the other which they are neither basically trained nor equipped to do? The idea of an appropriately balanced defence force remains at the heart of this idea, as implicitly perhaps as the idea of the balance between *yin* and *yang*.

But can this rebalancing be done with moxa?

This is a particularly interesting question given that the incidence of auto-immune disease is accepted by most to be on the rise, particularly in the industrialised nations, that its treatment is so difficult to manage and that there is still no comprehensively accepted explanation of its causation. At best we can speculate that the causative factors may be multiple, possibly with a single tipping point as a trigger. If it were all down to genetic disposition, for instance, it would seem unlikely that moxa might play any sort of useful role. But other causative models are being proposed. Two of these bear due consideration in the terms of our *wei qi/ying qi* model of immunity.

One is the so-called "Clonal Ignorance" theory, according to which host immune responses are normally directed to ignore self-antigens but fail to do so. From the perspective of an operational defence force, we can reframe this idea simply to be a fundamental break down of communication, inadequate training, and subsequent mis-instruction resulting in systematic friendly fire.

The other is the "regulatory T cell" theory, wherein regulatory T-lymphocytes fail to prevent, downgrade, or limit auto-aggressive immune responses in the immune system. This might be reframed as a failure of discipline, a neglect of duty, or a mistake in basic training.

Further causative models are proposed – one concerns toxic overload, and another long term stress, both of which could be construed as being directly accessible to moxibustion treatment. Recent speculation has even implicated the increased usage of vaccines as being at least partly responsible for the apparent increasing incidence of auto-immune disorders. All three can be blended into the *ying/wei* interdynamic model of auto-immunity to a greater or lesser extent.

It is quite arguable that the use of moxa at a point like St36 is largely self-regulatory in nature although it may be challenging to conclusively prove this. In support of this idea, there are strong suggestions in the modern Japanese literature on moxibustion that moxa mini-cautery, whilst promoting the immunological defensive functions of the body, does not excite an existing auto-immune condition, and in fact actually attenuates it – although the research evidence is sketchy. If this is indeed the case, it raises fascinating possibilities. Certainly, its use is judiciously endorsed for treating diabetes. It is also indicated in the modern literature for use with rheumatoid arthritis, indeed it is reported that insurance companies in Japan will actually pay for its use in treating this condition. Actuarial evidence, of course, can be as fundamentally persuasive as any controlled research data.

But it may also be that simple modifications of technique might best serve to develop special applications for treatments for auto-immune conditions, and that these have yet to be properly explored. Given that auto-immune diseases are often seen as a more "modern" phenomenon which may be quite possibly triggered by vaccines or atmospheric toxins, we will find little in the traditional literature to give us pointers for best practice. Possible indicators do exist, however, particularly because moxa has been used to treat both rheumatoid arthritis and diabetes (in both cases primarily using points on the back).

Moxibustion and the Immune Response – the Research Evidence

It is in the nature of scientific research that observed parameters should be reduced to an absolute minimum to maximise control and potential meaning in any results observed. A review of the published moxa research is unfortunately a wonderful example of the problems which arise from this approach because different methodologies produce different results. While it is clear that the immune system is complex, multi-facetted and interdependent upon its different parts, it is a commonality of the available literature that only particular discrete changes or markers are looked for or reported upon in each investigation. Whilst this accords with the nature of scientific research and certainly gives us interesting pointers, it makes it difficult to provide us with a more comprehensive and informative picture of what either a specific or non-specific response might be. But we can at least have a look at what is available to us, and see what we can conclude.

To gain any sort of reasonable picture we need to go back to basics – which in this case are to blood cells – once again borrowing the lens of bioscience.

All blood cells are created from stem cells within bone marrow. These stem cells create two different types of blood cells: the myeloid progenitor cells, and the lymphoid progenitor cells. Using this basic division is helpful in understanding much of what follows.

The myeloid progenitor cells provide the building blocks for the innate (or non-specific) immune system, as well as for both red blood cells and platelets. This evolutionarily ancient system is common to plants and fungi, as well as more evolved autonomous life forms.

The lymphoid progenitor cells provide the components of the more complex adaptive (or acquired) immune system. As we have already seen, in general this extra level of immune protection is afforded only to more recently evolved vertebrate life forms.

Whilst it is important to understand that overall immune function depends upon basic inter-connections between these two systems, this simple division of the system into two discrete parts is helpful in unpacking its general functionality. Keeping this division in mind also enriches our understanding of moxibustion's potential influence on immune response.

The older myeloid progenitor cells produce what are now seen as being discrete types of white blood cells: granulocytes (including basophils, neutrophils and eosinophils), Natural Killer (NK) cells (which are aggressive types of lymphocytes) and macrophages. Each of these types of cell has certain strengths in terms of their effect: on bacteria, fungi, parasites, some viruses and tumour cells, as well as removing dead cell debris. All of these cell types belong to the innate immune system.

In contrast, the lymphoid progenitor cells produce the more sophisticated white blood cells – including both the helper and cytotoxic T cells (among them both CD4 and CD8 cells), and the B cells which make antibodies to specific antigens to create a memory of prior pathogenic events with which to respond in more comprehensive defence of the organism. These cells belong to the adaptive immune system.

The actions of the immune system are also defined by how they work – as either "humoral" or "cell-mediated". Elements of each of these are found in both the innate and adaptive systems. Their regulation impacts on how the immune system responds to different pathogens. Humoral immunity is predominated by the actions of circulating antibodies formed from B cells, whereas cell-mediated immunity works through the actions of the T cells and the NK cells. It is principally with this cell-mediated action in mind that we must review the literature and develop our hypotheses.

In 1981, fifty years after his influential early research on moxa and WBC count described earlier in this section, Dr Shimetaro Hara was still working in moxa research – being involved in two papers which were published that year in Japan which helped to enrich the picture of WBC response[188]. The authors concluded that moxibustion could be accepted as a supplementary therapy to promote immune response, and that this activation of the immune system was specifically through T-cell function (meaning an adaptive and cell-mediated immune response), although they reported in this instance that a period of at least four weeks was required to create these effects. Their research was done this time on rats, although it remains frustratingly unclear which points were used in this research, as also unfortunately are the dosages.

It should also be noted that this research used what is described as "electronic moxibustion", a perfect example of the general inconsistency of moxa research approaches. Such techniques, using a controllable electronically pre-heated tool in lieu of processed moxa to mimic the sudden heat of a small moxa cone, are attractive for the scientist in that they take out some of the vagaries and variability created by using processed moxa. But is this the same thing as classic small cone direct moxibustion?

---

[188] Watanabe S, Hakata H, Matsuo K, Hara H, Hara Shimetaro 1981 "Effects of Electronic Moxibustion on Immune Response 1." Journal of Japan Society of Acupuncture and Moxibustion;31(1): 42-50. (Japanese); and –

Watanabe S, Hakata H, Matsuo K, Hara H, Hirose K, Hara Shimetaro 1982 "Effects of Electronic Moxibustion on Immune Response 2." Journal of Japan Society of Acupuncture and Moxibustion;32(1): 20-26. (Japanese)

It almost certainly isn't, as we will see later when we discuss the synergistic absorption of chemicals at the site of the moxa burn and their possible involvement in immune response. Because of this these results cannot be generally accepted as being typical of moxibustion, unfortunately, but they do give some indication of what may be taking place at the cellular level in response to the localised heat stimulation.

Other research from Korea in 2004[189] deepens this perspective. Here changes in NK cell population were investigated in rats treated with classic small cone moxibustion at St36 *Zu San Li*. The effects confirmed increased splenic NK cell cytotoxicity (this time provoking an innate and cell-mediated response).

So here we have two papers both supporting a general conclusion that moxa can improve cell-mediated immune response. However these results fail to complement each other in that one paper suggests a response from the adaptive immune system, the other from the innate, with neither attempting to measure the wider range of immune parameters.

This very observation was made in Japan in 2006[190] in a thorough review of the published research. This paper described a basic difficulty in drawing conclusions simply because inconsistent methodology has been producing different outcomes. By "inconsistent methodology" we can include (at the very least) variations in cone size, numbers of cones burnt, different points used, types of moxa used (including electronic moxibustion), the number and frequencies of application, and the relative size and mass of subjects.

The two papers quoted above do, however, provide productive food for thought. Since they separately demonstrate effects of moxa on both the innate and adaptive immune response, we can at least surmise that moxibustion can, either directly or indirectly, have an effect on the immune system and that the differences in response which were reported might actually depend exactly upon these "inconsistent methods". If we keep bearing these inconsistencies in mind whilst reviewing some of the other papers, however, we may still be able to draw some useful tentative conclusions.

---

[189] Choi G S, Han J B, Park J H, Oh S D, Lee G S, Bae H S, Jung S K, Cho Y W, Ahn H J, Min B I 2004 "Effects of moxibustion at Zusanli (St36) on alteration of Natural Killer Cell activity in rats." American Journal of Chinese Medicine; 32(1): 303-312.

[190] Tohya K, Fukazawa Y, Kasahara Y, Okuda M, Tahara S, Kuribayashi K 2006 "Literature Documentation of Basic Research on Immunological Effect by Acupuncture and/or Moxibustion Treatment". Immunological Research Committee for Acupuncture and Moxibustion. Japan Journal of Acupuncture and Moxibustion; 56 (5); 767-778. (Japanese)

Whilst reviewing some of the following papers it is also worth recalling the relative mass of a "half-a-grain-of-rice sized moxa cone". This is practically speaking the maximum cone size which might be used clinically in direct moxa techniques in the West if we are allow it to burn to the skin. Such a cone weighs in at around 1 milligram.

As discussed previously, reports exist of moxa being used in Japan to treat radiation effects following the bombings of Hiroshima and Nagasaki suggesting that the effects on immunity from radiation might be a useful field for moxa research. A Taiwanese paper[191], examined the effects of moxibustion on the splenic function of leukocytes (WBCs) in gamma-irradiated mice under general and local anaesthesia. Six "grain sized" cones were burnt on six points (bilateral Bl23, Bl27 and Bl28) every other day over a period of twenty-six days. The numbers of leukocytes (which had crashed as a result of the gamma-radiation) recovered positively with moxa, although intriguingly the effects were disabled when anaesthesia was added. (This may be a highly significant factor and is something we will review further shortly). Similar research five years later by the same authors[192] confirmed that moxa helped the recovery of what they described as "cellular incompetence caused by radiation", this time **without** any anaesthesia.

These studies were both done on animals, but the general results of human recovery from radiation effects using moxibustion were circumstantially endorsed elsewhere in a report from the Czech Republic following the Chernobyl disaster in 1986[193]. This study used both acupuncture and acupuncture-and-moxa, and suggested that the adjunctive moxa treatment made a significant positive difference to the recovery response.

A 1983 study compared phagocytic responses on mice using only three cones (2.5mg) at Liv14 in different treatment regimes[194]. The researchers observed increased phagocytic (cell-mediated) activity of the non-granular WBCs (macrophages) of the innate immune system, although this varied quite markedly

---

[191] Hau D M, Wu J C 1983. "Effects of moxibustion on splenic function of leukocytes and in gamma-irradiated mice under general and local anaesthesia"

[192] Hau D M, Wu J C, Chang Y H, Hwang J T 1988 "Effect of moxibustion on the cellular immunocompetence of gamma-irradiated mice." American Journal of Chinese Medicine; 3: 157-163

[193] L.Kravrechenko 2007 "Immunity deficiency caused by the Chernobyl disaster and its treatment"– International Council of Medical Acupuncture and Related Techniques (ICMART) Symposium (Cyprus)

[194] Okozaki M, Furuya E, Kasahara T, Sakamoto K 1983 "Effect of moxibustion on the phagocytic activity in mice." American Journal of Chinese Medicine. Vol XI; No. 1-4: 112-122.

between different strains of mice. Compared with the Taiwanese study cited above, however, the dosage was relatively large in terms of cone size, but fewer points were used and the total number of cones used was comparatively modest.

A 1988 study used smaller 0.7mg cones at a single unspecified *jing* well point on mice, rats and guinea pigs (five cones at each point)[195]. In this case a direct comparison was being sought between moxa and acupuncture stimulation. The paper confirmed that localised immunocyte activity was much higher after moxibustion than it was after acupuncture. The regional lymph nodes of the moxa treated animals, moreover, were recorded as being **five times** larger than those of the animals treated with acupuncture, suggesting a significant difference in immunological effect. Electron Microscopy revealed "peculiar cell-to-cell interaction" between immune cells after moxa treatment but this did not happen at all after acupuncture. This cell-to-cell interaction was interpreted as suggesting a complex developing immune response as a result of the moxa stimulation.

A Japanese study from 2001 used 1mg cones on humans (ten cones on eight points)[196]. It revealed a relative percentage decrease in NK cell numbers (innate immune system) and a relative increase in the CD4 and CD8 cells (adaptive immune system) with an altered ratio between them. A similar regime performed on rabbits, using cone sizes of 2mg (curiously twice the size as those on the human subjects), at only four points instead of eight, resulted in a slower and less marked change in CD4/8 ratio. Relatively, of course, the same cone size may represent a higher dose for a rabbit than a human, and, with the cone size of the rabbits being twice that applied to the human, these results suggest that a focused adaptive response may be achievable with smaller cones.

The 2004 Korean study which we referred to previously used nine rice-grain-size cones at right St36 for three days on rats. It identified a clear increase in NK cell cytotoxicity on the final day which fell away four days later. In this instance comparison was made between four groups of rats – one receiving no treatment, one receiving simple holder stress, one receiving non-specific burns at a similar temperature to moxibustion, and one receiving moxibustion. The moxa group showed the highest increases, closely followed by the burn group. Perplexingly, in contrast to the 1981 and 1982 studies (the ones in which Dr Hara had collaborated) with which we began this review, no significant T-cell differences in either group were recorded. In those earlier experiments, however, no change had

---

[195] Kimura M, Mastrogiovanni F, Toda S, Kuroiwa K, Tohya K, Sugata R, Ohnishi M. 1988 "An electron microscopic study of the acupuncture or moxibustion stimulated regional skin and lymph node in experimental animals." American Journal of Chinese Medicine. 16(3-4): 159-167.

[196] Yamashita H, Ichiman Y, Tanno Y 2001 "Changes in peripheral lymphocyte subpopulations after direct moxibustion." American Journal of Chinese Medicine; 29 (2): 611-621.

been noted until daily treatment had been maintained for more than four weeks, whereas in this case treatment was ended after three days only.

Many possibilities exist within these variable results from this selective group of papers. We have to recognise that the variables within them are huge. The smallest cone size encountered was 0.7mg, the largest 15mg. The number of cones used per treatment ranged from one to eighty, the number of points used from one to twelve. Treatment periods ranged from a single day to three months. Since immunological effects (albeit variable) were reported in all of the studies, we might at least suggest that this might help explain why less specific immunological effects have been observed with both the older aggressive treatments from China as well as the more delicate small cone moxibustion of Japan – but we can also suggest that they are most likely not the same immune responses. Whilst the evidence is far from conclusive we might also wonder, however, whether dosage (at least in respect of cone size) may have a more consistent specific effect on the immune system than has previously been proposed.

One further added complication has been identified by Professor Hitoshi Yamashita, which is the problem of maintaining a neutral control group. There seems no way that the control group can avoid the trauma of having blood removed in order to provide this basic control data. What is quite obvious from some of the research results is that the action of drawing the blood creates enough stress to generate a WBC response of its own. This makes for real challenges in recovering really accurate data since blood simply must be regularly drawn for comparable serological results to be collected[197].

Professor Abo's Theories of Immune Response and its Implications

One possible mechanism for the observed effects of moxibustion reveals itself through consideration of the theories of Professor Toru Abo, a prominent Japanese immunologist[198]. His intriguing ideas, based on years of research, propose specific ways in which the efficacy of the immune system is mediated through the dynamic balance within the autonomic nervous system (ANS). This is not a controversial idea; complex interactions between these systems are well established. Lymphocytes are known to respond to signals from the autonomic nervous system (ANS) and endocrine system via neurotransmitters such as histamine, serotonin and a host of other peptides released by the brain. These can act as immune-stimulators or suppressors and are essential in regulating inflammatory response.

---

[197] Professor H. Yamashita. Morinomiya University, Osaka. Personal communication.

[198] Toru Abo 2007 "Your Immune Revolution" (Kokoro Publishing, New York)

Where Abo departs a little however, is in his hypothesis that an imbalance of the autonomic nervous system might lead directly to an imbalance in the immune system which can critically favour or hinder a vertebrate's response to particular types of disease. Even this, however, may not be so controversial: a paper published from as long ago as 1919 (but which was largely ignored at the time) demonstrated the correlation between stressors and progression of TB[199]. It is also now known that stress affecting the hypothalamus and pituitary gland can initiate complex pathways that result in the release of corticosteroids which inhibit the inflammatory response. Abo posits that an imbalance in which the sympathetic nervous system is relatively "dominant" will result in a corresponding hyper-activity of theinnate immune system which in turn creates a correspondingly negative dampening of the adaptive immune system.

Bacteria (larger)	Tubercle bacillus (medium)	Viruses (smaller)
Increased granulocytes	< bodies defense >	Increased lymphocytes
Sympathetic nerves in charge	Autonomic nerves	Parasympathetic nerves in charge
Bad	Blood circulation	Good
Many	Granulocytes	Few
Few	Lymphocytes	Many
Causing suppurating inflammation, tissue damage, cancer	If over long term imbalance	Causing allergic problems

Table illustrating some of Abo's ideas.

The size of pathogen predicts the type of cellular response; this is also predicated by an autonomic nervous system state which also has an effect on blood circulation.

A dominance of the parasympathetic system has an opposite effect. He employs this theory as a model with which to explain many of the diseases which modern medicine finds so difficult to treat, including cancers, auto-immune disease and allergies, as well as proposing ways in which they might be better treated.

His hypothesis hinges on an axiomatic idea that the WBCs operate with maximum benefit to their host when in particular proportions – his operational optimum being 65% granulocytes, 30% lymphocytes and 5% macrophages. His resultant understanding of most types of modern diseases is that they are either predicated or accompanied by specific imbalances in these proportionalities of white blood cell types. He believes that such imbalances from this norm are common

---

[199] Ishigami T 1919 "The influence of psychic acts on the progress of pulmonary tuberculosis". Am Rev Tuberc; 2:470-84.

consequences of modern life and, if uncorrected for long periods, they can actually cause disease associated with them. He observes that cancer patients exhibit higher than average proportions of granulocytes in relation to lymphocytes, for instance. This he identifies as being a causative factor for cancer which he sees as a disease which is predicated by a hyper-sympathetic response to a constantly stressful environment, resulting in an increase in proportions between granulocytes and lymphocytes (> 65%/ <30%). He controversially proposes that simply rectifying this imbalance back to around 65/30/5 can reverse the disease which is associated with it. His theories promote a radical model of immunotherapy as a way to correct the imbalance and thereby treat the most challenging of diseases.

Accepted Normal Adult Total 3,500-10,000 cells/cc

CELL TYPE	RANGE (AVG)
Neutrophil (granulocytes)	2000-7000 (3700)
Lymphocytes	1500-4000 (2500)
Monocytes/ macrophages	200-1000 (400)
Eosinophils (granulocytes)	0-700 (150)
Basophils (granulocytes)	0-150 (30)

Table showing generally accepted "normal" ranges of cells

CLINICAL CONDITION	DIFFERENTIAL COUNT FINDING	ABSOLUTE CELL COUNT
acute infection	granulocytosis	>9000/Ul
chronic inflammation	monocytosis	>1000/Ul
parasitic infection	eosinophilia	>700/Ul
viral infection	lymphocytosis	>3500/Ul
aplastic anemia	neutropenia	<1500/Ul

Table showing typical differential cell-count responses exhibited as a result of different conditions

Using Abo's hypothesis as a template for exploration, we may wonder whether moxa need necessarily have a direct effect on the immune system at all to create its immunoligical responses – perhaps its more systematic immunological effect may primarily be mediated by the autonomic system, which then improves the integrity of the host immunity. In other words, we can wonder whether moxa, particularly if used judiciously, may thus serve to rectify exactly the imbalances that Professor Abo has recorded. If this is the case, it may even go some way to explain moxa's historical record of being most useful in treating difficult and intractable disease.

We can suggest that larger cones, supplying stronger heat and clearer pain, will most likely stimulate the sympathetic nerves and thus, according to Abo's theory, activate cellular components of the innate immune system. Smaller cones may rather stimulate the parasympathetic, thereby enhancing the adaptive immune system. It is certainly true that small cone moxa treatments can be profoundly relaxing in their effect, and can create reductions in levels of chronic anxiety states. This response is also often accompanied by spontaneous borborygmus caused by relaxation in the smooth muscle in the abdominal cavity – a further sign of parasympathetic activity.

In both cases, however, moxa appears to stimulate a cell-mediated response. Since the immune response to most pathogens requires a combination of humoral and cell-mediated systems complementing one other, this does not of course complete a picture of comprehensive immune response.

These suggestions concerning the autonomic nervous system's involvement in the immune response to moxibustion are actually strikingly supported by particular instances in three of the papers which were quoted from in the earlier review of the research papers, instances which otherwise remain perplexingly inexplicable. The 2004 study in Korea explicitly claimed that a sympathectomy (in other words a severing of the sympathetic nerve) effectively shut off the immunological effect. This would seem not just plausible, but actually predictable if the moxa which was used on rats was acting directly through their ANS. Another study tends to support the idea as well: a Japanese study from 2005 disappointingly reported that the immunological effects of long-term moxa on rats were "not statistically significant", but the twice weekly treatment over three months was accompanied by anaesthesia on each occasion [200]. Again an accompanying absence of a statistically significant immune response could be considered predictable given a lack of ANS response because of the anaesthesia, and therefore the lack of significant immunological response would make perfect sense. In fact, the Taiwanese research from 1983 had similarly found the moxa-induced increase in lymphocytes to be absent whenever anaesthesia was involved.

So did anaesthesia disable the parasympathetic response and thus the adaptive immune response in both studies? Did the sympathectomy disable the sympathetic nervous system response and therefore the otherwise clear effect on innate immunity in the Korean research in 2004?

---

[200] Matsuo T, Kasahar Y, Kuibayashi K 2005 "Assessment of the Function of Peritoneal Macrophages in Rats treated with long term direct moxibustion." Journal of the Society of Acupuncture and Moxibustion;1:36-42.

Modern understandings of the interactions between the nervous and immune systems give further weight to these possibilities[201]. Sympathetic nerve stimulation is known to activate anti-inflammatory Th2 cells and inhibits the pro-inflammatory Th1 cells, whilst the parasympathetic neurotransmitter acetylcholine potentially modulates several classical immune reactions via the vagus nerve. Chemically blocking these neural activities with anaesthetics would thus be highly likely to affect the immune response. This would certainly make sense of some of the results, although, as we will see, it is unlikely that the mechanisms of moxa are quite that simple.

If we accept Professor Abo's hypothesis about an appropriately balanced ANS being a precursor for a healthy immune system, however, we can at least suggest that these tentative conclusions deserve further investigation. They could be very useful, in fact, in developing a simple approach to further more coherent moxa research, as we will propose later.

Animal Research

A cursory review of the publications on moxa and immune response listed in Appendix 2 bears witness, unfortunately, to the fact that a lot of animals have been sacrificed in the name of moxibustion.

Animal research is generally accepted as a first line of research in order to minimise risks to subsequent human research subjects as well as to gain ideas of dosage efficacy. It is quite clear that this avenue of research has been viewed favourably by many of those involved in moxa research in most of the studies. We can wonder, however, whether either justification is valid at all in investigating the immune response to moxibustion for two reasons. Animal research is particularly suited to new types of medical intervention with relatively unknown effects: this can hardly apply to moxa considering its long history. Furthermore, the dosage disparities which we have already examined add particular complications for any really useful interpretations to be made from any such research results.

The dosage issue deserves a short review at this point. In terms of cone size two separate factors bear consideration – one of which is constant and one of which is variable. The constant factor concerns the cone's size relative to the size of the cells it affects at the treatment point; the variable one concerns its size relative to the overall mass of the subject on which it is being burnt. Both factors may be significant, and in relation to smaller mammalian experimental subjects this latter

---

[201] Steinman L 2004 "Elaborate Interactions between the immune and nervous systems." Journal of Natural Immunology;5(6):575-81.

relationship is really large. A rat is around 1/250 the weight of a human – and a 2.5mg cone on a rat is of totally different consequence to a 2.5 mg cone on a human, one very good reason (we can assume) why anaesthesia was used in some of the research experiments (another being that it may have been an ethically humane requirement for conducting the experiment).

It seems quite reasonable to suggest, therefore, that the results from animal experimentation (unfortunately the majority of the research) should at best be treated with caution – and furthermore there is other evidence to support this view. It is clear both from Doctor Hara's early research from 1933[202] and from research fifty years later that signs of general fur loss and intermittent diarrhoea are not uncommon in small mammals subjected to long term moxa treatment and this can readily be interpreted as signs of over dosage.

Immune Response and Specific Acupoints

It is a characteristic of the general reports concerning moxibustion and immune response, and also of the associated claims made in the acumoxa literature, that little attention is paid to the differing reactions resulting from use of different acupoints.

There may be fundamental reasons behind this. Many of the more biomedical researchers may simply not be so attached to explanations of body changes based on the channel system. The use of small mammals may also have practically affected the matter of point selection: it is far easier to apply moxa to the back of a mouse than to its hind leg for instance, and it is far more difficult to be as specific about point location on a tiny mammal as on an adult human.

This variation in the selection of points used in different research protocols, of course, presents one more hindrance to drawing any unifying conclusion about moxibustion's mechanisms. Yet point selection would seem to be so fundamentally important for effect.

Efforts to get modern master practitioners of moxibustion to disclose their personal ideas about which points they instinctively favour to create different degrees of immune responses have unfortunately resulted in frustratingly vague answers. We can certainly still wonder, however, whether experienced practitioners might favour their own specific empirical points for different infectious or inflammatory conditions, and that these may well reflect their point-specific response. Analysing their instinctive empirical gravitation towards specific points for treating conditions such as acute tonsillitis, the common cold, post-viral

---

[202] Dr Shimetaro Hara 1933 "Moxibustion Therapy effective for all Diseases" (Old Japanese) out of print.

fatigue, or chronic acquired immune deficiency syndrome might provide us with useful pointers for point selection – both for more refined research and also for enhanced clinical treatment.

Over previous centuries, certain points have been identified as being especially responsive to moxa therapy, and have also been associated with treating intractable disease. The following favourites come up again and again: St36, Bl43, Ren4, the Four Flowers (which are variously interpreted) and Sp17. Within this list some points may well have very much more direct influence on immunity than others. Of these, only St 36 has been used with any frequency in modern research, being used in 23% of all the research reports according to one Japanese review[203].

Regarding St36, however, we see in both old and newer references that it has been used in widely differing ways. Yang Jizhou in Ming times in the 17th century, for instance, repeated the long held endorsement of "keeping the point wet" (i.e. at least some blistering) for longevity. Hara in the twentieth century endorsed St36 with rice grain cones on a daily basis (but without blistering) as being effective for long term treatment of practically any condition except cancer, and also for promotion of health and longevity (surviving himself, as already mentioned, to become a centenarian). The Korean research used cones on St36 to induce raised levels of NK cell cytoxicity. Dr Yoshiaki Ohmura endorsed small cone moxa for the supportive treatment of both lung and colon cancer[204]. My own experience leads me to believe that daily applications of small cones at St36 can supplement anti-retroviral ARV drugs and significantly raise CD4 count in chronic HIV/AIDS patients above what would normally be expected. It can also raise WBC counts in neutropenic patients undergoing chemotherapy. With Moxafrica[205], we have even witnessed a tiny single 1mg cone applied bilaterally just on this point to have significant beneficial effects on an extremely weak patient co-infected with both HIV and TB – a treatment which we will review in more detail later when we look at dosage. Such a wide range of responses suggests that St36 must either be a very versatile moxa point, or offers us a possible gateway to a deeper understanding of immune response from moxibustion. There are, of course, other points which may deserve similar further investigations.

---

[203] Tohya K, Fukazawa Y, Kasahara Y, Okuda M, Tahara S, Kuribayashi K 2006. "Literature Documentation of Basic Research on Immunological Effect by Acupuncture and/or Moxibustion Treatment Immunological Research Committee for Acupuncture and Moxibustion". Japan Journal of Acupuncture and Moxibustion; 56 (5); 767-778. (Japanese)

[204] Ohmura Y, Uichiro T 2001. "Interview – St36 and its effects on Cancer." Journal of Japanese Acupuncture and Moxibustion; Vol. 60, No. 10 129-150.

[205] Some more detail on Moxafrica will follow later. Moxafrica is a charitable not-for-profit organisation set up specifically to investigate whether small cone moxa might be applicable today in the desperate fight to contain drug-resistant TB, especially in resource poor environments bedevilled with high rates of co-infection with HIV-AIDS.

Medical research has yet to unravel some of the immensely complex pathways and interactions between the neuroendocrine and immune systems. A host of chemical messengers tie these systems together and have wide-reaching effects on metabolism and behaviour. Immune cells have been demonstrated to make, store and secrete some of the very same neuropeptides (including endorphins) as do brain cells, effectively providing functional links between the brain (behaviour, mood and appetite) and immune system. But it is not just the brain and the immune cells which share these peptides, because the spleen and gastrointestinal system, for instance, also contain common receptors for certain peptides, suggesting the existence of an almost impenetrably complex multi-directional information system in which it is hard or impossible to distinguish which part ultimately controls which. It seems quite feasible, however, that direct moxa might provide a momentary influence on this information network which might have a determinable effect on the whole, and might start to explain how heat stimulation at a point on what is defined as the "Stomach" *yangming* channel of the leg might simultaneously have an effect on the immune system, and also on the emotional well-being of the patient.

We have already touched on the idea that moxa may elicit different responses depending on the point locations used. Combinations of these points might prove even more interesting – combining specific acupoints has been a fundamental part of acupuncture for centuries.

Clearly more research on human subjects is needed – but it is a difficult area to develop. Enormous problems in designing approvable models for research exist both in terms of ethics, and of legislation and control of substances used for medical intervention, as we will see in Part 5 the Leaves. For most in the field of acumoxa in the West, moreover, animal testing is in any case an unacceptable avenue for investigation.

Bearing in mind the negative impact that poor levels of nutrition have on the immune system, it might also be worth investigating further the positive effect of moxa on digestive response, an idea originally identified to us by an experienced researcher into moxibustion, Professor Hitoshi Yamashita of Osaka, Japan.

If we were simply to begin, however, by adopting Abo's hypothesis about the immune system, accepting that it may be largely mediated by the state of the autonomic nervous system, we may learn a lot even though we can assume that it is not the whole story. We could simply assess different subjects' relative balances of granulocytes, lymphocytes and macrophages before during and after courses of treatments using different points and dosages. In particular we could assess them in instances of disease. In this respect it might also be very interesting to compare Japanese 1mg direct moxa techniques with the semi-direct "snatch moxa" method using 10-20mg cones lifted off as the patient feels the heat (as is taught at some UK acupuncture schools).

A clearer picture might also emerge through simultaneous analysis with electrocardiography or analysis of heart rate variability before, during and after moxibustion, again comparing differing dosages and points, since doing so might offer an illuminating wondow of moxa's influence on the sympathetic and parasympathetic nervous systems. No-one yet appears to have attempted any of these. Simultaneous measurements of skin blood flow at various locations on the body might also provide indicators of some of the wider mechanisms of direct or indirect moxa application.

There seems to be a massive scope for systematic experimentation using small cone moxa over different periods, varying the points, point combinations and dosages and comparing electronically generated burns with moxa burns. What is required is simply a more systematic approach than has yet been attempted whilst keeping wider parameters in view.

We can seriously consider safely investigating the use of small cones of direct moxa with a view to confirming or disproving the conclusions of the moxibustion masters of the past. We can consider whether moxa might indeed be particularly applicable for treatment of intractable diseases including tuberculosis, particularly in the light of the fact that it is transforming into a modern plague which is drug-resistant on a scale never seen before in a life-threatening infectious disease. The nature of these types of disease has significantly changed in the modern era as the treatments have developed but their effects in terms of their capacities to kill are the same, and may in fact be increasing. The incidence of TB in Africa, for instance, increased a staggering five-fold in a recent period of fifteen years and in the company of HIV/AIDS this disease has shown itself to be more lethal than ever.

In discussing tuberculosis, we are unquestionably confronting a bacterial disease of a challenging nature. Viral diseases are also highly challenging, however, and are very clearly more challenging to the acquired immune system. They are also often similarly characterised by an insidious capacity for dormancy and latency. With viral disease, as well, we do not have the resort of antibiotic treatment to fall back on, and many of them present a huge challenge to modern medicine as a result. It may be that the nature of some of these newer challenging viral illnesses makes them particularly suitable for judicious small cone moxa treatment.

But the picture is still far from complete. Our next step is to take a hard-headed look at the temperatures at which moxa burns, and consider what effect this may have on the skin and the sub-cutaneous tissue.
.

Moxa and Temperature

Other possible mechanisms of immune response reveal themselves when we look at both the varying temperatures at which moxa burns, and also at its chemical constitution, both of which may have a significant effect on immune response. Moxa contains many chemical components (dependent upon both strain of plant and its source) which might have some sort of impact on the effects of the heat, particularly since some of these are now also known to affect immune response.

With this in mind, Jenny Craig and I designed a set of simple experiments to attempt to clarify some of the statements that have been made across the decades regarding temperatures reached by burning various different moxas.

In the initial experiment, different types of moxa were formed into cones of similar weight and size (approximately 20mm across the base and 20mm height) and burnt on seasoned softwood, for the purpose of comparing relative charring of the wood in terms of colour and depth, as well as measuring the different overall burning periods. No really significant differences in terms of the depth and characteristics of the charring were observable to the naked eye after combustion, although it was clear that the more refined moxa took slightly less time during its "smoking" phase implying that it generally burnt somewhat quicker.

In a second experiment, an infra-red thermometer was used to measure the surface temperatures of 20mm diameter balls of different moxas burnt on the handles of needles. A simple cooking probe thermometer was also used in an attempt to measure the maximum temperature as near as possible to the core of the ball. Slightly conflicting measurements were recorded with each device. The core temperatures were generally less reliable and it was quickly realised that they deserved re-examination with better equipment. With the infra-red thermometer, however, it quickly became clear that ALL the samples burnt at far hotter surface temperatures than the claims made in most of the commercial literature. At their surface, this was generally between 400 and 450° centigrade. It was clear that the more refined the nap, the slightly lower the temperature at which the material burnt although the largest difference was less than 12%, suggesting that the quantitative temperature differences between moxas of varying degrees of refinement might not be of the significance that some of the literature suggests.

Chinese moxa	450°C
Wakakusa ibuki moxa	430°C
Yomei gold mountain ibuki moxa	400°C

It seemed likely that some of these apparently erroneous claims in the literature reflected parts of the mythology of the therapy itself, but they also pointed towards a more general lack of clarity or rigour in some of the science associated with moxa temperature research. A gross example of this occurs in the current commercial literature for a smokeless moxa product where a claim is made that the material burns at a "maximum" temperature of 40°C. This is patently impossible and might just be because of an unfortunate omission of a zero, but requests for confirmation or clarification of this claim have disappointingly been met with a lack of reply. (Surface temperature measurements of this product actually suggested that it burns at around a much less modest 350°C.)

Dr Shimetaro Hara, however, suggested that the optimum heat for direct moxa to exploit its histological effects (examined later) is between 70 and 80°C. His idea was that, at these temperatures particular histological changes might be taking place in the proteins beneath the skin which could have a systemic effect through the body.

Professor Stephen Birch, a modern acumoxa practitioner-researcher, has hypothesised that this potential effect may possibly occur through "hormesis". This is the term used to describe generally favorable biological responses to low exposures to toxins as stressors. A toxin which might promote a hormetic effect thus has the opposite effect in small doses as in large doses.

Hara was investigating moxa under research conditions so patently was not making his claims fancifully. For this low temperature to have been measured, however, certainly with any of the finer grades that we examined, the only conclusion that we could draw was that his results were more dependent upon the relative size of the cone burnt than on the strain of moxa. We speculated that this might be the case because a smaller cone results both in a reduced period of burn with a lower peak of heat, and a larger relative kinetic transfer of heat to the surrounding environment (of both skin and air) with immediate consequent dissipation. For us, this would have to result in a lower maximum temperature at skin surface at the point of burn.

So we attempted to investigate this idea using bi-metallic type K thermocouples (made from chrome and aluminium) to see whether Doctor Hara's data could be reproduced. Various types of thermocouples were used from the most fine and delicate ones to slightly more robust types each of which were hooked up to electronic data-loggers in order to record, in graph form, the real-time temperature curves in intervals of one hundredth of a second, something which had clearly been beyond Dr Hara eighty years ago. Therefore it became possible to monitor the temperature continuously from the time of lighting and to establish not just the maximum temperature, but also the rate of combustion and cooling.

The graph below compares the combustion rates and peak temperatures for 10mg balls of moxa of four different grades. In this instance, the thermocouple was placed in the centre of each ball, the sizes of which were typical of what might be used on the handle of a needle.

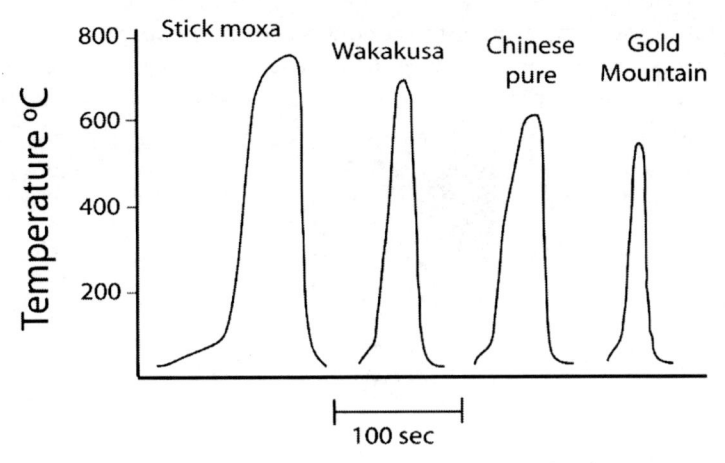

The burning curves of 10mg balls of different grades of moxa.

Four types of moxa were used –

1. "Whole" raw moxa from a moxa stick (typically 100% of original leaf matter)
2. Japanese "wakakusa" moxa processed especially for moxa-on-the-needle-head techniques (approx. 20% of original leaf matter, processed when unmatured)
3. Chinese pure grade moxa (approx. 20% of original leaf matter and also aged)
4. Gold Mountain pure Japanese moxa (approx. 4% of original aged leaf matter).

The "100 second" measurement on the horizontal axis offers graphic indications of the relative length of time that the moxa burnt at any significant temperature, the incrementally purer the moxa the less time there was heat.

The very coarse "whole" moxa taken from inside a Chinese moxa stick burned the slowest and also reached the maximum temperature of over 750°C. More refined Wakakusa moxa also burnt very hot – so it is worth noting that the handle of a needle may also be being heated to above 700°C. Chinese pure grade moxa reached a maximum of 695°C, whilst the purest Japanese moxa had quite easily the shortest burn time with a sharp peak and a maximum of 620°C lasting only a fraction of the time of the others. This last fact may explain why other studies using less sensitive equipment have reported much lower maximum temperatures when measuring combustion of small cones.

To match such measurements as closely as possible to clinical reality, we next tried to adapt our approach, taping the thermocouples to human skin, and then placed varying types of moxa and cone sizes on the tips of the thermocouples. In such a way, it became possible to record the typical actual peak temperature reached at the surface of the skin when moxa is burnt.

The traditional way of measuring moxa cone size is to compare its size in relation to the relative sizes of beans, seeds and threads, but this seemed scientifically too vague for us and is no doubt subject to great variation between practitioners.

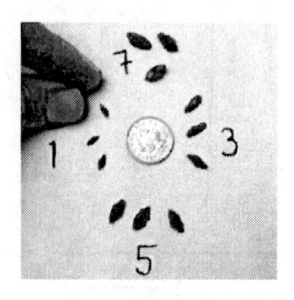

Indications of sizes of moxa cones of different weights (in milligrams). The coin is a UK 5 pence piece.

To try to be more consistent, we used a fine microgram balance and weighed out portions of moxa of 1, 3, 5 and 7mg. These were shaped into loose cones and used as templates for future cone size standardisation. Rice grain size is somewhere around 1 – 2 mg.

The temperatures recorded were somewhat higher than those of Doctor Hara. The most obvious explanation for this was that we were using slightly more sophisticated methods of measurement than were available to Hara in the 1930s. He had no access, for instance, to real-time temperature measurements as recorded by a datalogger. The only way that his temperatures could in fact actually be replicated was by using slightly larger cones and lifting them off as the subject first felt the heat – something which was not the method Hara described, since he was clearly using direct techniques. Since Doctor Hara's theoretical model of the mechanisms of moxibustion are predicated on the relatively low temperature at the base of the cone, however, our findings immediately called into question part of his explanation of the possible mechanisms of moxa treatment.

It was the treatment protocols which we were developing for the Moxafrica project which initially drew us to this field of research. These were distilled from the 20th century Japanese literature on direct moxa, which described tiny cones of 1-2 mg being burned on the skin, very similar to the cone sizes used by Dr Hara. It was important for us to be able to discuss the sorts of temperatures that the skin of potentially immune-compromised patients might be subjected to with some sort of authority, particularly if we seriously intended that our ideas might be accepted by other more orthodox medical practitioners.

To investigate this kind of temperature exposure, the burning curves for 1mg cones of several different types of pure grade Japanese moxa were compared. Burning curves of 15 replicate 1 mg cones of each type were used to calculate average maximum temperatures. In this case a "control" of Wakakusa was used, and this was compared to different grades of aged and refined moxa from Japan. For a simple indication of the general impact of increasing cone size on peak temperatures, we also chose to use 2mg cones of Gold Mountain moxa as well (shown at the bottom of the table). We selected Gold Mountain because it is a refined moxa for use in direct techniques and is also commercially available in western countries from importers outside of Japan.

Statistical analysis by Student T-test showed that the maximum temperatures of the purest grades (Saijo and Gold Mountain) were significantly lower than those of the two coarser grades, Wakakusa and Tokusen. It was also clear when comparing the data for Gold Mountain cones of 1mg, 2mg and 10mg (shown previously) - 189, 269 and 580°C respectively - that maximum temperature is also strongly dependent on cone size.

	Peak temp °C	Time above threshold temperatures (sec)			
		40°C	50°C	100°C	200°C
Wakakusa 1mg	247	14.0	10.7	5.2	1.8
Tokusen 1mg	235	11.9	8.8	4.1	1.0
Tenkyu 1mg	219	13.2	9.5	4.0	0.9
Saijo 1mg	186	11.6	8.4	3.3	0.3
Gold Mtn 1mg	189	9.3	6.9	3.0	0.2
Gold Mtn 2mg	269				

Mean values of 15 replicate cones showing analysis of burning curves

Also shown in the above table is a further analysis of the same 1mg cones to show the duration of time the temperature at cone base remained above certain thresholds. Student T-tests again revealed significant differences between moxa types especially at the lower temperatures – thus the Wakakusa cones stayed above 40°C for almost 5 seconds longer and above 50°C about 4 seconds longer than Gold Mountain cones. As we shall discuss later, this could have more physiological significance than the very briefly attained maximum temperatures.

The above measurements were taken under standardised draught-free conditions. In practice many environmental conditions such as skin moisture, humidity and air movement might be expected to affect the temperature, and cone sizes will be subject to some variation in density depending on practitioner skill. It was found that doubling the cone weight (using Gold Mountain) had a highly significant effect on heat production, raising the average temperature by 80°C, clearly showing the importance of standardising cone size if a consistent dosage of heat is intended. However, it is also possible that part of this effect was due to the larger cones being more densely rolled. Hitoshi Yamashita conducted a thorough study in 1996 of the influence of cone weight, shape and density on combustion temperatures[206]. Using 1–4mg cones he and his colleagues concluded that density was the most important factor in determining the rate of combustion and the duration of time above 45°C. The late Toshio Yanagishita, former president of the Toyohari Association in Japan, was similarly explicit that density is fundamental to effect, and made his assistants practise assiduously by burning cones on paper and comparing burn and tar residues.

We have found that using small rolling boards whilst applying minimal pressure to prepare the moxa creates worm like lengths of moxa. This is easily the simplest and most efficient method to ensure multiple cones of equal base diameter as well as of minimal density.

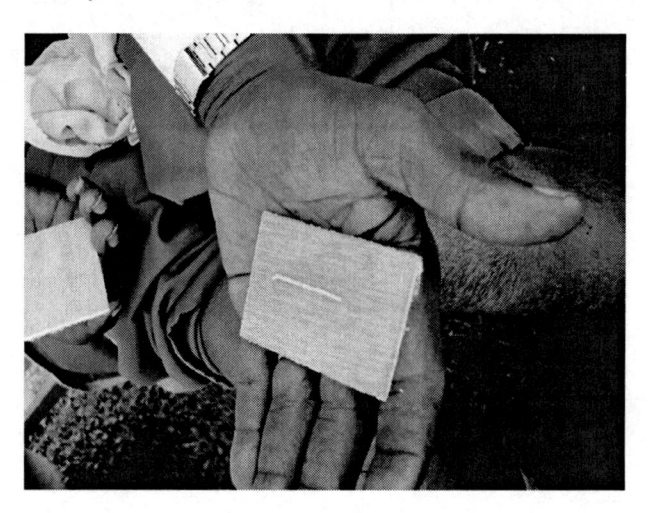

Of course, there are also various ways of modifying technique to control the amount of heat as has been discussed earlier, and these need further elucidation.

The graph immediately following, for instance, shows how placing a bamboo tube over three burning cones (dotted lines) slowed down the rate of combustion and reduced the maximum temperature compared with normal unprotected cones (unbroken lines).

---

[206] Yamashita H & Egawa M 1996 "A measurement of direct moxibustion temperature" (in Japanese) Journal of the JSAM; 45;3:203-7.

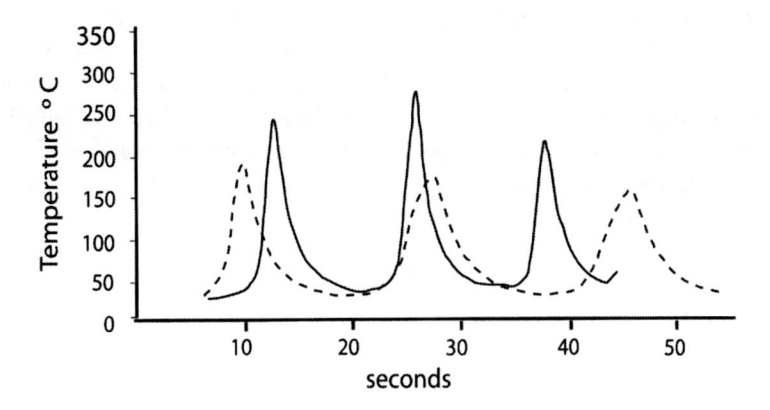

A passage from *Lingshu* 73 mentions the practice of blowing on the cones:

> "When the *qi* is full, disperse; when hollow, tonify. When using fire to tonify, do not blow on the fire. In a moment it will go out by itself. When using fire to disperse, quickly blow on the fire to propagate the action of the mugwort, then extinguish the fire."

As discussed in Part 3 the Branches, this text has been interpreted quite widely in the modern era to suggest that hotter moxa is more dispersive (because blowing on moxa would be expected to make it hotter), whilst in contrast warm moxa is more tonifying.

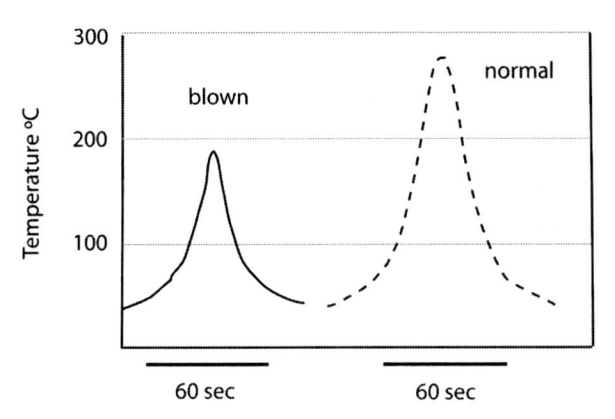

The effect of blowing on 2mg moxa cones (average curves for five cones)

It was simply not possible for us to confirm the idea that blowing makes moxa hotter; in fact, more to the contrary, it was found that cones burned faster when blown on, and maximum temperatures *at the base of the cones* were significantly ($P<0.01$; Students T-test) lower than cones burned in still air. This revelation is potentially quite troubling, since it serves to challenge some quite fundamental ideas which are current in moxa literature. Unfortunately, we could draw no useful conclusions from this anomaly.

Experiments with finger cowling were also tried as a means to alter the rate of burning, but results were inconsistent. Sometimes the cowling reduced burn time and temperature (as the cone is extinguished due to lack of oxygen), but sometimes it increased the heat, perhaps by forming a tunnel through which a draught of air could flow, feeding the combustion. It can be concluded from this that the effects from cowling may, in practice, be quite variable and are clearly dependent upon consistent technique.

Moxa on Skin

It was still not possible to determine, however, what temperature was actually being reached at the skin surface with direct moxa treatment. Up to this point investigations had focused just on the temperatures found at the centre of a burning ball of moxa, or at the base of a 1mg cone. These are the *potential* doses of heat, but we knew that the actual temperature of the skin under a burning cone is much lower, due to simple heat dissipation into the tissues.

We found two Japanese papers describing experiments on rodents where thermocouples were used to measure the temperature under moxa cones on the skin surface and in the subcutaneous tissue. One paper found that a single 5mg cone produced a maximum temperature of 65°C on the skin surface, 55°C in subcutaneous tissue and 48°C in the muscle layer[207]. Multiple cones led to an increase in temperature at deeper levels but not on the surface. A more elaborate study examined the effects of applying up to 20 cones and compared sizes of 0.5 to 10mg[208]. This study found that a single 1mg cone (the size of most interest to us) gave a peak temperature of 80°C on the skin surface, which was very close to Dr Hara's stipulated heat of 70-80°C. This same cone size also produced a temperature of 40°C in subcutaneous tissue. Peak temperatures, however, increased rapidly as more cones were added, but after about 5 cones there was no further increase, due to the effects of heat dissipation. Using these 1mg cones the subcutaneous temperature in fact never rose above 45°C, even after adding up to 20 cones. However, this subcutaneous temperature was maintained between successive burns, so that a dose of 10 x 1mg cones on the same point gave a longer period of sustained temperature rise than a single 10mg cone.

We then wondered whether the fact that a constant temperature of around 45° was being maintained in a multi-cone treatment might be significant and whether this degree and duration of temperature could be indicated specifically for certain

---

[207] Sugata R, Tohya K, Ohnishi M, Kuroiwa K, Toda S, Kimura M. 1988 "A study on temperature changes in vivo with moxibustion" (in Japanese)

[208] Aizawa S, Ohtsuki A, Usami K, Sakamoto K. 1985 "Effect of moxibustion on skin tissue" (in Japanese)

desired effects from the moxa – i.e. to maximise effect when moxa is burnt over indurations or perhaps even to invoke an immune response.

According to these papers, increasing the cone size to 2mg or more caused higher surface temperatures but this did not seem to proportionally increase subcutaneous temperatures. Their authors logically suggested that this was due to increased blood flow in the dermal layer as blood vessels dilated in response to the heat. This, of course, may also be an important part of the response mechanism. It also suggests that (if the temperature at the subcutaneous level is assumed to be the most important part of the effect of direct moxa) the use of larger cones with higher risk of trauma at skin level is unnecessary.

No similar experiments have been carried out on humans to our knowledge. However, it was interesting for us to try to confirm some of these observations using (dead) chicken flesh. Three 1mg cones peaking at 200°C raised the skin surface from 25°C to 45°C but no increase at all was detected 2mm below the surface, demonstrating a large effect of heat dissipation from the surface. Using bigger cones (3mg) subcutaneous temperature did rise to 36°C with a long retention time. Of course, in this dead tissue there would be no warm blood flow to aid the dissipation of heat. It should also be noted that the base temperature of the chicken (25°) was lower than what would be the normal temperature of human skin.

With the benefit of this data we returned to the thorny question of wondering exactly how moxa might work. What might actually happen on the skin surface, just beneath it, and within the whole body when small cone moxas are being burnt therapeutically?

Body Temperature and Immune Function

Within the world of biomedicine, some of the clinical ideas which emerge within this particular section may well be considered a little controversial, and should therefore naturally be treated with caution. Nevertheless, from the perspective of the heat-generating mechanisms of moxa, they are of definite interest. They are influenced by the published studies of Professor Toru Abo, who we have already encountered while discussing the relationship between immune response and the autonomic nervous system, and of Dr Nobuhiro Yoshimizu, a former Director of Yokohama General Hospital. Both of them choose to challenge some of the accepted methods for treating cancer, a dangerous thing to do since such challenges invite an instinctive backlash from the medical status quo. Both base their theories on body temperature.

Professor Abo suggests that a 1°C drop in body temperature below normal results in:

36% reduction in immune function
12% reduction in basic metabolic function
50% decline in enzyme activity

Both suggest that raising the body's temperature back to normal can rectify many diseases, including improving cancer recovery rates – although it should be noted in the case of cancer that such a suggestion is not intended to preclude the use of the orthodox treatment. Such treatment if used alongside chemotherapy may, in their opinion, mean that lower doses of the toxic treatment can be used, however. But it is particularly in the case of what Dr Yoshimizu refers to as "medical refugees" – patients who have failed conventional cancer treatment – that he really strongly endorses this approach for cancer. In other words, he does not advocate his thermotherapy as an alternative to conventional treatment unless everything else is failing, but rather generally advocates it as a complementary treatment to increase recovery rates and reduce suffering – so perhaps some of the responses from more orthodox medical practitioners to these ideas may be over-reactions.

The normal body temperature of a human is said to be 37°C, although this fluctuates a little during the day. This particular temperature was pegged by a german doctor, Carl Wunderlich, in 1861. He claimed to have taken over a million armpit measurements from 25,000 patients before deciding the figure. The generally accepted "normal" range today is in fact between 36.1° and 37.2°, suggesting that today'saverage may actually be a little lower than Wunderlich's original assessment. Intriguingly, some practising doctors today observe that they see many patients with temperatures beneath the accepted "norm". It may well be that the average human temperature, therefore, has already dropped a little in the last one hundred and forty years.

Yoshimizu is quite clear that, as far as he is concerned, if oral temperature is below 37°, it is in the best interests of health that something is done to raise it – either by life style changes, dietary changes (which he considers to be a main cause of hypothermia) and/or thermotherapy. He claims specifically, for instance, that many cancers activate if the body temperature drops to 35°C. Extensive surveys of his patients have confirmed for him that cancer patients almost always have lower than average body temperatures – although he is far from definitive as to whether this is a cause of the cancer or an effect of it.

Linking up with those ideas that we have already identified which lie behind Professor Abo's work, we also can recognise that body temperature drops when the sympathetic nervous system is dominant, often, of course, because of stress levels. Abo also linked stress with pedisposition to cancer, so it is very tempting to link up the two theories, and consider them both in relation to moxibustion.

We can suggest from this, for instance, that moxa, while it cannot treat cancer, may well be able to play a simple role in helping to raise the average body temperature back to around 37°C, and quite clearly some of the treatments which are described within these pages may serve to do this. One of the simplest ideas, actually, might be to intensively use the basic Korean Hand Therapy moxa treatments discussed at the end of Part 3, and to monitor the response of the body temperature.

But small cone moxa is recognised as stimulating immune response not just raise temperature so we need to further consider what actually happens within the dermis which might promote this effect, and whether there may be other effects apart from that of simple warming. It certainly would seem to be asking an awful lot of the exothermic energy from a 1mg cone to raise the body temperature of a 75kg human being by one or two degrees.

What happens in the skin when it heats up and burns?

Certainly everyone knows that warmth can often relieve pain, and a scientific explanation for this was in fact revealed by research which found that internal heat receptors responding to temperatures over 40°C block the effect of chemical pain messengers[209]. This is perhaps easier to imagine if a relatively large area of the body is heated up, but how much effect could a tiny 1mg moxa cone really have? Studies suggest that when using multiple cone applications to the same point it is possible to maintain a subcutaneous temperature above 40°C for several minutes. We needed to consider the implications of this.

Skin consists of two layers. One is the thin epidermis which is made up of five layers of cells, constantly migrating from the basal layer outwards to the surface where they die and are sloughed off. The other is the dermal layer which is much thicker, containing connective fibres and many kinds of cells: blood vessels, hair follicles, sweat glands, sebaceous glands as well as nerves that transmit sensations such as heat, pain and itching.

Burns can be categorised into first degree which affect only the epidermis and cause redness and pain, and second degree which penetrate the dermis causing pain, redness and oozing blisters. Most direct moxa treatment will barely amount to a minor first degree burn, although repeated burning of even 1mg cones to the skin frequently causes a small blister, and can leave a pale scar which may indicate damage to the pigment layer at the base of the epidermis and dermal injury.

It is well known that severe burns damage the immune system. However there is plenty of available evidence from the research already discussed that small burns from direct moxa can enhance and/or balance various aspects of immune response. Once again, this reminded us of the possible hormetic response

---

[209] King, B.F. 2006 "Heat blocks body's pain signals"
http://news.bbc.co.uk/1/hi/health/5144864.stm. retrieved 10/12/ 2010

suggested to us by Professor Birch arising from Dr Hara's ideas about denatured proteins from small cone moxa trauma.

What Dr Hara could not have known in the 1930s is that any sudden temperature increase in the skin triggers the production of Heat Shock Proteins (HSPs) which are able to protect other proteins from heat damage. They can also act as antigens, activating specialised dendritic cells in the epidermis. These serve as messengers between the body tissues and the immune system, migrating to local lymph nodes, where they activate lymphocytes. HSPs are also thought to have cardiovascular effects, promoting vascular dilation and thus increasing local blood flow. So, even by just heating a small area of epidermal cells to a non-physiological temperature (>40°C) we can begin to see how small cone moxa could possibly have wider effects on the whole body.

As heat penetrates deeper into the dermis it will stimulate sensory nerve cells directly. Special proteins known as Transient Receptor Potential (TRP) channels within the cell membranes serve as versatile sensors that allow individual cells and entire organisms to detect changes in their environment. This is of potentially enormous significance to a better understanding of the mechanisms of moxibustion, since some TRPs are known to be sensitive to particular temperature thresholds – for example TRPV3 responds to innocuous warm temperatures (24°C to 39°C), whilst TRPV1 triggers a response to temperatures above 42°C, which causes us to experience a hot sensation. TRPV2 is activated by temperatures above 52°C resulting in a sensation of painful heat. These reactions trigger complex biochemical pathways involving both the nervous and immune systems, which might be important to a better understanding of moxa treatment.

These TRP thresholds are particularly interesting in relation to our moxa temperature data and suggest that the length of time that tissue is maintained over 42° but under 52°C may be most important (activating TRPV1). Could it be that a larger cone, causing painful heat and activating TRPV2 gives rise to quite different effects in the body compared with a milder heat only triggering TRPV1 or TRPV3? And, if this is the case, might this also help explain some of the accepted temperature-dependent "tonifying" and "dispersive" effects which may be valid to some degree but may have been misconstrued from the passage in *Lingshu* 73?

When using larger cones, such as "snatch" heat perception moxa taught in some traditions when bean size cones are burnt and then lifted off the skin, it is usual to remove the cone as soon as the patient reports feeling the sensation of heat. Using a thermocouple to measure skin surface temperature under 4mm diameter cones which are typically used for this technique, we found the point of removal to be between 50-60°C at the skin surface. In this case the temperature within the actual skin layers would be highly unlikely to exceed 50°C due to heat dissipation, and the temperature in the tissue below would barely be raised at all.

Some larger cones, such as are used in *chinetsukyu* techniques in some Japanese traditions, may be removed by some practitioners even before the patient feels the heat – as soon as a good pulse change is observed. So a brief investigation using *chinetsukyu* on TB4 whilst monitoring the pulse was carried out and we concluded that a palpable pulse change corresponded with a cone base temperature of 45°C, so skin temperature would hardly have reached the 42°C threshold and might at best only be activating TRPV3.

The Additional Impact of Chemical Components on Immune Response

Pure moxa contains a complex mixture of natural chemicals as was discussed at the end of Part 2 the Stalk. It will be recalled that an analysis of *Artemisia princeps* leaves (a premium strain of mugwort used for refined moxa in Japan), using two methods of chemical extraction, identified 192 volatile substances[210]. The most abundant were borneol, cineole, artemisia acetate and alpha thujone. It is not known how many of these 192 substances are lost during the processing and ageing of moxa, but the strong fragrance of pure grade moxa such as *Ibuki* Gold Mountain is said to be evidence of its remaining high cineole content.

Borneol and cineole belong to a large and varied group of chemicals called monoterpenoids, which form the basis of essential oils derived from plants, and are used in many traditional herbal formulae. Borneol, closely related to camphor, has anti-inflammatory and antiseptic properties, and has many uses when applied topically, such as to treat burns, skin diseases, rheumatism and haemorrhoids[211]. Cineole (also called eucalyptol) is a common ingredient in mouthwashes and cough suppressants. Its anti-inflammatory action controls mucus and when applied to the skin it reduces pain and inflammation.

Among the less volatile components of moxa are tannins. These are classified as polyphenols – complex organic molecules that have known antioxidant properties. Low volatility alkanes (paraffins) are also important constituents, particularly in their influence on the combustion qualities of moxa. Japanese research has revealed that during the refining process of moxa there is a significant decrease in tannin content, whilst the amount of the major alkane, heptatriacontane, remained much the same[212]. Moxa from which the alkane had been removed burned much

---

[210] Umano K, Hagi Y, Nakahara K, Shoji A, Shibamoto T. 2000 "Volatile chemicals identified in extracts from leaves of Japanese mugwort (*Artemisia princeps*)" Journal of Agricultural Food Chemistry 48(8): 3463 9.

[211] Dharmananda, S. 1998. "Relationships of borneol, Artemisia and moxa" Institute for Traditional Medicine, Portland, Oregon. (Online article) http://www.itmonline.org/arts/borneol.htm retrieved 3/1/2012

[212] Kobayashi K. 1988. "Organic components of moxa" American Journal of Chinese Medicine. 16:179-85.

more slowly, so variations in the ratio between the tannin and heptatriacontane (alkane) may help to explain differences in the rate and temperature of combustion of different moxa grades, as well as some of the attributed therapeutic effects.

It is highly likely that, in addition to affecting the combustion properties of moxa, some of these chemical constituents have some direct effects on the body if they are absorbed into the skin, some of which might support or complement the initial effects of the heat from the moxa. We might expect their penetration into the tissues to be determined by factors such as the quality of moxa, mass and basal area of the cone, burning temperature and the degree of tissue damage from heat.

Another factor that we have already discussed is how we can vary the dosage when using multiple direct moxa cones if we remove the ash each time or if we burn the next cone on top of the existing ash. In the latter case the patient will feel less heat (which, of course, may or may not be desirable depending upon intended response), but we can also suggest that this procedure will allow more of the tar components to penetrate the skin. In many moxa techniques we are advised that heat/pain must be felt in order for the treatment to be effective (although it has to be said that there are differences of opinion on this issue). This idea is certainly supported by some of the research discussed above. Some patients, however, are much less sensitive to the heat from direct moxa than others, and so may need more or larger cones, providing a higher dosage of chemicals. Indeed, some locations on patients' bodies appear almost thermoceptively inert, sometimes possibly pathologically so. We began to suspect that the relative importance of heat versus chemical effect is far more significant than the amount of available research on the subject suggests, and so we began further research to uncover possible circumstantial evidence that the chemical actions of moxa at the site of the burn may even be critical for some effects.

Most of the studies investigating the effects of moxa chemicals have been carried out *in vitro* (using cell cultures on which individual chemicals are tested under carefully controlled conditions). Whilst these studies provide information about the potential effects of chemicals on biochemical processes in the body, they are far removed from the real situation of direct moxa application on skin, and the results cannot be extrapolated to predict tissue or whole body responses to moxa. However, some information about tissue penetration of moxa chemicals was provided by Professor Tohya and his colleagues from Kansai College of Oriental Medicine. Professor Tohya has specific interest in moxa's possible mechanisms concerning immune response. His team burned 0.5mg cones on rats for 20 consecutive days and observed the changes in the skin cells[213]. After 3 days they

---

[213] Tohya K, Urabe S, Igarashi J, Tomura T, Take A, Kimura M. 2000. "Appearance of peculiar vessels with immunological features of high endothelial venules in the dermis of moxibustion-stimulated rat skin"Am.J.Chin. Med. 28:425-433.

noticed an influx of inflammatory cells into the surrounding dermis, although only the epidermis appeared to be damaged by heat. After 20 days there were changes in the blood vessel walls of the dermis that allowed further infiltration of lymphocytes into the area. However, when they used moxa that had been treated with alcohol in order to remove the major components of the moxa tar, these effects simply did not occur. They therefore hypothesised that moxa chemicals permeating the skin were able to stimulate cell growth in the blood vessels and somehow act as attractants for migrating immune cells into the area. In a later study using similar methods, these same authors observed enhancement of the immune cells in regional lymph nodes after moxa treatment, but again, not when the moxa had been alcohol treated.

Analyses of biochemical components of moxa and demonstrations of their antioxidant and anti-inflammatory qualities have been reported by several groups[214]. In particular, caffeetannins have been confirmed as being present in high concentrations in pure grade moxa (and these can also be removed by prolonged soaking of the moxa in alcohol, supporting the ideas of Professor Tohya and his team). Caffeetannins are recognised antioxidants and free radical scavengers; it is likely that these compounds, as well as affecting the combustion temperature of moxa, are able to have some biochemical impact as they penetrate the skin.

But it was in connection with the Transient Receptor Potentials (TRPs) discussed above regarding their being triggered by specific temperature ranges that a more coherent picture of potential chemical absorption began to emerge.

As discussed, Transient Receptor Potentials are sensory receptors found in skin cells and some sensory nerve cells. They play a vital role in the perception of temperature and other stimuli, but fascinatingly their activation is also known to be involved in certain immune responses, triggering systemic effects on the whole body. In particular, four of these receptors (TRPs) act as molecular thermometers, each being activated by a different temperature threshold. Previously, it was considered how the effect of temperature stimulation by moxa cones might depend on the relative activation of these TRPs, but it was then unexpectedly discovered that, in addition to temperature, TRPs are also receptive to some plant chemicals – indeed, a whole field of pharmacological research is exploring the

---

[214] Aizawa S, Menjo Y, Tohya K, Nakanishi H, Toda S. 2003 "Present research on moxibustion". JJSAM.53(5):601-613 (in Japanese)

[214] Ozaki A, Aizawa S, Toda S, Kumamoto K, Ebara S, Koike T. 2008. "Study on moxibustion: Elucidation of characteristics of moxa" JJSAM 58(1): 32-50 (in Japanese)

potential of these sensing channels as targets for the development of new phytopharmaceutical drugs, particularly with respect to analgesia[215].

Monoterpenoids are amongst the plant derivatives which are known to activate TRPs, as demonstrated in a number of *in vitro* studies. For example, in one study TRPV1 (the receptor that is sensitive to temperatures between 42° and 52°C) was found to be activated by camphor, although repeated applications cause desensitisation, something which may perhaps explain the analgesic action of camphor[216]. This study also found that the effect of camphor on TRPV1 was stronger at a slightly elevated temperature or in the presence of irritant chemicals, suggesting that camphor may be a more effective counter-irritant under conditions of tissue inflammation. These results strongly suggest a synergistic effect of temperature and chemical stimulation on TRPs, which could be very relevant to the use of direct moxa.

TRPV3 operates in the temperature range of 39° – 42° C and is also activated by many monoterpenoids, including the most abundant chemical found in refined moxa – borneol, which was actually shown to be much more effective in this activation than its close relative, camphor[217]. In another study, cineole (the second most abundant chemical found in moxa) was found to sensitise TRPV3 with short term repeated applications, but long term application caused desensitisation, again possibly explaining its analgesic effects[218].

Some interesting links can be made here, which may help explain how moxa may work on the body, although we should remain cautious about doing so. For example, TRPV3, which has been shown to play a key role in the maintenance of healthy skin and hair growth, is strongly activated by borneol, the most abundant chemical in moxa. Both borneol and camphor have long been used in topical treatments for hair loss, and direct moxibustion is also recognised as a local treatment for hair loss by some practitioners. Another example links moxa use with vasodilation, and as discussed elsewhere moxa has been indicated widely for treatment of hypertension. Carvacrol, isolated from oregano plants (but also

---

[215] Vriens J, Nilius B, Vennekens E. 2008. "Herbal compounds and toxins modulating TRP channels" Curr. Neuropharmacol.6 (1): 79-96.

[216] Xu H, Blair NT, Clapham DE. 2005. "Camphor activates and strongly desensitises the Transient Receptor Potential Vallinoid subtype 1 channel in a vallinoid-independent Mechanism". J. Neurosci 25 (39): 8924 – 8937.

[217] Vogt-Eisele AK, Weber K, Sherkheli MA, Gisselmann G, Hatt H. 2007."Monoterpenoid agonists of TRPV3". Br J Pharmacol 151(4):530-540

[218] Sherkheli MA, Benecke H, Doerner JF, Kletke O, Vogt-Eisele AK, Gisselmann G, Hatt H. 2009 "Monoterpenoids induce agonist –specific desensitisation of TRPV3 ion channels" J Pharm Pharm Sci. 12(1): 116-128

found in moxa), has been found to relax arteries and cause vasodilation by activating TRPV3 in artery walls[219].

In contrast, TRPV1 is activated by capsaicin (from hot chilli peppers) and extracts of ginger, which may be an important aspect of the mechanism of action of these natural substances in the traditional treatment of more systemic conditions such as gastric problems and arthritis. This same response (or one like it) might be involved in local moxa treatment near inflamed arthritic joints. One study found that exposure to ginger extract promoted adrenaline secretion via the activation of TRPV1 in rats[220]. This finding might suggest that the practice of indirectly burning moxa cones on slices of ginger on the skin may actually stimulate TRPV1 and thereby directly affect the neuroendocrine system, even if the subcutaneous temperature does not reach the 42°C threshold. The overall effect on the body, however, may be the result of a potentially complex combination of temperature and chemical stimulation.

The overall implications from these speculations are both intriguing and challenging. What seems likely is that, even in the limited area of immune response to moxa, two or more mechanisms may be at work simultaneously and they may even be synergistic. We initially were wondering whether a more coherent and enlightening picture might emerge by cheaply and effectively investigating measurable effects on the balance within the immune system through consideration of Professor Abo's research, but we were now coming to realise that results from this might be compromised by our dawning awareness of a second possible mechanism through Transient Receptor Potential Channels triggered in the skin tissue.

There may, of course, be other factors working synergistically. Despite knowing that there is documentation which claims that moxibustion reduces acidosis, we have yet to address the known impact of acidosis on the immune system, but we can speculate that this may also be part of the bigger picture.

One conclusion which does seem quite reasonable to draw, however, is that, whilst suggestive evidence of immune response from aggressive blistering techniques does quite clearly exist, this approach seems far from necessary. This is something which might open up a more welcome avenue for further research, and may also open up opportunities for more widespread application of direct moxibustion in the clinical environment.

---

[219] Earley S, Gonzales AL, Garcia ZI. 2010 "A dietary agonist of Transient Receptor Potential cation channel V3 elicits endothelium-dependent vasodilation" J.Mol. Pharmacol. 77(4): 612-620

[220] Iwasaki Y, Morita A, Iwasawa T, Kobata K, Sekiwa Y, Morimitsu Y, Kubota K, Watanabe T. 2006 "A nonpungent component of steamed ginger--[10]-shogaol--increases adrenaline secretion via the activation of TRPV1"Nutr Neurosci. 9(3-4):169-78

The Moon over Matsushima

These investigations began simply as an exercise to confirm and perhaps refine some of the accepted dogma concerning the temperatures reached in the use of small cone direct moxa. However, it became clear that it was simply not possible to confirm some of what has become accepted in the literature, and much of what was found has stimulated still more questions which need better answers than those found thus far. There is clearly much ground for further investigation in this fascinating field to help explain much of moxa's self-evident effects, and some of the challenges such research may face will be looked at in Part 5 the Leaves.

Smokey versus Smokeless

We are faced in the West with problems regarding smoke which may not currently face our colleagues in the East, particularly as a result of recent widespread legislation concerning smoke-free working environments. Notwithstanding such legislation, and in spite of patients often expressing their liking of the smell of burnt moxa, a heavy day of *kyutoshin* moxa-on-the-needle-head acupuncture, for instance, leaves one with clothes smelling stale and smokey, and a chest that can feel a little congested.

So the so-called "smokeless" methods may have something going for them.

Generally, smokeless moxa, whether with moxa stick, indirect mini-moxa or needle-moxa, is said to consist of charcoal "impregnated with *artemisia*". We must accept that some *artemisia* is in there somewhere, but how much and in what proportion we can only guess (and exactly what strain of *artemisia* is it?). Can we even assume that it is the main component, and that this is somehow carbonised and compression-moulded into shape? No list of constituent ingredients is listed on any proprietary brand seen to date by the author, and no information has been forthcoming in response to requests. The resultant fumes from a burning smokeless moxa stick are quite acrid, and it has even been suggested that they might contain an unhealthy proportion of carbon-monoxide[221].

Eric Brand, formerly of Blue Poppy Press, has helpfully clarified some of the issues in a recent blog on their website [222]. Having visited the factory of a manufacturer of smokeless moxa in China, his account actually challenges the idea that it is charcoal "impregnated with *artemisia*" at all. He describes it as definitely beingmade purely from mugwort but explains that it is mostly from its stems after the leaves have been removed from the stalks and used for raw moxa floss production. "The process", he wrote, "is similar to that of making charcoal, and one traditional method involves burning the moxa [stalks] in a small stone

---

[221] Gordon Peck 1993 "Moxa smoke and the acupuncturist" Journal of Chinese Medicine no.41

[222] http://www.bluepoppy.com/blog/blogs/blog1.php/moxa-grading retrieved 30/6/11

structure while sealing off the air vents to let it smolder in a low oxygen environment...Once the powdered charcoal has been obtained, it is stored and mixed with water before putting it into a machine not unlike a meat grinder or an industrial version of a play-doh toy. The machine turns the wet charcoal into a long tube of smokeless moxa, which is sliced and then dried on racks."

According to this account, we can at least be assured that the smokeless variety comes from the mugwort plant, although it will almost certainly be chemically different from raw smokey moxa not only because of the changes resulting from the low oxygen burning but also because it comes from a different part of the plant, a part which has none of the important down or nap which is considered the essential component of the floss. We also certainly cannot be completely confident that additives are not introduced in the process, particularly because he tellingly states in his blog that "most facilities outsource the manufacturing of the [moxa] charcoal".

This product certainly provides controlled heat – but is it as good as the real thing? My own subjective view is that it is not, but with indirect techniques it may be preferable to use it, either to protect the patient or the practitioner from irritants in the smoke. No-one has suggested that any of the components of "normal" moxa smoke are particularly noxious or carcinogenic, although when adulterated with *xiong huang* (realgar), as has been common in moxa sticks in the past, serious questions might arise. (Realgar is poisonous, and is added, it can be assumed to help keep moxa poles alight).

But whether adulterated or not, smoke is smoke.

"The risks of exposure to moxa smoke are probably similar to that for any other smoke, and total exposure time, particularly when it involves prolonged exposure, is the key concern. Occasional use of ordinary moxa would be associated with low risk, while routine exposure to moxa smoke during much of the day would be a moderate risk. Therefore, venting or filtering is an appropriate step when moxa is done regularly. There is no evidence that moxa smoke contains any unusually harmful substances[223]."

Recent research directed and funded by the British Acupuncture Council of the UK but carried out in the US indicates that the risks from moxa smoke are actually minimal[224]. In fact, in light of this research perhaps the most reasonable

---

[223] Subhuti Dharmananda 2004 "Moxibustion: Practical Considerations for Modern Use of an Ancient Technique" http://www.itmonline.org/arts/moxibustion.htm retrieved 3/1/2010.

[224] Wheeler J, Coppock B, Chen C 2009 "Does the burning of moxa (*Artemisia vulgaris*) in traditional Chinese medicine constitute a health hazard?" Acupunct Med **27**:1 16-20

cause for concern remains for the so-called "smokeless" products because unfortunately they were not included in this investigation.

Some fascinating, if rather heartless, animal research has been carried out in Brazil which supports the view that "smokey" may actually be best[225]. Three groups of rats with indomethacin-induced gastric lesions were respectively treated with indirect moxibustion using raw moxa, "*Artemisia vulgaris* charcoal" (i.e. smokeless moxa-stick), with a tobacco cigar, and with heated water pads at Ren12 (*Zhongwan*) St25 (*Tianshu*), and St36 (*Zuzanli*). The raw moxa was deemed by the researchers to be "significantly more effective". Other Chinese research, however, takes the opposite view. It may, of course, be that in Brazil the charcoal moxa was applied at a lower temperature because of relative distances of the lit ends of the sticks from the skin or because of an uncalculated difference in thermal output, and this alone might explain the result. More complex differences relating to different profiles of infra-red emission may also account for the result – a topic which will be addressed shortly in further depth.

Some other intriguing research from Shanghai, in fact, has attempted to compare the intensity of infra-red radiation emitted from (among other things) the lit ends of a traditional moxa stick, a smokeless moxa stick and a cigarette.

Material	*Intensity of radiation (mV)*	*Peak wavelength (μm)*
Traditional moxa pole	43,300	3.5
Smokeless moxa stick	31	7
Cigarette	37	3.5
Moxa on aconite	681	8
Moxa on ginger	520	7.5
Moxa on garlic	595	7.5
Moxa on cucumber	274	5
Moxa on carrot	51	5
LI4 (skin)	20	7.5

Chart showing the relative intensities of radiation and the peak wavelengths of each material studied by the Shanghai team

The results are astonishing and actually quite difficult to credit: the moxa stick, according to this research, emits a thousand times more infra-red radiation than the smokeless moxa (which is even outdone in turn by the lowly cigarette end).

Infra-red emission intensity directly relates to temperature so that, if the principle effect being looked for is simply from emissivity and intensity of heat (which is not necessarily the case, of course), then the smokeless moxa might seem to have

---

[225] Freire et al 2005 "Effect of moxibustion at acupoints Ren-12, St25 and St36 in the prevention of gastric lesions induced by indomethacin in wistar rats" Journal of Digestive Diseases and Sciences. Vol 50, Number 2

little going for it, and the Brazilian research is vindicated. Simply bringing the smokeless moxa pole closer to the acupoints on the rats in order to have allowed for this difference, however, might have produced a different result.

This dilemma takes us back to currently unanswered questions about the combinatory effects of the actions of moxibustion – the heat, the potential absorption through the skin of specific biochemicals, the secondary effect of moxa smoke inhalation, and the possible "vibrational" or other effects from the plant material itself.

A relatively unrecognised use of burning raw moxa in China is its apparent ability to reduce bacterial count and inhibit viruses in kindergartens and nurseries, no doubt as a result of the anti-bacterial properties of some of its constituents. It is said to have been routinely used in Chinese hospitals, for instance, for this purpose in the past. Claims have also been made of a reduction in the transmission of all common childhood diseases by routine burning of mugwort incense. If this is true, there has to be some possibility of complementary effects to general acumoxa treatment from the smoke created in the treatment room if raw moxa is used.

Certainly, after I have treated a patient whom I consider to have been potentially infectious, I have no hesitation in floating a large chunk of moxa wool in a saucer of water and lighting it, then leaving the room for it to burn itself out before admitting and attending to the next patient. In fact, if I have treated a patient whom I consider to be, in any real sense, seriously emotionally disturbed, I find myself sometimes choosing to do the same - subconsciously, perhaps, repeating the older superstitions of using moxa smoke to dispel evil spirits.

The Possible Mechanisms with Indirect Techniques

This is an intriguing area that begs more than a little discussion, if only because there is so little written about it.

If a moxa stick is used, as it is most commonly with indirect techniques, we can assume that there may be clear differences in effect, dependent upon the method of application. The most common ways are by "sparrow-pecking" (bringing the tip of the pole repetitively close to the point to warm it), holding the pole statically over the point at a distance, or quite literally waving it around to warm an area. The Brazilian research referred to in the last section[226] compared different heating protocols at differing temperatures (60°C at skin compared with 45°C). The higher

---

[226] Freire et al 2005 "Effect of moxibustion at acupoints Ren-12, St25 and St36 in the prevention of gastric lesions induced by indomethacin in wistar rats" Journal of Digestive Diseases and Sciences. Vol 50, Number 2

temperature was significantly more efficient in preventing artificially triggered gastric lesions. In terms of the possible triggering of TVRP response, this may be significant, and at the very least this suggests that the temperature produced by the indirect technique at the skin surface may be of importance.

We touched earlier on the probability that the biochemical components of mugwort might add some effects to the localised heat. Logically, these seem less likely with a less direct technique, but modern sources nevertheless frequently invoke mugwort's bitter and acrid properties as playing specific roles in penetrating the channels and drying cold-damp or resolving damp-heat. Where such factors may well come into play with indirect moxibustion use, however, is when other materials are placed between the mugwort and the skin. Traditionally these have been slices of garlic, slices of ginger, *fuzi* aconite cake (monkshood), salt, miso paste, tangerine peel, loquat leaf. Each are utilised from different rationales, based on the perceived properties of the materials themselves. Sources also repeatedly advocate the puncturing of the intermediary material so that the moxa smoke will also permeate to the skin, so there are clear implicit suggestions of quite complex chemical mechanisms at work with these techniques. Pharmacological effects from the intermediary substances have definitely, for instance, been reported in Japan[227].

The same research from Shanghai which compared infra-red intensities of moxa and charcoal moxa has additionally suggested that some fascinating and complex interactions may be taking place when these particular indirect techniques are utilised. The researchers used multi-spectral imaging technology, something more normally reserved for space research, and measured the spectra of infra-red radiation emitted from various moxa samples in addition to the relative intensities described above. Their findings scream out for further investigation, since they imply that a complementary or completely discrete mechanism to some of the serological ones discussed above may well be taking place when these indirect intermediary methods are applied.

Infra-red is a form of wave energy which comprises wavelengths from 0.7μm up to 1000μm (microns). Any object in the universe above absolute zero in temperature emits some form of infra-red radiation. Similar to general white light which is a composite of varying wavelengths of visible light energy, any sample of infra-red radiation will be composed of a unique composite of varying wavelengths of infra-red energy making up a whole. A multi-spectrum measurement graphically represents the relative densities of the various wavelengths in the particular emission being tested. With these densities plotted in graph form, each source provides individual visually identifiable patterns.

---

[227] "Research on Indirect Moxibustion" 1988 Journal of Japan Society of Acupuncture and Moxibustion; 38 (4): 420-422.

Far Infra-Red (FIR) is variously defined – often as consisting of wavelengths of more than 3μm. Medical research into this field of interest was stimulated by efforts to obviate health problems for astronauts exposed to weightlessness for long periods. The recorded negative responses from weightlessness deserve listing: they include immune-deficiency, sluggish wound healing, muscle and bone atrophy, pituitary insufficiency and hormone imbalances. The initial NASA experiments involved plant experiments which showed that plant cells exposed to particular wavelengths of infra-red grew as much as 200% faster than cells not exposed. Subsequent research has suggested that wavelengths of between 4 and 14μm have particularly beneficial effects on human cells, with recorded benefits in the treatment of diabetic skin ulcers. It is understood that FIR penetrates deeply into tissue with a very uniform warming effect, and it has even been widely claimed by the infra-red sauna industry that tissues needing a boost in input selectively absorb the energy by a process of "resonance absorption" although this may well be challengeable. It is also suggested that this helps reduce body acidity by expanding capillaries, and increasing the flow of both blood and lymph.

The Shanghai team measured the spectra of infra-red radiation emitted when raw moxa from a moxa stick was burnt over three different intermediary materials under controlled conditions. The materials they chose were those most often used in traditional practice – on aconite, ginger and garlic. The results were compared with each other.

These were then compared to the similarly measured spectra emitted from moxa burnt over slices of cucumber and carrot as controls. These findings in turn were then (rather imaginatively) compared to the spectrum of infra-red emitted from a typical acupoint location (LI4 *hegu* was used), since, of course, infra-red radiation is also continuously naturally emitted from human skin. (In fact they compared the emission at LI4 to other skin surface and found no major differences, so no particular significance need be attributed to the selection of this point).

The initial resulting comparisons provide us with provocative food for thought – because the profiles of the graphs for moxa burnt over each of the three traditional sample materials (ginger, garlic and aconite) reveal themselves to be almost identical. In stark contrast, the control samples of carrot and cucumber, and indeed of the raw moxa stick as we will shortly see, bear no resemblance to them at all. These general spectral profiles are shown above in Graph 1.

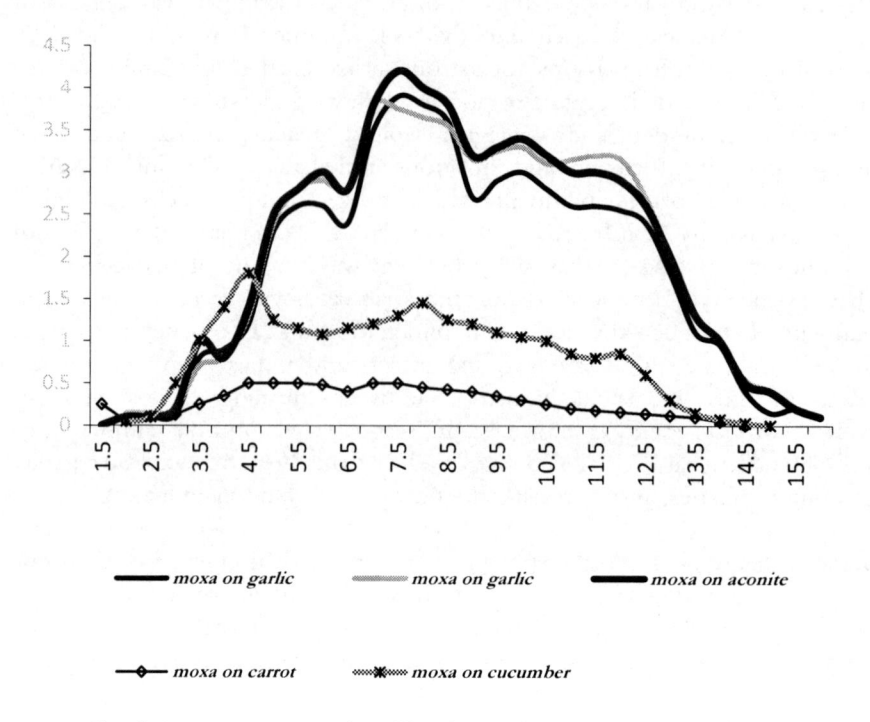

*Graph 1 comparing spectral profiles of moxa burnt on five intermediary materials
(The figures across the base are in microns; the vertical axis have been unified to a relative value)*

Such similarities in profile might well account for the selection of these particular traditional materials based on perceived responses across the centuries. But what was even more remarkable is shown in Graph 2. This was that these particular spectral profiles (what can best be described as profile fingerprints) when moxa was burnt on ginger, garlic and aconite almost exactly also matched the spectral profile which revealed itself when infra-red emitted from the surface of human skin at LI4 *Hegu* was also analysed and mathematically unified. The intensities of the emissions, of course, are dramatically different, but the profiles are uncannily similar.

It should additionally be noted that the spectrum recorded spreads between 1.5 and 16μm, but that all the peaks occur within the 4 to 14μm range that have been identified as the "vital range" of infra-red radiation for cell health.

Indeed the peak lay right in the middle of this range.

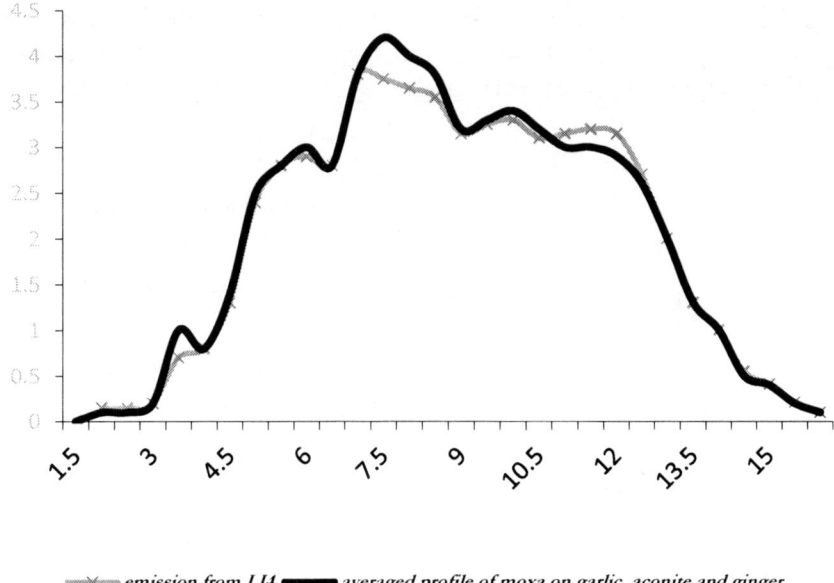

[Graph: x-axis 1.5 to 15, y-axis 0 to 4.5]

—x— emission from LI4   —■— averaged profile of moxa on garlic, aconite and ginger

Graph 2 showing the almost identical unified graphic spectral profiles of infra-red emitted through human skin, and of moxa on garlic, aconite and ginger.

The quantity of radiation is hugely different, but the relative ratio of wavelengths is almost identical, peaking at 7.5μm[228].

The hypothesis proposed by the researchers from this finding is that moxa burnt over these intermediary materials, because of an almost identical profile to the radiation emitted from the body itself, might create some type of sympathetic vibration in the organic molecules around and under the moxibustion site because of its easy absorption.

Any molecule is known to have single or multiple modes of oscillation. A sympathetic vibration may sometimes lead to a change in dipole in a molecule which, in itself, may alter ionic composition resulting in absorption or release of photons. Most organic molecules in the body consist of ones which are either positively or negatively charged, and the predominance of some of these are associated with both good and/or ill health. The tentative suggestion which arises from this study, therefore, is that the effect of moxa smouldering on these intermediary materials might promote a sympathetic vibration in local molecules in the tissue beneath which might in turn lead to changes in dipoles which might

---

[228] In order to show the differences in infrared radiation between the four different sources within the same figure, a complex mathematical formula was utilised (ej=xj x n/Σn i_1, j=1,2,3,…) in order to unify the data.

help correct metabolic dysfunction and pathology[229]. As shown in the graph below, however, the therapeutic effect of a moxa stick, whether smokeless or smokey, however, would not be due to such a vibration, but would rather be simply due to its potent infrared radiation.

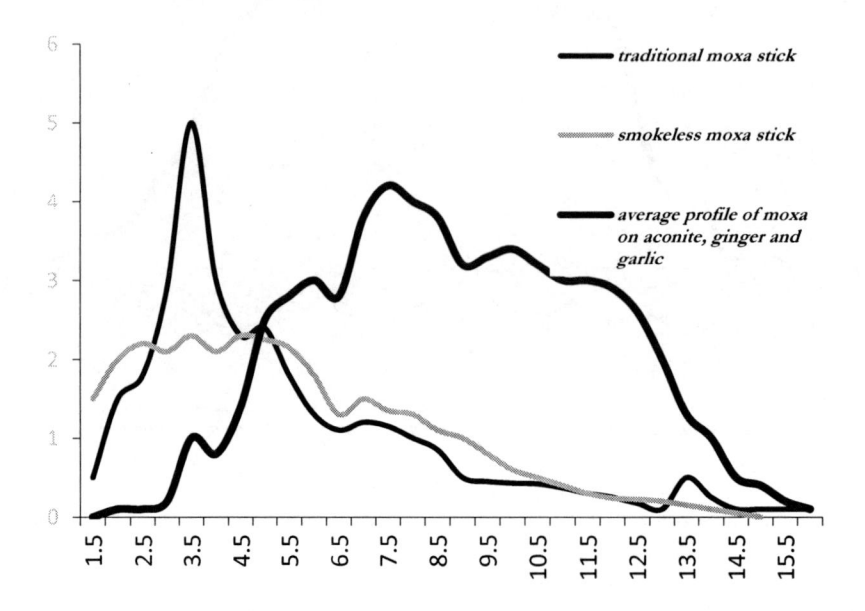

Graph 3 showing the significant unified differences between both profiles and emissions between a traditional moxa stick, a smokeless moxa stick, and moxa burnt on traditional materials.

Frankly, this is a huge assumption to make from the data available, but the similarities in some of the profiles in Graphs 1 and 2 are so strikingly similar that further research should surely be undertaken to look at this in more detail.

Certainly, when the wavelength range of a source of infrared radiation is so similar to that of the infrared radiation emitted from the body, it seems reasonable to suggest that body metabolism may, in some way, be affected. Elsewhere it has been previously suggested that moxibustion might induce a sympathetic vibration of molecules which may help to correct metabolic dysfunction and pathological conditions[230]. This study certainly would suggest how this might happen. The

---

[229] Ma J 1998 "Effect of middle-far infra-red electrical-magnetic irradiation on biochemical reaction" Ziran Zashi 21(2):85-8

[230] Yang H, Liuy T-Y 1996."Preliminary study on biophysics mechansims of moxibustion therapy." Chinese Acupuncture and Moxibustion 16(10):17-8

questions which arise from this research, in fact, are practically limitless, with enormous therapeutic implications as well.

The moxa (whether stick moxa or raw moxa) used in this research all came from the same source to maintain quality of control. It is interesting to note that the frequency at which this raw moxa peaked (around 3.5 μm) is similar to the frequency of infra-red radiation which is most transmissible through air..This clearly may be an advantage in the application of the moxa stick indirectly in the air above the skin, particularly given its relatively potent infrared radiation

In contrast, the higher frequency elicited by the use of the traditional intermediary materials (at around 7.5 μm) is similar to frequencies of infra-red radiation which conversely are *least* transmissible in air. Since the materials, of course, are placed directly on the skin, this implies no adverse efficiency in the transmission of the energy. It does, however, suggest that in the cases where the spectrum of infra-red radiation is so similar to that which is transmitted through or emitted from human tissue, the possibility exists that this "familiar" profile might find itself allow the more transmissible infra-red to pass deeperinto the connective tissue, a little like the interaction between a key and a lock.

We can recall that research has suggested that wavelengths of between 4 and 14μm have particularly beneficial effects on human cells. The peak for the traditional moxa stick actually falls just outside this waveband. The peak for a smokeless moxa stick does fall within this range, however, and it will be quickly recognised that its total profile presents no similarity at all to any of the startling similarities mentioned above so would also be unlikely to induce any sort of vibrational response.

Since it is almost certain from the report that the moxa used was not aged in the traditional fashion, but in contrast was more "raw" (fresher and relatively unprocessed) it begs the question as to what frequencies aged and refined moxa may burn at. It is fairly safe to assume that the infra-red "profile" of aged moxa will be different to the moxa used in the research (certainly the intensity may be significantly reduced).

It would clearly be rash to conclude too much from the above or to extrapolate these propositions of effect to aged moxa when used alone, or indeed to more aged or refined moxa samples on the same intermediary materials since significant variables would have been introduced. The question arises, however, (particularly in view of the whole body photonic response provoked from the mildest possible *chinetsukyu* aged moxa application to TB4 & TB5 which we will come to in the next section) whether the infra-red profile may be of major significance to response in some methods of moxibustion, particularly since the process of ageing moxa goes right back to its earliest recorded references as shown in Part 1 and indeed possibly to its very pictographic etymology.

Of additional interest in this research is the fact that no differentiation at all is made in this study between these respective traditional intermediary materials, and yet in the literature, of course, there are clearly identifiable differences of individual actions.

Moxa and the Channel Pathways (or Photonic Release)

In 2005 some research was published intimating that the holy grail of acumoxa research, the demonstrative proof of the existence of the *jingluo* channels, had been revealed[231]. Indirect stimulation using moxa (or "similar light stimulation") at the 3-5 micron infrared wavelength spectrum typical of a moxa stick revealed channels of light appearing on the body when photographed with a biophotonic camera. This clearly seemed to imply something not only about the energetics of the human body, but also about the property of moxa.

Unfortunately it appears that the research has been difficult to replicate[232] (something which seems to be a common characteristic of the quest for proof of the meridian system).

But some secondary research to this, currently unpublished, using the same camera equipment and using refined moxa, may have produced some possibly even more fascinating results amounting to recordable whole-body effects resulting from the lightest stimulation by moxibustion. The Inoue-style tonifying "*chinetsukyu*" moxa technique was used, consisting of large loosely formed cones of aged moxa burnt only until the merest hint of warmth was felt. These were burnt on principle key acupoints, reportedly on TB4 and TB5. The biophotonic camera in this instant revealed, not the lines of light in the earlier research, but an unexpected whole body effect from this tiny heat stimulation[233]. The camera captured an instantaneous release of photons across the body.

Since this is an emission of energy, initially this might suggest that the body is losing something energetic in response to the slight stimulation from the moxa, something which would seem counter to the idea that moxibustion gives some type of energetic sustenance to the whole system. But if the photonic emission might be a sign of a general ionic discharge reflective of a rebalancing response in

---

[231] Schlebusch, Maric-Oehler & Popp 2005 "Biophotonics in the infrared spectral range reveal acupuncture meridian structure of the body" J Altern Complement Med. 2005 Feb;11(1):171-3

[232] Gerhard Litscher 2005 "Infrared thermography fails to visualize stimulation-induced meridian-like structures"Biomed Eng Online. 2005; 4: 38
http://www.ncbi.nlm.nih.gov/pubmed/15958163 retrieved 27/5.2009

[233] International Toyohari News 2006 (Toyohari Association)

the body, the implication is that there may well be significant potential therapeutic effects at work.

It will be recalled in the previous discussion on FIR profiles that particular bands of infra-red might create a sympathetic vibration which in turn might lead to a change in dipole in a molecule which may alter ionic compositions resulting in the release of photons. This may possibly be what occurred in this instance but, as ever, much more work needs to be done before we can be more definite. Unfortunately we have no record of the wavelength spectrum of the moxa when it was burnt on this occasion but, if we could review these two pieces of research together, something really exciting might be revealed.

Direct Moxibustion – Dosage and the Issue of Scars and Blisters

When using direct moxa techniques, one inevitably runs the risk of creating blisters, and therefore possibly scars. This is certainly why the method is avoided by many of us in the West and, therefore, with the potential effectiveness of this particular part of moxa treatment, is an issue which needs careful review.

Firstly, it is quite possible, with only a little practice, to use direct moxa techniques without causing burns or blisters. The best way to develop maximum confidence is, without doubt, to practise on oneself. This way one can build up a clear idea of how the moxa burns down, and how the heat is perceived, and one can monitor any noticeable benefits at the same time.

Nevertheless, it will quickly be realised by a novice user of direct moxa that a huge range of variation in nociception and thermoception exists between patients. Indeed it will also be found that some indicated or reactive points can actually be relatively insensitive when one starts to treat them with moxa, so it is always wise to be wary.

The uncomfortable reality exists, unfortunately, that it may even be essential that some tiny blistering takes place to maximise effectiveness, particularly with some intractable conditions for which moxa has been endorsed in the past. Almost certainly, some of the effects recorded in the Japanese research using small mammalian subjects must have been accompanied by major blistering given the cone sizes used, and many of the descriptions of treatment effects in the older Chinese literature are clearly thought to depend upon this for their effect.

Sun Simiao in his "Thousand Ducats" (*Qianjin Yao Fang*) of 652 wrote: "People who tour Wu and Shu [modern day China south of the Yangtze extending right down to the Tropic of Capricorn] should moxa some points regularly and leave the sores unhealed for some time. This will keep the toxic *qi* of miasma, leprosy, and warm malaria away from them." It should be borne in mind that these geographical areas would have been prone to infectious summer sub-tropical disease, and the self-evident degree of risk from infections from blistering was obviously considered to be sufficiently outweighed by the positive effects of the sores, certainly enough in Sun's experience to warrant this endorsement.

It is also noteworthy that Sun Simiao was writing in a time of frequent epidemic, and that the "toxic *qi* of miasma" speaks clearly to us of airborne infectious pathogenic disease. To some extent, one might surmise therefore that this was conceived as the seventh century Tang dynasty equivalent of travel inoculation. In similar vein the "Great Compendium" of 1601 says, "If one intends to be safe and sound, one should keep *zu san li* (St-36) wet" – implying quite clearly that mild suppuration from constant moxa sores at this particular point is a guarantor of health.

We can feel fairly confident, therefore, that a tradition of blistering moxa survived across at least the millennium which separated these two highly influential texts. It is also indisputable that there existed a strong tradition of suppurative moxa, whereby a point is allowed to blister and is then encouraged to suppurate by the application of herbs, which reputedly is extremely effective with really intransigent conditions[234]. This tradition still survives in Japan, and was described by Doctor Yoshio Manaka as a means of treating extremely difficult-to-treat disease. It is known as *Danokyu* but it is rarely used today.

Even in the modern era in China, specialists such as Wang Kenliang have proposed that blistering of the skin was and is essential to the success of moxibustion when treating serious ailments[235]. Further research right up to the present supports this view.

A complementary tradition developed in which moxibustion on a specific channel was restricted to the times of day at which that channel might be replete with *qi* according to the midday-midnight circadian circulation of qi. This tradition suggested that, unless moxa was burnt on a channel at a time when its *qi* was full, suppurative effects would be less likely to occur[236]. Thus treatment on St36 *zu san li*, for instance, might most effectively be applied between 7am and 9am to maximise effectiveness in this respect.

Such blistering approaches, however, cannot today be considered remotely safe or responsible practice in the West, although it is interesting to consider that a

---

[234] Yoshio Manaka et al 1995 "Chasing the Dragon's Tail" (Paradigm Publications) p351.

[235] Wang Kenliang 2000 "Several diseases treated by suppurative moxibustion therapy." International Congress on Chinese Medicine, Beijing

[236] Lorraine Wilcox 2008 "Moxibustion, the Power of Mugwort Fire" (Blue Poppy Press) p209

somewhat similar (and even more extreme) tradition of "laudable pus" existed in western medicine right up to the advent of antibiotics.

This particular tradition is originally attributed to the ancient physician Galen (c.130-200 AD), who coined the phrase *"pus bonum et laudibile"* (the good and praiseworthy pus). Known as a Roman although he wrote in Greek, Galen was actually born in Pergamon in Anatolia (modern-day Bergama in Izmir, Turkey) and was immensely influential in the development of medicine in both Europe and the Middle East. In later years he wrote passionately about his concern over the growth of sects within the medical world of his time, believing strongly in the importance of cross-fertilisation of ideas and disciplines. It is a message which, as students of East Asian medicine, we can do well to heed today, not only in the world of integrative medicine, but also in the world of traditional acumoxa bearing in mind the field's propensity to devolve into something which could sometimes perhaps be described as acu-sectarianism. Galen encouraged the physicians of his time to take ideas from wherever they might find them, otherwise he saw them as being destined to commit themselves to intellectual slavery.

Galen's ideas concerning the healing values of pus were enthusiastically adopted in the later middle ages, and English medicine at the time ascribed the dubious term "laudable pus" to these less attractive side-effects of the body's immune response, considering it for centuries to be an essential component of wound-healing. From the time of Joseph Lister in the nineteenth century, however, pus was more generally seen as an indicator of infection rather than one of healing, although exceptions still occurred. In the Spanish Civil War, for instance, casualties were reported to have had their infected wounds wrapped in plaster casts for lack of any better available treatment despite their wounds being predicted to suppurate, and were then summarily evacuated to France. On arrival doctors were reported as being frequently amazed at the absence of the predicted infection when the casts were opened and the wounds inspected.

In the East blistering moxibustion can be traced back to a time not much later than Galen's – at least back to Huangfu Mi's third century Systematic Classic. At different times in the development of East Asian medicine, the practice flourished, and it is indisputable that across the centuries this seemingly barbaric approach had many advocates, often endorsing different methods with which to induce the suppuration. It seems that the sores were seen as a way to help expel the pathogenic *qi*, as well as being a means to allow the *qi* of the moxa to penetrate more deeply into the patient.

Notwithstanding such anecdotes, both occidental and oriental, two colleagues have independently come across Tibetan refugees sporting large scars from moxibustion treatment, and both of these were reported as the result of treatment for life-threatening illnesses from which both individuals believed they would otherwise not have survived. One has to wonder.

Few references, however, are made to these techniques in modern literature. One example is in the treatment of asthma which, as suggested by some Chinese sources, cannot be cured completely without this technique. It is advocated that this should be done in summer when there are no acute symptoms. Cones are described as being about 7mm across at their base. It is advised that not more than two or three acupoints are used each year, with suppuration being encouraged over a period of forty or fifty days[237].

Alternative Views on the Necessity of Blistering

Doctor Hara, however, had very different views on the matter of blistering, and thankfully they fly contrary to the idea that aggressive blistering is of such importance. They are certainly remote from the belief that blistering is vital for effect. Hara's stipulations are clear: if blisters form with visible pus, the treatment should be stopped. He considered the formation of pus to be associated with what he called "ignorant" practice: he is quite clear in his belief that it is not the pus which creates the therapeutic effects, but rather the associated systemic effects from the tiny burns. Mild blistering, on the other hand, he considered to be not so problematic, with mild scarring a necessary side effect for effective treatment. In consideration of his ideas we should remember that he always advocated tiny grain-sized cones.

In fact, without any real visible blistering forming, repeated daily treatment almost invariably results in a tiny scab. Since this creates something of a barrier to the penetration of the heat, in Doctor Hara's opinion this often required that the number of cones should be increased, and/or the cones should be formed more densely by twisting them hard to make them hotter. The size nevertheless should remain the same – the size of a grain of dried rice or less.

In stark contrast to the classical Chinese descriptions of multiple numbers of cones, Doctor Hara was fastidiously cautious when describing dosage and possible ill-effects. He proceeded from the quite reasonable premise that burns create toxins, and that it is actually these toxins resulting from more substantial cases of burning which create the many fatalities in burn victims, and not the burns themselves. Whilst he based this idea on research which is now nearly a century old, it is far from disputed in more recent research[238]. Hara then adopted the conclusions drawn by contemporary homeopathic doctors that, dependent upon tiny dosage, specific toxins create opposite effects to those observed in normal

---

[237] "Suppurating moxibustion – Yan Dingliang's Experience." "Essentials of Contemporary Chinese Acupuncturists Clinical Experiences" 1989 (Foreign Langauages Press, Beijing) pp 200-202

[238] K. Städtler, M. Allgöwer, L.B. Cueni, G.A. Schoenenberger 1972 "Formation of a Specific 'Burn Toxin' in Mouse Skin by Thermal Injuries
Experimental Results" Journal of European Surgical Research Vol 4, No 3

pathological doses. We have today an alternative model to the homeopathic one suggested by Hara himself that might be more scientifically acceptable. This model is that of "hormesis", which describes a generally favourable biological response to low exposures to a particular toxin which creates an opposite effect in small doses to that seen with larger doses. Whilst there is no uniform acceptance of the hormetic model among immunologists, there is some evidence of it. In a paper discussing the action of bacterial toxins on immune response it is suggested that, "While in the past major emphasis on bacterial protein toxins was directed towards their cytotoxic role, it is increasingly evident that toxins can also modulate various cellular functions at non-cytolytic concentrations[239]." For Doctor Hara, the key to such effects seems to have been, not in the huge number of cones of moxa as described in the Chinese literature, but in the tiny cones and the low numbers described in the Japanese literature[240].

Doctor Hara is specific that the cone should be rice grain sized, though its temperature can be further moderated by the density of the material in the cone. Whilst his treatments were carried out on humans, his research was done mainly on guinea pigs. We can at least conjecture, in respect of this, that the size of the cone really should not matter at these dosages whether carried out on a mouse or a human although the risk of overdosage is probably more acute in a small mammal than an adult human. Hara himself successfully conducted experiments on guinea pigs infected with TB, subjecting them to differing moxa regimes in order to monitor their recovery tendencies. It would be rash to draw any general conclusions about dosage from this, however, particularly as Hara suggested "millet-sized" cones for children in lieu of the rice-sized ones, although this may well have been merely to accustom them to the experience of moxa rather than because of dosage concerns. Fifty years later, however, Doctor Yoshio Manaka similarly advocated "thread-sized" cones for children.

What is clear is that Hara witnessed evidence of toxic-type effects in some of the guinea pigs on which he conducted his experiments and he put this down to over dosage. Typical effects which he considered to be dosage related were loss of fur and failure to thrive, and reducing the dosage seemed to put the treatment back on track. Instances of fur-loss are recorded elsewhere in more recent moxa research, invariably occurring when relatively larger doses are recorded as being utilised than those under current discussion.

---

[239] Backert S, Konig W 2005 "Interplay of bacterial toxins with host defence: Molecular mechanisms of immunomodulatory signalling" International Journal of Medical Microbiology Vol 295, issue 8, pp 519-530

[240] It should be noted that hormetic theory is not the same as homeopathic theory. With hormesis measurably low doses of a toxin are observed to have an opposite effect to the larger dose; homeopathic doses are immeasurably smaller – homeopathy's immeasurability is why its theories have presented such a challenge to current scientific thinking.

The Moon over Matsushima

Hara generally attributed risks of over dosage to the number of points used – too many and the risks become much higher. His conclusions were that fewer points are safer as well as being more effective as a basic approach.

Regarding the number of cones per point, Hara believed that systematically building up the quantity was both the safest and the most effective option. His ideal number of cones for health maintenance at St36, for instance, was seven on each side daily. His basic approach, however, was to build up to this number over days or even weeks, starting with one, two or three, increasing to five and then to seven. In this way, any ill-effects could be easily monitored. He was also clear that the condition of the patient determines the numbers of cones likely to be used – the weaker the patient the fewer the cones.

Moxafrica's very first patient

To illustrate Hara's point, we have to allow the Moxafrica project to be properly introduced for the first time in this study. It was set up in 2008 to investigate whether the small cone direct moxa – recorded as being effectively used in Japan in the 1930s for the treatment of tuberculosis – might be applicable today in resource-poor environments where TB is rife, particularly in the context of developing strains of drug resistance which present such an immense challenge to treatment in such situations.

Our very first African TB patient, who was also co-infected with HIV/AIDS, provided us with a startling object lesson apparently confirming Dr Hara's advice. We found the patient languishing on a dirty mattress under a grubby blanket in a hospital in Lyantonde, Uganda, during a trip when we were assisting the Pan African Acupuncture Project in the training of some Ugandan health workers in basic acupuncture. We had been discretely observing him for several days – being as he was the first HIV-TB co-infected patient we had ever encountered. He was quite clearly dying, unable to take in food or keep down the medication which his sister desperately tried to administer to him. We unexpectedly found ourselves being asked to treat him as part of a demonstration for the health worker trainees the day before we were due to leave the town, and frankly the prospect was far from a welcome one for us since he seemed so ill and beyond any sort of help. We were quite familiar with Hara's cautions concerning dosage, so, after a brief discussion (particularly bearing in mind not only our complete inexperience of treating such a patient, but also our lack of evidence for treating a TB patient co-infected with HIV/AIDS – and most importantly one in such advanced stages of illness) we decided to play it quite literally as safely as we possibly could. Instead of using the ten point protocol we had developed for African patients, we elected to use just two points with a single moxa cone on each. For us, this seemed a ridiculously tiny token treatment, but we did it anyway, feeling at least that it was safe, with little hope of it having any effect but doing it with the best of intention.

What we observed there and then was an immediate conscious re-engagement of the patient with his environment. It was far from dramatic, but it was quite enough for his sister, who was with him at his bedside, to notice. She was instantly keen to know more about what her brother had just experienced, so we taught her there and then this diminutive two-point protocol, how to locate the points and how to prepare and apply tiny cones, and we gave her some moxa so that she could continue the treatment. The next day the patient was eating again, and two days later he was walking in the ward. Soon afterwards he discharged himself. We had left Lyantonde the morning after the first treatment so we were not present to witness these subsequent quite startling improvements, but we heard about them later from Richard Mandell, the Project Director of the Pan African Acupuncture Project with whom we had been working in the hospital. "I will never forget," he wrote to us later, "the joy associated with that treatment."

Just two cones as a total treatment for a dying man – and definitely no blistering involved. We had to accept that Doctor Hara may have been right.

The story, unfortunately, did not end in final triumph. We heard through others several months later that the patient had subsequently died – where or how we never learnt, however. Did the treatment positively extend his life or did it prolong his agony? We hope the former. Did he and his sister continue the treatment? We just do not know – and in Africa, as we have come to learn since, it is best to get used to such uncertainty.

What we can be pretty sure of, however, is that he was the first HIV-TB patient anywhere in the world to be treated with a moxa TB treatment adapted from one used in the 1930s in Japan. For us his treatment constituted a milestone event. It also comprehensively and dramatically confirmed Doctor Hara's ideas about dosage, and particularly demonstrated that blistering is not necessary for effect, at least in the treatment of tuberculosis.

It also confirmed for us that moxa might yet be reviewed as a possible tool with which to confront one of the oldest and deadliest diseases on the planet, one that is now morphing into untreatable forms and combining with a modern counter-plague, HIV/AIDS – two deadly diseases which in combination are unconscionably difficult to treat in any resource-poor environment.

With less aggressive direct moxibustion using the smallest possible cone sizes, what may occur is that small "dots" of blistering may in fact be produced at the site of the moxibustion. This is something which any moxibustion practitioner should expect as a likely result from repeated application of moxa cones. Based on our experience, two factors clearly mitigate the risks from such blistering if this does occur: firstly the size of such a blister is 1-2mm in diameter so is of no serious consequence. Secondly, some of the research we have reviewed does suggest that particular immunological reactions occur at the site of the moxibustion which may serve to counter the risks of infection from the tiny blisters. Our experiences to date suggest that, even in very immune compromised individuals, this research is quite correct in its conclusions because we have yet to see a problem arising from daily treatment, even in co-infected patients with very low CD4 counts.

Nevertheless, blistering should definitely be avoided if at all possible, and clearer evidence of the effectiveness of the treatment must be shown before blistering can possibly be considered to be in any way essential to the treatment effect as has been proposed in the past.

The risk from blistering does seem dependent principally upon the size of cone, something which of course directly impacts upon the temperature at the skin. Early twentieth century research as referred to above suggested using larger cones of between 3 and 5mg for an adult human to activate the immune response. Pragmatically, however, and deducing effects from other research results, it would seem prudent to use maximum cones of 1mg (half rice grain size), and work up to 5 cones of this size per day, with applications every other day if considered appropriate because of a perceived sensitivity of the patient. This would still capitalise on the apparent cumulative effect of the treatment as well as maximise the chance of the reported histological or hormetic effects taking place, whilst minimising the risks from blistering.

As we become more familiar ourselves with small cone direct moxa treatment, we should become especially alert to the fact that, for almost all of our patients, this will be a completely unknown and very foreign treatment. Unless a patient has come to us specifically asking for moxa treatment, we should make every effort to explain why we consider that such a treatment might be particularly beneficial for them, and how it might work. We should teach them carefully and ensure that they leave our clinics confident in the technique. We should also make them understand that tiny blisters may result but that they will heal, and actually that this healing process may even help the effect of the moxa. Such an effect is medically known as an "eschar", similar to a vaccination scab[241]. If patients seem at all shocked by this, we should be very cautious and seriously reconsider whether moxa is the best treatment option for them.

One further fact deserves mention concerning scarring. The fairer the skin, the faster the moxa "scars" tend to disappear. With darker Afro-Caribbean type skin, tiny scars may actually end up as a permanent reminder of their treatment, whereas with fairer skin they will almost certainly fade away completely.

The following strategy is also worth considering if either practitioner or patient has issues about pain or discomfort from moxa. Dr Yoshio Manaka experimented

---

[241] The principle of escharring is at the heart of the eradication of one of the world's previously most virulent killers – smallpox – and most of us alive today bear testimony to this on one of our upper arms.

by asking particularly sensitive patients to listen to the ticking of a metronome set to specific frequencies dependent upon the channel on which he was applying the direct moxa. With the metronome set to particular frequencies, he recorded that patients reported feeling heat but no discomfort.

A further clinical application is suggested from this idea. Dr Manaka also claimed that just having a metronome beating at any of these frequencies would activate the *qi* in the respective channel, and that a point on the channel could be effectively treated by simply tapping it at the appropriate frequency.

The following is a table of the channels and the frequency of beats per minute for each:

Channel	BPM	Channel	BPM
Ren	104	Du	104
Lung	126	Large Intestine	108
Spleen	132	Stomach	132
Heart	126	Small Intestine	120
Kidney	120	Bladder	112
Pericardium	176	Triple Burner	152
Liver	108	Gallbladder	120

Adapting the idea that moxa on a specific channel might be particularly effective at a particular time when the *qi* of the channel is said to be at its most active (i.e. say for the Stomach channel between 7am and 9am) then applying direct moxa at St36 *zu san li* at 8am whilst using a metronome beating at 132 beats per minute might quite possibly maximise this effect at the same time as minimising possible discomfort from the heat. This is not an approach that I have personally tried but would certainly theoretically seem worth investigating.

Some of the techniques referred to previously in Part 3, however, using tubes or cowling with the fingers may produce equally good results.

The twentieth century Japanese moxa master Isaburo Fukaya has left us some further insights on the subject of dosage from his writing – particularly precious because of their possible relevance if we aim to adapt earlier treatments in any way successfully for western patients. "The patient needs to feel a comfortable heat, this is one of moxa therapy's most important points," was his clear advice. "Soft/sunken points require few cones, hard resistant points require many cones." Generally, his views are not dissimilar to Doctor Hara's, who stated that the weaker the patient, the fewer the points which should be used.

Fukaya also suggested that a characteristic of an "ill" patient is that they are less likely to be particularly sensitive to heat. He qualified this further by suggesting that, if a patient experiences exhaustion after a treatment, it should be considered a clear indication of overtreatment. He further stipulated that if the pulse should become hurried this was a sign of mistaken treatment and moxa should be immediately stopped[242].

Fukaya also offered his opinion on the changes he was observing in post-war Japanese society, an opinion which may serve to enrich some of our wider understandings of acumoxa today. He was clear that urban living and rural life require different levels of stimulation within treatment – and quite different approaches. Urban patients need much less in the way of dosage, he believed. Fukaya began his career at a time when the vast proportion of Japanese lived in the countryside – a situation which was in transition and which reversed during his lifetime. As a rule, he deemed urban patients to require lighter stimulation, and rural ones stronger treatment, and we wonder whether he might well feel even more strongly about this if he were alive today, now that life styles are even more sedentary and the urban working environment has so dramatically changed with the advent of computers.

This idea, incidentally, has similar expression in the field of acupuncture itself, being suggested as one of the reasons for the current disposition in Japan to much lighter needling techniques when compared with those developed in the late twentieth century in China. In fact this idea was actually mentioned as far back as the *Neijing*. Essentially those individuals hardened by manual work and natural weather were likely to require much larger doses of treatment than those involved in civil work indoors.

Might this explain what seems to be a clear contradiction across the centuries between the tiny doses advocated in the twentieth century in Japan and the huge dosages endorsed across earlier centuries in China? If only it were that simple! It is a tempting idea, but it is far from totally convincing. The differences are too huge – so huge in fact that one might almost be describing two completely different therapies.

Contra-Indications around Heat and Hypertension

Here we come to a subject that is awash with conflicting ideas. As mentioned in Part 1 the Roots, at acupuncture schools in the West it is regularly taught that moxa is contra-indicated in conditions of heat, and particularly with hypertension – sometimes even summarily defined in this respect as being when the difference between systolic and diastolic counts is more than fifty rather than by using any conventional biomedical definition. But if we care to look through the indications for moxibustion in both Chinese and Japanese modern texts, we will find that they

---

[242] Isaburo Fukaya "*Kyu ni yoru chiryu*": 'Treatment with moxa' Vol 1, section 2. In Japanese.

both recommend moxibustion for treatment of hypertension[243]. Despite this, it is pretty clear that a persistent aversion to using moxa for this condition prevails in the West[244].

Certainly the idea of using moxa cautiously in case it might exacerbate existing heat goes back a long way. In the *Jue Gui Yao Lue*, an Eastern Han text edited by Wang Shu He, there are clear cautions against using "fire moxibustion". It remains a little unclear as to exactly what this term means, however, and the cautions are hardly comprehensive.

It also seems quite possible that some of the more modern conceptions may arise from integrating the herbal properties of mugwort when taken internally with the mechanisms and effects of burning the processed mugwort at or near the skin. Some of the traditional descriptions of the actions of moxibustion clearly support such possible misconceptions, often invoking mugwort's "acrid and bitter" properties as enabling it to penetrate to the channel level. In fact such ideas may erroneously reflect the properties of the herb when ingested internally as much as or more than the empirical effects of the therapy itself when the herb is burnt on or near the skin surface.

The fact that such penetrative properties of, not just mugwort, but also moxa are very clearly discussed by Li Shizhen, one of the indisputable giants of Chinese medicine, however, should at least make us cautious of making too hasty a judgement on the matter. The idea that, at least for the herbalist, *aiye* mugwort is simply a "hot" herb might just have clouded the issue enough as far as moxa practice is concerned, however. At the very least it offers arguable evidence of the political pervasive dominance of the herbal canon over the practice of acumoxa, not only in the current incarnation of *Zhong Yi* Traditional Chinese Medicine but also back then in the Ming Dynasty.

In fact definite discussions concerning the different properties of mugwort when taken internally or when used in moxibustion exist in the literature of the Ming dynasty, and they certainly show that there was no agreement at the time, as is also implied by some modern sources.

The fact remains that many points are regularly indicated for moxa treatment for hypertension, and some sources would argue that, in certain cases, it is a preferable treatment to needling – particularly when acupuncture is having no effect, as is unfortunately often the case. Some published research from China supports this view.

---

[243] See Appendix 1.

[244] Lee H, Yu Y, Kim s, Kim K 1997 "Effect of moxibustion on blood pressure and renal function in spontaneously hypertensive rats" American Journal of Chinese Medicine 25 (1), 21-26

In the modern era Chen Dazhong, for instance, prescribes "wheat grain sized cones" of moxa at Du20, St36 and GB39 for hypertension (applying plaster afterwards at St36 and GB39 to create mild suppuration)[245].

Another modern reference to the use of Du20 provides an interesting window into its possible mechanism with respect to hypertension. Using a moxa stick, the following points are indicated: Du20, Ki1 and LI11, with St36 and GB 39 used as "subsidiary points". The main points are used singly or are rotated in successive treatments. With Du20, however, it is suggested that each sparrow-peck should be held until the patient (in a seated position) feels a burning sensation, and that this should be repeated a full ten times in one treatment. For the other points a mild technique is employed simultaneously on both sides with the patient supine. There is a clear dispersive intention with the application of heat to Du20 in this protocol, and a contrasting warming and tonifying intention for all the other points[246].

The only caution which seems worth adding to this is Shudo Denmei's from Japan[247] – that, based on his personal experience, he is very cautious of using moxa on the head at all for hypertension (even though indications for using moxa at Du20 for hypertension occur in the Japanese as well as the Chinese literature). He favours the use of more distal points. In the light of the possible consequences of ill-effects from such treatment, his advice is well worth keeping in mind.

My own view is that, rather than liberally adopting a cavalier approach to the treatment of hypertension with moxa, one should use as much evidence for the basis of employing it as is possible. I personally am in no doubt that 1mg cones at St36, LI11 and perhaps special points either midline on the proximal crease of the palmar surface of the big toe or on the Small Intestine channel, can, when cumulatively used, often bring down blood pressure. The basis of this approach is derived from a study of the literature, but my confidence in it comes from clinical experience and observation. But I would not hesitate to qualify this statement by saying that it far from works in every case.

If I were to employ an alternative moxa method, however, say the style of "snatch moxa" which I was taught as an acupuncture student, I would feel far less comfortable in its application for hypertension if only because of mismatched methods. The first method (small cone direct moxa) is clearly defensible on the basis of the literature (and the fact that it often works); the second (snatch moxa) is an adapted treatment from a source which considers the use of moxa inadvisable with hypertension with no record of efficacy in any case. If problems

---

[245] "Essentials of Contemporary Chinese Acupuncturists Clinical Experiences" 1989 (Foreign Langauages Press, Beijing) p316

[246] Zhang Ren and Xu Hong 2006 "Of Acupuncture Treatment for Hypertension" (Shanghai Scientific and Technical Publishers) p161

[247] Shudo Denmei 2002 "Finding Effective Acupuncture Points" (Eastland Press)

arose in the latter instance, the practitioner concerned might find him or herself in a very vulnerable position. In such a case, if a supposedly authoritative expert were called to question the use of moxa in the treatment of hypertension in the case of a complaint being made, and that expert was only familiar with the questionable dogma contra-indicating moxa with hypertension, then there would be no grounds to challenge such expert opinion. If, however, such treatment had been modelled on recorded and recommended treatment technique using small cone moxa, such "expert" opinion would be entirely challengeable on the grounds of alternative evidence.

It is also worth considering that there are multiple causes for hypertension, and therefore there are almost certainly many possible ways to help reduce it, some of which may be only effective in certain circumspances. Expecting one single protocol-type approach to succeed when there may be such complex causation at work is certainly expecting too much of any protocol treatment. If one of the underlying causes of hypertension, however, is that of long-term stress, and if cumulative moxa treatment can help a flexible treatment get right to the heart of this, then it certainly would seem a very sensible treatment to employ.

When it comes to simple conditions of heat, however, the line gets a little more distinctly drawn across the East China Sea. In Japan the only contra-indication for heat would be direct moxa on a hot joint, but moxa **around** the joint, or at points near to it would likely be indicated. In fact, in China in the Yuan dynasty there were ideas being proposed of guiding heat out with the heat itself and these were being actively propagated as being effective.

Such ideas have also clearly survived into the modern era: treating fever at Du14 *Dazhui* dispersively with moxa that is allowed to burn hot, for instance, is discussed in both Japanese and Chinese sources. Modern Chinese sources, nevertheless, are more guarded than Japanese ones; indeed they explicitly generally advocate against treating hot conditions with moxa. In spite of this, however, a debate seems still in progress on this issue in the PRC and we should best watch this space.

Perhaps the core of this dilemma again concerns the method of moxa used. As stated previously, moxa use in the PRC today consists mainly of stick moxa. As demonstrated by the Shanghai research, this gives off a massive intensity of infrared radiation (in other words it gives off an awful lot of heat). Moxa in a pole is also generally fairly fresh and unrefined. In contrast, moxibustion in Japan uses both more refined and more aged moxa, and is used in small sizes, one of the properties of which is a reduction in its combustion temperature. This in itself may account for the variations in interpretation.

But one very important contra-indication which is not frequently cited does deserve a mention: Junji Mizutani lists a contra-indication for moxa in cases of leukaemia. Whilst utilisation of moxa as an adjunct to cancer therapy is potentially extremely beneficial it should, nevertheless, be carried out with a lot of care. Moxa as support for chemotherapy can be highly effective and actually in some cases is far more effective than acupuncture; it is even, in some instances, essential in preventing neutropenia if the intention is to enable the patient to complete a cycle of chemotherapy treatment. But a cancer specifically of the blood, particularly with symptoms of over-production of white blood cells, does deserve far more careful consideration. Without more specialist advice or better research it seems that this particular contra-indication is highly advisable.

Moxa in Needle-Shock

Moxibustion can be considered as a useful antidote to fainting from needling, although, of course, the preferred option is to avoid the patient fainting in the first place.

Dr Shi Jimin suggests that needle fainting is caused by collapsed *yang qi* in which case moxa can be seen as being the perfect restorative. He considers lower body points best for fainting caused by needling in the upper body, and vice versa, which certainly makes some sense. If fainting seems caused by needling in the middle of the body, either upper or lower points can be selected, but points from the same area from which the needling provoked the faint are to be avoided. The favoured points he lists are Du20, Pc6 and Pc5, St36 and Ki1. With typical Chinese pragmatism, Dr Shi has apparently even been known to use an ignited cigarette in lieu of the moxa stick when carrying out such a remedy[248].

Moxa and Warts

There is very little in the English literature on East Asian medicine on this subject, although it has been a treatment of choice in the past. A scientific paper, however, has been published on the topic in an acumoxa journal in Japan[249].

The treatment principle is quite simple and is one of cauterisation directly on the wart. On plantar warts of either the foot or the hand the treatment is the same. Cones with bases of the same diameter as the wart are burnt repetitively directly on the wart. Thirty or forty cones can be burnt repetitively at each application – and the treatment should be done daily.

---

[248] "Essentials of Contemporary Chinese Acupuncturists Clinical Experiences" 1989 (Foreign Langauages Press, Beijing) "Essentials of Contemporary Chinese Acupuncturists' Clinical Experiences" p432

[249] "Clinical Effect on Two Cases of Warts by Moxibustion Treatment and Application of Burnt Moxa Products" Journal of Japan Society of Acupuncture and Moxibustion. 1987; 37(3): 188-193.

If the wart becomes uncomfortable or tender the treatment should be stopped, but generally the treatment will incrementally destroy the wart which becomes blackened in the process before dying off.

In cases of wart clusters it is reported that the correct selection of what might best be described as a "mother wart" can effectively see the entire cluster dying off in some kind of sympathetic response. The only problem in such a case is simply the correct selection of the mother wart.

Moxa with Breech Presentation – and also in Pregnancy

The subject of moxa and breech presentation has been well addressed in other books. Indeed it is probably responsible for the most widely held appreciation of moxibustion in the West[250]. It certainly is likely to be the only published references to moxibustion treatment which can be found in online medical reference resources such as the Cochrane database or MedLine. Some further observations are worth making on the subject however.

Firstly, there are, yet again, varying approaches in technique.

Some use direct moxa on the points. This would certainly have been how the treatment began. Some use moxa sticks, whilst (quite understandably in smoke-free environments) many use smokeless moxa sticks. Some even just use large incense sticks. As we have already discussed above, there are possible significant variables in effects from each of these approaches, any of which might have impact upon efficacy. Interestingly, all claim some levels of effect, but the fact remains that the results claimed from studies done in East Asia generally exceed the results obtained in what trials there have been in the West. Before resorting to the standard and simplistic "therefore the Chinese trials cannot have been rigorously controlled" critique, however, it would seem wiser briefly to consider different possibilities.

Bearing in mind the measurements in terms of quantities of Far Infra Red radiation recorded by the Shanghai study mentioned previously, particularly in comparing smokeless moxa with standard moxa sticks, it might be reasonably proposed that one of the reasons that Chinese studies appear to significantly outperform Western ones is that in the Chinese ones standard raw moxa sticks were used, whilst in the Western ones they would be considered unacceptable. If the density of warmth/heat in the context of Infra Red is any part of the component of efficacy for this particular part of the moxa repertoire, then this might well explain the difference. Timings and regularity of treatments might well also play a part.

---

[250] Yoichi Kanakura 2001 "Moxibustion Treatment of Breech Presentation" American Journal of Chinese Medicine, 29(1):37-45

Another possible explanation, of course, may well be that different techniques or dosages were being used in China from those used or even considered acceptable in the West.

The best we can do is to search out the most respectable or acceptable study available to us. In the Cardini study of 1998, which has become the study most frequently referred to in the western literature, smokeless poles were used and they were applied daily to each Bl67 point for fifteen minutes over a period of two weeks[251]. One group used this protocol twice a day, another once only. Initially, version rates in the "twice a day" group was somewhat higher, but this tended to equal out in the second week to an insignificant difference.

The general opinion is that version with moxibustion can be safely attempted from week 33, and that the later the start from this point, the less likely the treatment will result in successful version. The optimum time may be at around 34 weeks [252] although opinions vary. The Cardini study also suggested that moxibustion is more likely to succeed when used on multiparous women than with primaparous. One report even suggests that version is more likely to occur in the afternoon [253]. For many acupuncturists, this finding might encourage capitalising on the traditional idea that the *qi* of the Bladder channel is at its fullest between 3pm and 5pm, and that this would thus be the optimum time for this treatment.

What seems incontestable is that heating this point on the little toe promotes foetal movement, one report recording that foetal movement increased on average after seven minutes of moxa warming and that this persisted after the treatment stopped. The general probability is that, the greater the foetal response, the greater the likelihood of successful version. The frequently expressed concern about all of this, of course, is one of safety for the baby. Concerns are raised about "nuchal" cords (when the umbilical cord becomes wrapped around the baby's neck resulting in stillbirth). The particular concern raised is that, if the cord is already wrapped around the baby's neck, any efforts at encouraging the baby to turn might have fatal effects.

The concern may be a little overestimated. Firstly, it is generally accepted that a third to a quarter of all deliveries have the cord round the neck, and even when this is seen before delivery on ultrasound no action is normally taken.

---

[251] Cardini F, Weixin H 1998. "Moxibustion for Correction of Breech Presentation" JAMA, 280:1580-4

[252] Habek D, Habek J.C, & Jagust M. 2003 "Acupuncture conversion of Fetal Breech Presentation" Fetal Diagnosis and Therapy, 18:6; 418-421.

[253] Grabowska C, Manyande A 2008. "Management of breech prespentation with the use of moxibustion in women in the UK". European Journal of Oriental Medicine, 6:1;38-43.

Furthermore, there is no evidence of any general increase in mortality associated with such wrappage, and only rarely is it considered a causative factor of stillbirth[254][255].

Expert opinion in fact suggests that cord problems in childbirth are probably grossly overestimated. It has actually been suggested that, in reality, medical personnel are often tempted to attribute death to the most obvious feature at hand – which may appear as a twisted or knotted cord simply when there is no other more obvious cause.

In the current litigious climate of medicine, however, the possible liabilities from a hasty and erroneous explanation for a cause of unexplained stillbirth following attempted moxibustion version should rightly make practitioners a little wary. A recent systematic review of effectiveness and safety in breech version which looked at eight studies involving a total of 411 women, however, concluded that no significant harmful effects of moxibustion on women or their infants were reported during or immediately after performing the treatment. Apart from the risk of minor skin burns if the moxa is applied at all clumsily or with too much zeal, no adverse effects on either mothers or infants have reportedly been observed in the West[256].

This may still not serve to satisfy some. "During or immediately after" may not be good enough ultimately, since it is also not necessarily to be expected that a baby will turn either during or immediately after a moxa treatment. The version is most likely to take place some time in the next few days if treatment is pursued regularly.

But despite the claims of between 74 and over 90 per cent success rates from the Chinese studies, it is indisputable that the modern Chinese approach to breech presentation resorts more and more to Caesarean section and actually ignores the moxibustion approach. Without further explanation of this policy, it seems right, therefore, to be a little wary of accepting their figures on the subject of version with moxibustion too glibly. There seems no clear reason for this trend towards Caesarean section, given that the moxibustion technique is apparently so successful and relatively safe, apart from the ubiquitous modernisation of China

---

[254]Reed, R, Barnes, M & Allan, J 2009, 'Nuchal cords: Sharing the evidence with parents', British Journal of Midwifery, 17(2) pp106-109

[255]Sheiner E, Abramowicz JS, Levy A, Silberstein T, Mazor M, Hershkovitz R 2006 "Nuchal cord is not associated with adverse perinatal outcome" Arch Gynecol Obstet. 274(2):81-3

[256] Milligan R, Hannah V, and Donohue BM 2003 "Breech Version by Acumoxa". Washington: Georgetown University Medical Center, www.akupunktur-aktuell.de retrieved 30/3/2009

since the 1990s. More generally, hospital scheduling has been a factor of the increased frequency of Caesarean procedures in the West, so the same may well apply in China and this trend may be spilling over to affect responses to breech presentation; but there may also be cultural factors at play – babies can be selectively born by scheduled Caesarean at the most auspicious times on the most auspicious days.

One of the principle problems with the western studies seems to be that of lack of compliance as much as failure of version. This non-compliance, of course, is most probably explicable by the fact that it is a treatment which is culturally "acclimatised" in the East, but relatively unknown and considered bizarre in the West. In the UK, however, an 11 year audit by acupuncturist and midwife Sarah Budd found a 20-25 per cent increase in spontaneous version rates at 34 weeks after using a moxa stick[257]. This is far from insignificant. Furthermore, in contrast to external cephalic version (ECV), which is the standard medical intervention after 36 weeks, the general experiences of the mother are certain to be considerably more comfortable if the moxibustion approach succeeds as the research suggests it probably will do, and the risks may well be much lower. The risks associated with ECV include both rupturing of the membrane and separation of the placenta, neither of which have been recorded as happening with the moxibustion treatment, and it is standard for the practice of ECV to be only attempted when the facility for emergency section is right at hand. Indeed, if ECV is considered to be the only option, it is at least arguable that moxa treatment beforehand may well make this more comfortable and safer for both mother and baby, and quite possibly more prone to success. However, there is little more than circumstantial information on this subject, so it certainly would seem to warrant more penetrating research.

There is some significant variation in general approach between practitioners. Some suggest that treatment should not be started until 35 weeks – the logic being that before this the baby is likely to revert to the breech position. Others endorse starting from week 32, exactly because there will be more room for the baby to turn and this will make turning more probable. Treatment from 32-35 weeks does seem possibly to be the optimum period for best results, but babies can turn later.

The bottom line, as ever, is that further RCT's seem necessary to convince anybody of power and influence in orthodox medicine. Of course, this constitutes the standard and simplistic retort to this and other similar scenarios where inadequate resource is available to finance the requisite larger scale trials – "It is recommended that further randomised control trials are required to evaluate outcomes", etc, etc. We read this *ad infinitum,* and our profession's failure to respond adequately to this challenge is then incorrectly assumed to be a failure of

---

[257] Budd S 2000 "Moxibustion for breech presentation" Complementary Therapies in Nursing and Midwifery; 6:176-179.

the treatment itself to stand up to any sort of proper scrutiny – something we will look at more deeply in Part 5.

Some sensible contra-indications exist, however, for attempting to rectify a breech with moxa. A previous history of a Caesarean for breech should warrant a very cautious approach, but, more specifically, pre-enclampsia or raised blood pressure, bleeding, a low lying placenta, and the incidence of twins all mean that the treatment should not be considered at all. As a basic principle in any case, the treatment should be deferred until the appropriate consent has been obtained from a member of the mother's obstetric team.

Finally, however, we should review the general contra-indications for moxa use during pregnancy, something which is widely taught in basic acupuncture training.

It is worth mentioning the routine pregnancy treatment using Sp6 *Sanyinjiao* starting from the 5th month using small cone direct moxa techniques. This was developed by the obstetrician Dr Ishino Nobuyaso in Japan. The treatment, known as *An Zan Kyu* ("Easy Delivery Moxa"), recommends daily moxa on Sp6, 5 cones a day in the fifth month, 7 in the sixth, 9 in the seventh, and so on. This treatment is said to make for an easy birth.

I am also aware of practitioners who routinely use direct moxa at the master and coupled points of the *Chongmai-Yinweimai* and *Renmai-Yinqiaomai* (Eight Extraordinary Vessel) pairings on patients during pregnancy dependent upon palpable findings without concerns for safety.

Some Conclusions

We may conclude that we have partially consigned another sacred cow to the fire, but this conclusion comes with a caveat which applies to the adoption or adaptation of any moxa protocol. Varying techniques (and they do vary considerably) are frequently blurred into a single umbrella of "moxibustion". We have been reviewing and analytically examining, as best we can, these varieties of techniques – using raw moxa, using super fine moxa, using smokeless moxa, using moxa on intermediate substances, using large cones, using medium cones, using tiny cones, lifting off, snuffing out, letting cones burn down, cowling cones, blowing on cones. Whenever we come across a moxibustion treatment which seems to be accorded with general safety, it is really important that we satisfy ourselves that we understand the approach and technique which was used before replicating it on our patients.

The use of direct moxa for easy delivery is a classic example of this. The moxa used is half-rice grain size, and the moxa is highly refined. The technique is direct. Alternative techniques which might be more familiar to acumoxa practitioners generally in the West should be adapted with utmost caution, if adapted at all, since the normal cautions attributed to patients in pregnancy should then still be seen to apply. Applying a moxa pole to Sp6, for instance, may have a completely different effect to applying a tiny cone of direct moxa. In fact, based on the discussions in this part of this book, it would be unlikely if this were not the case. These discussions have proposed not only that different mechanisms be at work with different techniques, but even that synergistic mechanisms may even be at work within a single technique.

The only clear conclusion that we can really draw is that we have a lot yet to understand.

Part 5 – The Leaves

"ACTIVELY EXPLORE AND BROADEN YOUR KNOWLEDGE,
BUT STAND FINALLY ON THE PRINCIPLES OF WHICH YOU ARE
CERTAIN"
Sun Si Miao

"THE SLENDEREST KNOWLEDGE THAT MAY BE OBTAINED OF THE
HIGHER THINGS IS MORE DESIRABLE THAN THE MOST CERTAIN
KNOWLEDGE OF LESSER THINGS"
St Thomas Aquinas

"WHEN YOU KNOW A THING, TO HOLD THAT YOU KNOW IT; AND
WHEN YOU DO NOT KNOW A THING, TO ALLOW THAT YOU DO NOT
KNOW IT — THIS IS KNOWLEDGE"
Confucius

So finally…

In the previous sections, we have been attempting to tease some of what we might describe as the purer nap of clinical relevance away from the rougher chaff of myth or misunderstanding. In so doing we have hopefully clarified a little of what may or may not be clinically most useful for us as twenty-first century acumoxa practitioners – or indeed what may be of most interest to a more general reader. My hope is that the process has thrown up a few interesting possibilities.

For me it all boils down to duly considering the tensions between the certainties cited in the quotation above by "Wise Person" Sun, one of the major figures in Chinese medicine, and the more slender but no less valuable lesser certainties endorsed by the equally wise St. Thomas Aquinas, whilst trying to hold on to the honesty and clarity of the inestimably wise Master Kong[258]. In truth these very tensions lie implicitly as the sleeping elephant in the bustling room of modern scientific process as much as they far more explicitly exist in the field of acumoxa in the form of scientific uncertainty. Such uncertainties generally find themselves too easily discarded in a waste bin as non-science (albeit that they might more usefully be secreted for future reference by scientists of greater imagination or of more developed knowledge). The act of discarding them means that possible jewels of knowledge become no more than screwed up scraps at the bottom of a waste paper basket, something which is particularly sad if they are dismissed as

---

[258] Confucius, although still almost universally known by this name, should, strictly speaking, be transliterated (using the most universally accepted method by the Pinyin system) as Kong Zi.

discredited claptrap primarily because of a passing fad of modern science despite centuries of apparent empirical effectiveness.

As an example of this, under the aegis of Evidence Based Medicine (EBM) we are encouraged to clinically confine ourselves to the certainties revealed by relatively intensive reductionist research in order to demonstrate the efficacy and mechanisms of acupuncture. Some interesting findings have been revealed from this process. Most of this work has focused on its effects through the Central Nervous System. As a result we seem to be also obliged to dispose of the larger part of acupuncture practice as it has been conducted for two millennia, which hardly seems that intelligent an act – and acupuncture is questionably awarded a special privilege in the process by being given a place in the UN's "intangible cultural heritage list" as a result. And, somewhat ironically as well, we (as practitioners of "traditional" acumoxa) both welcome and readily quote any positive results that are reported under such controlled reductionist conditions as if they reflect what we do in our treatment rooms when of course they frequently do not.

So, with this in mind, exactly what can we agree has been revealed to be "certain" in this exploration of moxibustion?

Firstly, and most importantly, it is very clear that there are, and have been, widely varying approaches to the therapy across the centuries.

Secondly, whilst its mechanisms have been explored both in terms of the theories of traditional East Asian medicine and in terms of biomedicine, they are still far from understood to any conclusive degree.

Thirdly, many of the mechanisms, and therefore also the effects, may be dependent on the technique or approach applied.

Fourthly, some moxa techniques deserve deeper investigation because of their potential to be effectively and economically utilised in primary medicine when conventional modern medical techniques, for one reason or another, are failing patients.

Finally, even within the acumoxa community itself, it seems that moxa is often not well understood and may be largely underestimated, and that there may be enormous potential for us as practitioners to capitalise on the apparent actions of the controlled combustion of mugwort on acupuncture points to make our treatments significantly more effective for our patients.

In this section we will review how challenging it really may be to conduct rigorous double-blind randomised control trials on moxa techniques in the West (at least as far as direct techniques are concerned) and explore the reasons why this may be so. We will consider whether, if moxa fails intrinsically to stand up to the scientific gold standard of research, it risks being peremptorily consigned to the sarcophagus of non-scientific medicine.

Particularly if we look at those very less-certain and more slender claims that can be made on behalf of this fascinating therapy, things undeniably become altogether much more interesting. Several different actions may be separately or simultaneously taking place dependent upon the techniques applied. Changes in constitutional condition almost certainly occur after prolonged cumulative application. There are probable baseline whole body immunological effects which can be accentuated in specific ways by the employment of moxibustion at specific acupoints. We have revealed evidence of serological actions alongside good evidence of neurological ones with indicators of neural dermatome reflex response from selective localised stimulation. Whilst there are indicators of simple thermological effects which might be obtained from any heat source, we have found tantalising pointers that moxibustion may also provoke subtle responses (including biophotonic adjustments) within the human organism as a result of sympathetic Infra-Red radiation; we have also identified possibilities of chemical absorption, of vibrational response, and even aromatherapeutic stimulation either through the skin or via the incumbent inhalation of moxa smoke.

Further investigation would seem at the very least to be desirable, especially since there already exists a significant overlooked body of research which appears both scientifically quite persuasive and also very relevant to our troubled age. Some of the older moxa literature, in fact, quite clearly reflects its use in situations of illness which were otherwise considered terminal. This is far away from moxa's more current application in the West as a complementary therapy, when it is more likely to be applied to assuage the day to day chronic discomforts of what might unkindly be described as the "healthier and wealthier" among us rather than to treat life-threatening diseases of the more needy. Today, such acute life-threatening situations are rightly treated using the powers of modern pharmaceutics, but it is becoming widely recognised that many of these in themselves do not hold the answers and some of them sometimes even create problems of their own. It is also indisputable that large parts of this treasure chest of modern medicine lies economically out of reach from as much as a third of humanity.

When we consider the above, we find ourselves facing something of a dilemma since, if we embrace the methodology of modern medical research we are left with an oxymoron: we may struggle to apply RCT research to moxibustion, as we will shortly see, and yet it is possible, in the interests of mankind, more research may well be necessary – as will hopefully also become evident later in this section.

Moxa and the Problems of Modern Research

We discussed in Part 4 the Stems how we, in the Complementary and Alternative Medicine (CAM) sector, find ourselves repetitively bombarded by the demand that "more research is needed" in order to better demonstrate evidence of the efficacy of our treatments. Such a comment accompanies nearly every evidence-focused report – as a mantra for any wider acceptance of a CAM treatment.

In fact we can start by clarifying things a little: any therapy which has plenty of persuasive case study evidence but lacks conclusive research data is by definition a CAM treatment, whereas any CAM treatment that actually breeches the outer walls of the bastion of Evidence Based Medicine (EBM) by offering conclusive research data automatically is no longer actually a part of CAM at all. It immediately then becomes *de facto* part and parcel of orthodox biomedicine.

We should also bear in mind that more research is needed" is not a mantra which is only applied to CAM, because it occurs frequently in the conclusions of many research papers in all aspects of medicine, particularly when promising but not entirely convincing signs of efficacy or safety are found. It certainly does not dismiss such findings out of hand. The word "inconclusive", moreover, often accompanies such judgements, meaning that the available evidence remains unconvincing to the implacable and supposedly impartial eyes of the systematic reviewers who present themselves as the primary bastion of defence for the proper scientific and safe practice of modern medicine. In more general lay terms, such judgements may actually indicate that the treatment does seem to be probably effective but that appropriately controlled demonstrations of mechanisms and of efficacy have simply not yet been satisfactorily completed or replicated.

"More research", however, also inevitably gets equated with more Double-Blind Randomised Controlled Trials (RCTs), which are considered by many to be the gold standard for modern medical research, and it is in this context that we encounter the real problems.

However circumstantially persuasive some alternative ways of presenting positive evidence may be, we appear for now to be stuck with a demand to design RCTs which provide conclusively convincing quantitative data to support clinical treatment. In essence, qualitative research, which forms the body of research in CAM, can be seen at best as an egg which might lead us to the chicken of more quantitative data. The problem we face is how to find a viable pathway from the one type of research to the other. This may not actually seem that problematic, but under the auspices of modern research methodology, we will now set out to consider how truly tricky this might be.

Within the practice of acupuncture, particularly when it is conducted according to more "traditional" principles (however we may choose to define such a problematic term), RCTs can present difficulties enough; but when it comes to moxibustion we have to confront the fact that it represents a minefield.

These difficulties can best be examined by considering once again the most common "biomedical" practice of moxibustion – for correcting breech presentation. We can use the word "biomedical" because the practice is of interest and is relatively familiar to midwives who comprise the front line of the orthodox medical force consigned to tackle the problems of obstetric complications. Extra Cephalic Version (ECV), is a common primary intervention to avoid the necessity of Caesarean section, but it is known to present risks to both mother and baby[259] so alternative ways of avoiding sections and promoting natural birth demand due attention from the obstetric profession. Clearer confirmation of the possible efficacy of moxibustion in such circumstances is needed, together with confirmatory evidence of safety. Without any doubt the general public requires reassurance on this issue before wider introduction of such a relatively unfamiliar procedure.

In fact, if the subject of moxibustion is looked up on the Cochrane online library, the following predictable conclusions will be found: "**There is insufficient evidence to support the use of moxibustion to correct a breech presentation...** *there is a need for well-designed randomised controlled trials* **to evaluate moxibustion for breech presentation which report on clinically relevant outcomes as well as the safety of the intervention**[260]."

In spite of this cautionary judgement, papers on the subject in English which can be regarded as being both credible and reputable have in general been rather favourable. A couple of exceptions exist but both are explainable: one in which the outcome was not demonstrably positive simply because of patient non-compliance (i.e. not treatment failure *per se*); and one in which the intervention may be reasonably considered to have been attempted both too little and too late (at 37 weeks with three treatments only). Not a single paper has recorded particular concerns regarding the safety of either baby or mother. Certainly, since the moxa protocol would seem to go some way towards bridging the gap between "scientific" and "traditional" acumoxa, one would think that the suggestion for a well-designed clinical trial would be a universally acceptable idea for all concerned – biomedical professionals, expectant mothers and acumoxa practitioners.

---

[259] McParland P and Farine D 1996 "External version: does it have a role to play in modern obstetric medicine?" Canadian Family Physician, 42: 693-698 and -

Salami R, Theiler R and Lindsay M 2006 "Uterine torsion and fetal bradycardia associated with external cephalic version". Obstetrics and Gynecology, 108 (3 Part 2): 820-822

[260] http://summaries.cochrane.org/CD003928/cephalic-version-by-moxibustion-for-breech-presentation retrieved 1/6/2011

But there is an evidence-based rub to this idea, unfortunately, because exactly such a trial has already been attempted. Mary Mitchell and Katherine Allen (a senior lecturer in midwifery and an experienced midwife respectively) applied for funding to carry out exactly such a proper RCT on moxibustion and breech presentation in the UK. They found their request rejected. The rather startling grounds given for the refusal was that the approval committee felt that there was "no evidence" available to them that moxibustion would be an acceptable intervention for Western women[261]. For most acumoxa practitioners who are regularly approached by expectant mothers confronted with an unwanted prospect of a probable Caesarean section, the idea that moxa might not be acceptable to Western women might seem a little perplexing. To any fair-minded and logical observer, however, such a judgement seems to render the Cochrane recommendation that "more research is needed" as something of a Catch-22. How can one conduct the appropriate requisite trial if one is denied the facility to do it on contentious or even judgemental grounds? And how can such an intervention ever be deemed to be "acceptable" to western women if they are not appropriately exposed to the option?

Of course, unlike most modern medical studies, there are no patents to be secured nor are there profits to be made, factors which more normally stimulate private investment or pressure to support research for the public good. Neither is there any promise of such patents which might provide a motive to massage approval processes through direct or indirectly connected subsidies to health trusts, universities etc.

The UK's Nursing and Midwifery Council's "Code of Professional Conduct" (2002 - Para 3.11) states quite explicitly that professionals "must ensure that the use of complementary or alternative therapies is safe and in the interests of patients and clients." This, of course, was *exactly* what Mitchell and Allen were attempting to do. Furthermore, the idea is widely promoted within the UK health sector that consumers' access to information regarding making their own choices for their healthcare is fundamental to the wider improvement of quality of care. As part of this process, in fact, the UK Department of Health has specifically highlighted the need for professionals to be better informed about CAM[262]. Clearly the response to Mitchell and Allen's application for funding strayed somewhat from these principles.

Such resistance may unfortunately not be unique. Christine Grabowska, another UK midwife, reported problems in obtaining funding for similar

---

[261] Mitchell M, and Allen K. 2008 "Breech presentation and the use of moxibustion" The Practising Midwife 11; 5: 22-24

[262] UK Department of Health 2001 "Government Response to the House of Lords Select Committee on Science and Technology's Report on Complementary and Alternative Medicine"

moxibustion/breech research – this time on ethical grounds[263]. This "unproven" but not entirely unfamiliar treatment in the field of midwifery is cheap, apparently safe and can potentially, in most cases, resolve a problem which confronts around 4% of pregnant women. Breech presentations have a major impact on mothers' experiences of giving birth and can indisputably also create dangerous complications. Caesarean sections are also associated with identifiable high incidence of post-delivery morbidity. That research into moxa use should meet with what appears to be such instinctive resistance from approval committees under such circumstances is clearly worrying.

Thi example, however, merely set out the store for the likelihood of a far greater challenge for moxibustion research relating to other conditions for which its application might be even less familiar to committees made up of orthodox professionals relying on such august reference points as the Cochrane database. When compared to acupuncture, for instance, moxibustion (aside from its use for treatment of breech presentation) is almost unknown in the West. If we were to contemplate attempting to research moxa for the treatment of any type of intractable disease (on which subject Cochrane will have absolutely nothing to say but on which there has been much written in traditional East Asian medical literature) it is hardly likely that any approvals for research will be readily gained.

In the particular cases quoted above, the responses seem to have focused on the perception of the unproven nature of the treatment, and the relative strangeness of it to the western culture which would be hosting the research. Since research by its very nature deals in uncertainty, such a response, when accompanied by an endorsement from Cochrane that "more research is needed" may seem an illogical criterion on which research should be fundamentally denied. If relative "strangeness" is the principle criterion, then arguably we might suggest that these committees entrusted with taking medicine forward for the benefit of all in the twenty-first century may not be exhibiting the creative insight which we trust they might have.

The argument against such accusations, of course, is that these committees represent a safety barrier for both public and patient, and they would be failing in their duty if they were not to take this responsibility very seriously. This is a valid point. The public is the first to become outraged when medical research goes wrong. The media can also cause embarrassment if much needed funds appear to be being wasted on pointless research.

There is clearly also a problem concerning smoke. Here we are –living in a society in the twenty-first century which has drafted complex legislation and spent billions expunging smoke of almost any kind from our environment – and now we are proposing to **incorporate** smoke **into** a medical intervention?

---

[263] Grabowska C.2006 "Turning the breech using moxibustion". RCM Midwives – December; 9(12): 484-5.

For direct techniques no alternative to creating smoke exists. For indirect techniques (such as for breech, of course) this sticking point may perhaps be obviated by using smokeless moxa, although we have already raised some uncertainties concerning both its comparative efficacy and indeed its intrinsic safety. As acumoxa practitioners we might try getting around the smoke problem by quoting the research which demonstrates the general non-toxicity of moxa smoke, but it will surely still be a difficult case to make.

One alternative might be to attempt to research the effects of moxibustion by attempting to replicate its effects using electronic devices – ones which create controlled heat that can be applied to the skin at specific locations. At face value this would seem a useful solution, and it is one that has been already attempted in Japan. We have already discussed, however, that there may be a complex combination of mechanisms at work with traditional moxa treatment: one of these is clearly the heat, but another may well be due to the chemical composition of the processed mugwort and its absorption, especially in direct techniques. Electronic moxibustion in this respect simply cannot be expected to replicate the normal treatment, and the results from the studies using electronic moxa (which were variable) may well be explained by this fact.

A far more insidious potential problem arises, however, at least in Europe, if processed mugwort is considered to be an "Investigational Medicinal Product" (IMP) as defined under article 1.1 of the EU directive 2004/27/EC. The definition includes the following:

> (a) Any substance or combination of substances presented as having properties for treating or preventing disease in human beings; or

> (b) Any substance or combination of substances which may be used in or administered to human beings either with a view to restoring, correcting or modifying physiological functions by exerting a pharmacological, immunological or metabolic action, or to making a medical diagnosis.

Under these definitions, it would be hard not to classify refined mugwort for moxa (or indeed smokeless moxa) as anything but an IMP. IMPs unfortunately are generally defined as such in order to temper the excesses of pharmaceutical research, and are clearly intended for purely pharmaceutical products, which it is quite arguable mugwort-for-moxa is not. But the definition above is unfortunate for the cause of moxibustion research, because as a result of it, any moxa used could have to be approved in terms of quality assurance, and in terms of available records of good agricultural practice. Moxa production, certainly for the more refined type which is a prerequisite for direct moxa treatment, is at best still largely a cottage industry, in which the prime mugwort is still discretely picked and processed according to "secret" family traditions, and is still harvested from the wild and not grown under any form of controlled cultivation[264]. This issue is further complicated by the fact that the same strain of plant when grown in different locations is known to have different constituents – and since these plants, unlike those which are processed for pharmaceutical use, are neither chemically reduced nor reconstituted as part of the production process, it will be impossible to provide any consistent breakdown of mugwort's chemical constituents if such were required. To my knowledge no-one has yet attempted to obtain approvals for moxa research in the light of such stipulations, and we must hope that they will never have to.

It is worth mentioning that most of the problems identified above apply to both direct and indirect moxa practice, but if one wishes to research direct moxa techniques (where the real jewels for research may actually lie) the ethical problems become increasingly challenging as the risks from accidental blistering will have to be considered as well.

Above and beyond such significant instinctive resistant forces confronting moxa RCT research, we must then consider the arena of the trial itself, which normally requires the implementation of some form of double-blind sham or placebo. This has proved a challenge enough for acupuncture, for which it is far from resolved as an issue, since the idea of "sham" using sliding needles or sham points are all far more complex and controversial than when the same model is applied for "simple" ingested pharmaceutical interventions.

But what might best be designed to be a sham in a moxibustion treatment? It either burns with heat or it doesn't (and things which burn *do* by their nature generally create heat). If heat is the dominant mechanism in the treatment (which at face value is a fairly acceptable proposition), what combustible substance could possibly provide an inert sham? At best one might expect a slightly modified response, but certainly not one which could be defined as being inert.

Possibly, one could compare processed mugwort with another spongy vegetable matter that burns evenly at an appropriate heat, but actually selecting and controlling such a substance would seem as much of a challenge as controlling the quality of the mugwort. In any case, of course, it is known that, in the history of moxibustion, other materials than mugwort have been used, so such comparisons may of themselves present no data of significance and will beg challenges which will not be dissimilar to those offered with sham needling.

---

[264] An enquiry made to one of the major Japanese producers as to whether mugwort for moxa was cultivated or picked from the wild was met with a totally perplexed response, as if it were the most stupid question imaginable: "Of course we pick it from the wild. Why not? It grows everywhere!"

In a similar vein, one might choose to control by selecting standard and non-standard points and comparing outcomes. In fact, it is eminently arguable that this would be a great idea. We can consider the 1983 study which compared the differing serological response using moxa applied to Liv14 and Sp15 in this context [265]. But, as with acupuncture research, agreeing on supposedly inert "sham" points and the location of "real" ones would be challenging, particularly as it is arguable that general responses may more probably occur with moxa applied anywhere on the body than may occur with acupuncture. Doctor Hara certainly believed so to a degree. So results from such research may prove as challengeable as they would be interesting, and unfortunately would almost certainly create as many questions as answers in the short term.

Double-blinding the action of burning moxa on the skin would appear to be practically very difficult, if not impossible. One might be able to successfully convince a research technician who is newly trained in moxibustion techniques that ground-up Scottish autumn heather, for instance, is actually processed mugwort; one might even manage to persuade him that a set of anatomical locations over which he has been trained to smoulder such sham moxa are "real" points when in fact they are not; but the likelihood of this being managed in a way that could be deemed conclusively controlled or effectively double-blinded is slim.

Ultimately, risk taking is often a necessary part of advancing medical knowledge, and it is to manage and mitigate such risks, of course, that such strict regulations have been designed to manage such research. The higher the stake for potential benefit for medicine (and of course therefore for the patient) the more kindly the risk should be viewed. In the case of the moxa and breech trials, unfortunately, it seems that the research was simply considered not worth it. The potential benefits to mothers and babies cannot unfortunately have been seen ultimately to outweigh the potential risks in researching the protocol, nor indeed to outweigh the known risks of manual version, so the proposal was sacrificed accordingly.

The implication for more general moxibustion practice from this situation is a worrying one. Ever increasingly we are being encouraged as acumoxa practitioners to be more research conscious and to become governed by the auspices of Evidence Based Medicine (EBM). We are accordingly exhorted to improve our act with more scientifically rigorous research. We must face the possibility that, as wider regulation of less orthodox medical practice grows, however haltingly, we may find ourselves proscribed from using certain acumoxa interventions precisely because we have such little scientific evidence on which to justify their application. For acupuncture, lines may well remain conveniently blurred and things may well

---

[265] Okozaki M, Furuya E, Kasahara T, Sakamoto K 1983 "Effect of moxibustion on the phagocytic activity in mice." American Journal of Chinese Medicine Vol XI; No. 1-4: 112-122

continue largely as they are, but regarding moxibustion we should consider the possibility that things may be far less certain.

The institutions which carry the torch of educating acumoxa practitioners for the future take such exhortations for more scientific research very seriously, recognising that ignoring them creates the possibility that acupuncture, or indeed moxibustion, might be biomedically discredited. If acupuncture research is by its nature that much easier to get approved to trial status than moxibustion research, however, it is easy to see why research into moxa has been instinctively avoided in the West. Aside from the intrinsic difficulties involved, we can also see that such research, whilst of potential interest to the wider profession, might not be of such interest to these institutions. Such institutions logically must focus their attentions on less controversial or challenging parts of the acumoxa canon at the cost of more marginal practices, of which moxibustion is clearly an example. This may well ultimately have a restrictive impact on the practice of acumoxa in the West, but it also will have an overall inevitable detrimental effect on the therapy itself.

One of the current strategies employed by those attempting to discredit CAM is to invoke embarrassment for such educational institutions by focusing on their more challengeable or curious therapeutic approaches. Challenging the fundamental ideas of homeopathy by focusing on the non-scientific basis of its primary mechanisms is a typical case in point and has resulted in curtailing funding to publicly funded teaching hospitals in the UK and compromising existing Bachelor of Science degree courses. The same strategy is being used against CAM in Australia.

It should be noted that this strategy contains a revealing flaw. The basic premise behind this tactic is that CAM equals quackery because of an absence of a convincing evidence base. We have already recognised, in fact, that CAM is in fact merely CAM because of this absence, not necessarily because it is ineffective. It does not necessarily follow from this therefore that CAM equals quackery. Those courses involved in CAM which have managed to associate themselves with a university have, at least, provided themselves with an opportunity to correct this issue of deficient research evidence by having access to the specialist researchers and statisticians who might help them construct the sort of trials which such critics claim the field so shamefully lacks. But at exactly this point in the story, these same critics endeavour to get these very courses kicked out the institutions they need to be a part of, effectively denying them access to the resources that they need to be able to properly satisfy such criticisms. Effectively they are attempting to deliberately confine these therapies to scientifically substandard research (and to their disdain) for ever! It's a "lose-lose" situation for CAM which is being disingenuously promoted by some hard-nosed and highly savvy members of the scientific community with quite evident axes to grind. In fact, such critics, if they were to operate more fairly, should properly allow the field the capacity at the very least to appropriately "test" their own unproven hypothesis that "CAM equals quackery" in a fair and unbiased way rather than dismissing it out of hand as they do because it lacks the evidence base that it has yet to get access to.

Notwithstanding such inconsistency, such a tactic of challenging acupuncture through drawing attention to the less-scientific and more traditional components of a Bachelor of Science degree may already have resulted in the closure of at least two acupuncture courses in the UK recently. It is not remotely far-fetched to imagine some similar campaign which could be equally effective and far more easily waged to ridicule moxibustion on the basis of it being a primitive treatment belonging to another age – whatever its potential applicability today might actually be. As a result of such pressures, moxa, which is already poorly understood and under-taught, could find itself simply removed entirely from undergraduate acupuncture training and become even more side-lined in post-graduate education. Acupuncture, in its more traditional forms, potentially suffers the same challenges of course, but for moxibustion practice, this risk is particularly acute: further research into moxibustion will almost certainly be avoided without really good cause, as will a wider promotion of its effectiveness.

This runs the risk of returning moxibustion to an even poorer status than it has suffered to date in comparison to its acupuncture sibling. It is something which should encourage us to think long and hard about alternative strategies to confer appropriate status on what we do – strategies which might not necessarily include the gold standard of the double-blinded RCT since, for moxa at least, it may largely lie *de facto* beyond our grasp.

The RCT itself, however, may not be the issue. The real issue may be that of systematic reviewer whio presides as ultimate judge and jury over the system of the Randomised Control Trial. In a field of research that involves hundreds of well-designed studies such a system has useful validity. Someone has to do the painstaking work of trawling through all the available data, weighing it up, and offering some sort of conclusive report on the state of play, although it has to be said that a systematic review of systematic reviews suggested that they are far from consistent in their conclusions. This study looked at three hundred systematic reviews and concluded that the quality of their reporting was inconsistent and that the findings from such reviews should not be accepted uncritically[266].

In a field where the research is limited, however, is less systematic and often less well-designed than is desirable, the ducks are well lined up for any reviewer with any sort of agenda. The proof is in the pudding. Recently in the UK the Advertising Standards Agency has ruled that UK acupuncturists can only publicly say that they "treat" (just "treat", not "help" or "cure") four conditions – nausea,

---

[266] Moher D, Tetzlaff J, Tricco A, Sampson M, Altman D 2007 "Epidemiology and Reporting Characteristics of Systematic Reviews".PLoS Med.; 4(3): e78. Published online 2007 March 27. doi: 10.1371/journal.pmed.0040078

dental pain, knee pain and lower back pain. Such a list is frankly ridiculous given the range of conditions which the WHO list as being potentially helped by acupuncture, but in spite of this the ruling remains purely because of the unwarranted power of the systematic reviewer. Since the systematic reviewer tends to stay pretty much in his or her academic tower never actively being involved in research itself or in the treatment, it's difficult not to see them as being something akin to the bankers of medicine, making money out of other peoples' industry with the least amount of effort whilst never taking off their suits or getting their hands dirty.

At the least, as the study suggested, the situation could improve if more widely agreep upon evidence-based reporting guidleines were determined. But it could also improve if the general strategy for researching CAM was more systematic itself to allow for and anticipate such opposition.

So, for the present, while more research is plainly necessary and is being quite logically (and apparently so reasonably) requested by the power houses of EBM, it seems unlikely that, without very compelling reasons, approval for any such research with moxa will be granted. In the extraordinary event that such approval were obtained, the consequential risk exists that the treatment would be bowdlerised into something unrecognisable as normal clinical practice simply in order that it might conform to the quirky geometry required by an RCT.

Moxibustion as a practice thus risks finding itself accused of being frightened of, or unable to, withstand rigorous examination by science – or alternatively may find itself asking for special concessions to allow our therapy to duck beneath the bar of acceptable scientific accountability. This, at least, is how the detractors of CAM generally see such situations. Such pressures may well prove too uncomfortable for those among us who do not embrace the practice of moxibustion that positively anyway. "Dump it!" might then seem like the most pragmatic answer, particularly if the cost of not doing so is seen to prove so limiting to acupuncture practice generally, or even to taint its image.

Moxibustion research, which has hardly begun in the West, thus seems to be already controlled by a double-bind as much as a double-blind. In fact, it is indisputable that we have yet to begin to understand the mechanisms or indeed the power of good moxa treatment. Whilst the same may well be true of acupuncture as well, it is unlikely to find itself under such a direct threat of practical extermination, so the glint in the needle will certainly continue to glisten, while the glow in the moxa cone may find itself snuffed out.

Attempts to further investigate moxa, by this definition, may simply confer upon it (hardly for the first time in its long history it should be said) an orphan status. Having been somewhat of a poor relative in the acumoxa relationship for centuries, this really should be nothing that the therapy cannot handle, but, given the times we live in, it presents challenges nevertheless. One of the most fascinating possibilities (concerning possible IR spectral densities and the implications of their relation to the equivalent human infra-red radiation discussed in Part 4 the Stems) could remain un-investigated as a result. The tools for such measurement are the domain of NASA scientists, and require funding which is quite literally astronomic compared to anything normally available to researchers in the field of complementary health. In fact, mention the words "complementary health" and "research" in the same sentence, and the funding shutters tend to roll down with alacrity as a matter of course anyway, as many have found already.

But things may even be a little more complicated still! Using our earlier definition of CAM (that it is a medicine of known reputed effect which is insufficiently confirmed by rigorous scientific research) then acupuncture as a wider therapy mayitself already have become dangerously fragmented: treatment for knee or back pain, for instance, which is now accepted to be supported by rigorous RCT research can already be defined as no longer being part of CAM at all, whilst acupuncture for IBS, for instance, is still very clearly a CAM treatment. We need to be far more aware that by researching acumoxa at all we are actually at risk of dissecting it in a way that many of us would instinctively consider to be abhorrent.

This may sound unfair, but digging around in the pages of Cochrane reveals this (very reasonable and carefully worded) definition of CAM which casts further light on an emerging dilemma: "Complementary and alternative medicine (CAM) is a broad domain of healing resources that encompasses all health systems, modalities, and practices and their accompanying theories and beliefs, other than those intrinsic to the politically dominant health system of a particular society or culture in a given historical period. CAM includes all such practices and ideas self-defined by their users as preventing or treating illness or promoting health and well-being. Boundaries within CAM and between the CAM domain and that of the dominant system are not always sharp or fixed."

It may seem reassuring to be reminded that boundaries between these different strands of medicine are not always that sharp or fixed, but we should also become wary when CAM is broadly being defined as any therapy that is not "intrinsic to the politically dominant health system of a particular society".

This makes scientific research in this field complex and potentially self-defeating, since any successful research could (and/or maybe should) render the treatment intrinsically more acceptable to the so-called "dominant health system" and no longer a part of CAM at all, otherwise the dominant health system itself would be scientifically flawed and certainly prejudiced.

Such an idea raises interesting challenges for both biomedicine and for CAM in terms of research. Achieving the sorts of goals for CAM research for breech treatment with moxa that are encouraged by Cochrane, for instance, would effectively leap-frog moxa (for this particular problem) from a fringe treatment for what is a recognised medical problem to an evidence-based one which would have become automatically intrinsically freshly acceptable to our "specific society and culture" (to requote the language of Cochrane). Perhaps this idea goes some way to explain why there was such clear implicit resistance to the idea of supporting such research.

But to extend this line of thinking even further, one has to ask a further essentially discomforting question as to why any professional CAM researcher would have any true interest in successfully completing any program of comprehensive research in CAM if he or she is truly wedded to many (or even any) of the ideals of CAM. Such ideals might include those of holism, and person-centredness rather than symptom-centred diagnosis and treatment. The success of the scientifically controlled "nothing but" of research is only likely to undermine such ideas or ideals. In other words, we might even speculate whether it is actually more in these researchers' professional interests to keep these therapies necessarily "fuzzy", and that, if this is in any way the case, such actions might be to the possible detriment of those very sections of society that might best benefit from them. To put it bluntly: whilst some opf the issues of developing good research into CAM are very complex, there are more than a few academics making a reasonable living from CAM research; but are they working under a leaky umbrella of conflicting interest? And, furthermore, does the "fuzziness" which already exists in the record of CAM research stand as proof of this concern?

We can even ask whether we, as traditional acupuncturists, are similarly suspect. Many of us, for instance, instinctively resist the idea that other medically-trained orthodox healthworkers should carry out simple evidence-based protocol treatments for lower back pain. We do so because we consider such healthworkers to be undertrained technicians because they have only undertaken short-course training. Those who manage modern medicine, of course, see this slightly differently – they see it from the perspective of simple economics.

We are genuinely convinced that such treatments undersell both treatment and therapy, and we instinctively believe (without too much genuine evidence it has to be admitted) that we could do a far better job than the technician since we have undergone (and, of course, invested in) lengthy and arguably sometimes irrelevant training – irrelevant in that much of it may have little or no ultimate impact on clinical effectiveness as far as bioscience is concerned.

This may seem unfair, but we have to recognise that it is exactly these chunks of our training which Cochraneand others select in order to place traditional acumoxa outside of the domain of orthodox medicine. Such parts of the training both embrace and explore what they consider to be scientifically-troubling "theories and beliefs". Meanwhile, we honestly and very sincerely profess and share such theories pretty much profession-wide, and many of our patients embrace them as well. Ultimately, however, we may be forced to confront the possibility that a much larger number of people might benefit from acumoxa if it was more widely carried out in the sorts of scenarios we consider to be anathema to what we consider to be "true" acupuncture (whatever that really is!) without some of its more philosophical accoutrements, carried out by under-trained technicians rather than by accomplished practitioners.

Such are challenging ideas, but we are facing challenging times.

Final Conclusions

From most perspectives, it can be quite reasonably argued that moxibustion deserves a decent-sized cabinet for veneration in the museum of the history of world medicine. From another perspective entirely, it is equally arguable that it actually deserves to be taken out of this cupboard, dusted off and objectively held up to the light of scientific investigation – but that this should surely be an investigation on terms which are at least fair and equitable to the therapy itself rather than on the general terms of modern medical research which is predicated by the power, politics and profit of the pharmaceutical industry with which it has so little in common. One of the therapy's handicaps, as well as it being one of its intrinsic strengths, is that there can be no patents associated with it, so no huge profits are to be made from its further development[267]. This is a handicap only in as much as this effectively stifles the commercial stimulus for appropriate enquiry; but it is a strength in that it imbues the therapy with a quality of innocence and simplicity of which the health industry generally is regrettably often deficient and of which it is instinctively wary.

Certain uncomfortable conclusions might be drawn from the above. Given the overall state of global health, medical scientific enquiry can justifiably stand accused of obsessively seeking out its knowledge whilst remaining negligently blinkered to the wider fundamental welfare of the majority of mankind. Using NASA as a prime example of the dynamic power of modern science, untold millions of dollars have been heaped into the debatable but very real goal of identifying habitable planets whilst the host planet itself is simultaneously being rendered less and less habitable by the waste and detritus of this self-same science. An obscene see-saw phenomenon seems to have developed: the technological and economic forces required to jettison mankind upwards and off from his natural home seems to have irreversibly thrown the larger part of mankind and much of the natural world it inhabits into a pit of despair. The policy of "nothing-butness" which is at the heart of Cartesian thinking seems to be sending us down nothing but a dreadfully perilous path.

---

[267] There are some who might challenge this assumption. A patent, however, is defined as providing the right to **exclude others** from making, using, selling, offering for sale, or importing the patented invention. If moxa remains processed and used in ways which are self-evidently traditional and historical (and not in any way invented), it is difficult to see how it could be ever construed as a therapy that could be patentable.

What appears to have been developing for the health of humanity are two very different highways of medical research, one which is primarily focused on the developed world, and the other more focused on the uncomfortable realities of the less-developed and developing ones. Realities on the one highway are defined by scientific certainties, and progress along it is fuelled by pharmaceutical profit; the realities on the other road are defined by just that – reality, and little progress is made. Along this highway lethal disease is quite literally "neglected".

Of the 1223 drugs globally licensed between 1975 and 1996, only 13 were for treatment of tropical diseases[268]. Two of these were an outcome of military research, six resulted from veterinary research, and two were merely modifications of existing drugs. Thus, over a period of more than 20 years, unbelievably **only three** drugs were developed specifically for the tropics (artemether, atovaquone and eflornithine) and one of these is no longer produced. That is some sorry story...

The Beijing Declaration adopted by the UN in 2008 attempted to address just this anomaly, recognising that, for the benefit of millions of human beings, realities had to be confronted which might necessarily have to include the wider recognition of traditional medicines. Amongst other things the Declaration recognises that:

- "The knowledge of traditional medicines, treatments and practices should be respected, and preserved, based on the circumstances in each country;
- Governments have a responsibility for the health of their people and should formulate policies, regulations and standards, as part of comprehensive national health systems to ensure appropriate, safe and effective use of traditional medicine;
- Recognizing the progress of many governments to date in integrating traditional medicine into their national health system, those who have not yet done so are called upon to take action;
- Traditional medicine should be further developed based on research and innovation.
- Governments, international organisations and other stakeholders should collaborate in implementing the global strategy and plan of action;
- The communication between conventional and traditional medicine providers should be strengthened and appropriate training should be established for health professionals, medical students and relevant researchers."

---

[268] Trouiller P, Olliaro P 1999 "Drug development output from 1975 to 1996: what proportion for tropical diseases." Int J Infect Dis; 3: 61-63.

So things could really still change, but it must readily be recognised that bridging the gap between these two highways may be the biggest challenge of all. Being awarded a listing on the UN's "intangible cultural heritage list" is certainly not going to be the answer.

Regarding moxa, we can conclude that there is likely to be no easy road towards better and more comprehensive research. The potentials from the research (and in moxa's case it is the potential which should provide both motor and fuel for fresh research) should, in fact, serve to motivate rather than to create despondency. Huge opportunities exist here. We have already established that the road of research in the field of complementary health and in traditional medicine is a stony and rutted one, running parallel to a metaphorically shinier multilane freeway for conventional profit-motivated pharmaceutical research. And we have also recognised that the double-blinded RCT model is not one which is necessarily bespoke to moxibustion, but similarly it is not that bespoke to acupuncture nor to many similar physical therapies, any and/or all of which face similar threats from the sledge-hammer of Evidence Based Medicine when applied in its more fundamentalist form. Alternative models **must** be found, developed and used to better investigate these or humanity as a whole will be worse off as a result – and these other therapies will also be destined to line up in cabinets on the same floor of the museum of medical history which is already potentially reserved for moxibustion.

If (and it is clear that this is a big "if") moxibustion can be shown to line up fair and square as a *bona fide* treatment to help combat an infectious scourge of the modern world, even if it finds itself merely with the status of sling-shot alongside the laser-guided missiles of modern medicine, important ground will have been broken. The rutted track for such research will at least have had some potholes filled in, so that any other wobbly-wheeled traffic struggling along it will find its going that little bit easier.

In the course of drawing these conclusions, the management and development of modern medicine has been shown up in a somewhat tawdry light. It is my considered opinion that the world of commercial medicine has a lot to answer for, but this is not to imply the same for the millions of health professionals who are using the theories and techniques of modern medicine to combat human suffering across the world. Indeed, in the field of medical research and development there have been, and still are, many extraordinary people. Jonas Silk, for instance, the man responsible for the discovery and development of the polio vaccine, saw it as impossible that his treatment, which has proved to have been of such value to humankind in the past fifty years, could possibly be patented. "Could you patent the sun?" he asked (naively perhaps by the standards of the world we inhabit today because some in the business would almost certainly argue otherwise...).

But perhaps we could say something similar about moxibustion, with its intimate association with the sun's energy – its *yang*ness, how the better strains are grown on the sunny south facing slopes, how they are associated with high summer, and dried in strong sunlight, and how it is burnt almost as an emblematic ceremony which echoes the power of the sun itself. Just possibly, should it be jostling for its own discrete position right in there in the front line of medical practice?

If the allopathic approach can be best described as an "outside-in" approach, some of the mechanisms of moxibustion might equally be described as being more "inside-out". It is incontestable that some of its more compelling actions in some way stimulate the host immune response. With such an understanding, it is quite feasible that moxibustion has real immuno-therapeutic potentials in primary care that may ultimately prove to be neither complementary nor alternative.

The fact is, unfortunately, that significant motivation may also be required to reverse the general tendency of CAM practitioners, many of whom are at best somewhat reticent or reluctant to engage in research, and at worst actively suspicious of it. Some similar motivation will be required to attract a more positive attention from the scientific community which is often dismissive of the apparent flakiness of the CAM world, sometimes quite rightly so. Raising awareness of larger issues may actually serve to help this process.

We began by identifying how moxa therapy was most probably the "older-twin" of acupuncture, and how it may have found itself sidelined over the centuries in favour of its sibling, at times giving it almost orphan status. It is my hope that the reader may now be left wondering whether we have, lying in the moxa jars in our treatment rooms, more of a reluctant prodigal son, whose proper return is now perhaps overdue.

In the pages above we have gently seen off a couple of acumoxa's sacred cows, if not to the market at least to the vet's for re-examination. In their absence, the tender fatted calf which has been left behind might be justified in feeling a little nervous. Moxibustion, acumoxa's prodigal brother, just might make a long-delayed return if we can help him find his way home – and the feast on his arrival could be a confounding one in that it may even serve to challenge some of the fundamentals of biomedicine (one of which is that medical therapies have to be both technologically complex and expensive to be effective).

Three hundred years ago, Bashō considered the islands at Matsushima to be the most beautiful sight in Japan. On his way there he had stopped in both Fukushima and Sendai, two place names that, since March 2011, have been painfully etched on to global consciousness. Suffering and beauty unfortunately often walk hand in hand across this earth.

On the 26th June 1689 Bashō arrived at Matsushima and was finally confronted with the reality of his vision – the vision that he had originally imagined before starting his long and hazardous journey after he had applied moxa to strengthen his legs back in Edo/Tokyo. On finally seeing the bay, the master poet simply found himself lost for words: "My pen strove in vain to equal this superb creation of divine artifice," he wrote. The only lines of verse which he could muster follow below to conclude our own journey. Including them at this point means that this book, which began with one of his beautiful poems, can now end with another: it opened with seventeen enigmatic syllables about the simple wayside weed mugwort, but now ends with a further seventeen which describe the ultimate reality of what Bashō had previously envisioned. They were the only words that the master poet could find at the time:

MATSUSHIMA YA,

A-A MATSUSHIMA YA,

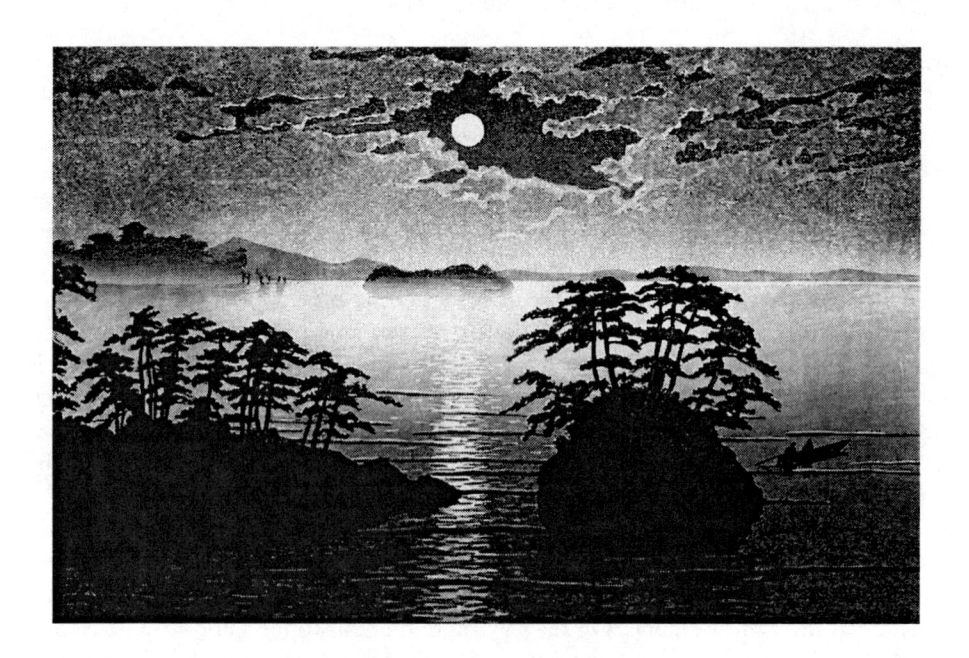

MATSUSHIMA YA....

Postscript:
Page 1 of the Story of Moxafrica

> "FADE FAR AWAY, DISSOLVE, AND QUITE FORGET
> WHAT THOU AMONG THE LEAVES HAST NEVER KNOWN,
> THE WEARINESS, THE FEVER, AND THE FRET
> HERE, WHERE MEN SIT AND HEAR EACH OTHER GROAN"
> **John Keats "To a Nightingale"**[269]

> "IF A MAN TAKES NO THOUGHT ABOUT WHAT IS DISTANT, HE WILL FIND
> SORROW NEAR AT HAND"
> **Confucius**

Reflecting on moxa's applications over the centuries for treating difficult or intransigent conditions, it is immediately difficult to resist the temptation of speculating whether some of what we might describe today as "modern-type" diseases which present such a challenge to medicine might be our own contemporary equivalent of the intractable conditions of the past. With clearer information on the reactions of different viruses to whole-body moxa stimulation, for instance, might there be possibilities for the integrated treatment of HIV/AIDS, or Post-Viral Syndromes with moxa? Could possibilities exist for the treatment of certain types of cancer, or for the treatment of patients with variously compromised immune systems, including auto-immune disease? Might a use be found for moxa in the treatment of what have come to be called "hospital superbugs" – those bacteria which have seemingly adapted and percolated the defensive super-systems of antibiotic medicine? Other "primitive" techniques such as the use of antibacterial maggots, have been successfully if somewhat begrudgingly accepted into the repertoire of modern medicine, so why not moxa? And might such possibilities even include the potential of preserving life?

Such are audacious thoughts – and are certainly not ones which often come into consideration in the field of Complementary and Alternative Medicine. In genereral CAM focuses on the supportive treatment of non-life-threatening chronic disease and disorder.

Based on the recognised challenges for moxa research, the possibilities of actually testing such ideas would seem hopelessly remote – but it was exactly one such idea which lit the touch paper for Moxafrica.

The taper itself was drug resistant tuberculosis………

---

[269] This was one of Keats' last poems, written whilst dying of TB. Keats' mother and brother also died of TB. This particular stanza relates to the death of his brother Tom who succumbed to the disease at the age of nineteen.

The Moon over Matsushima

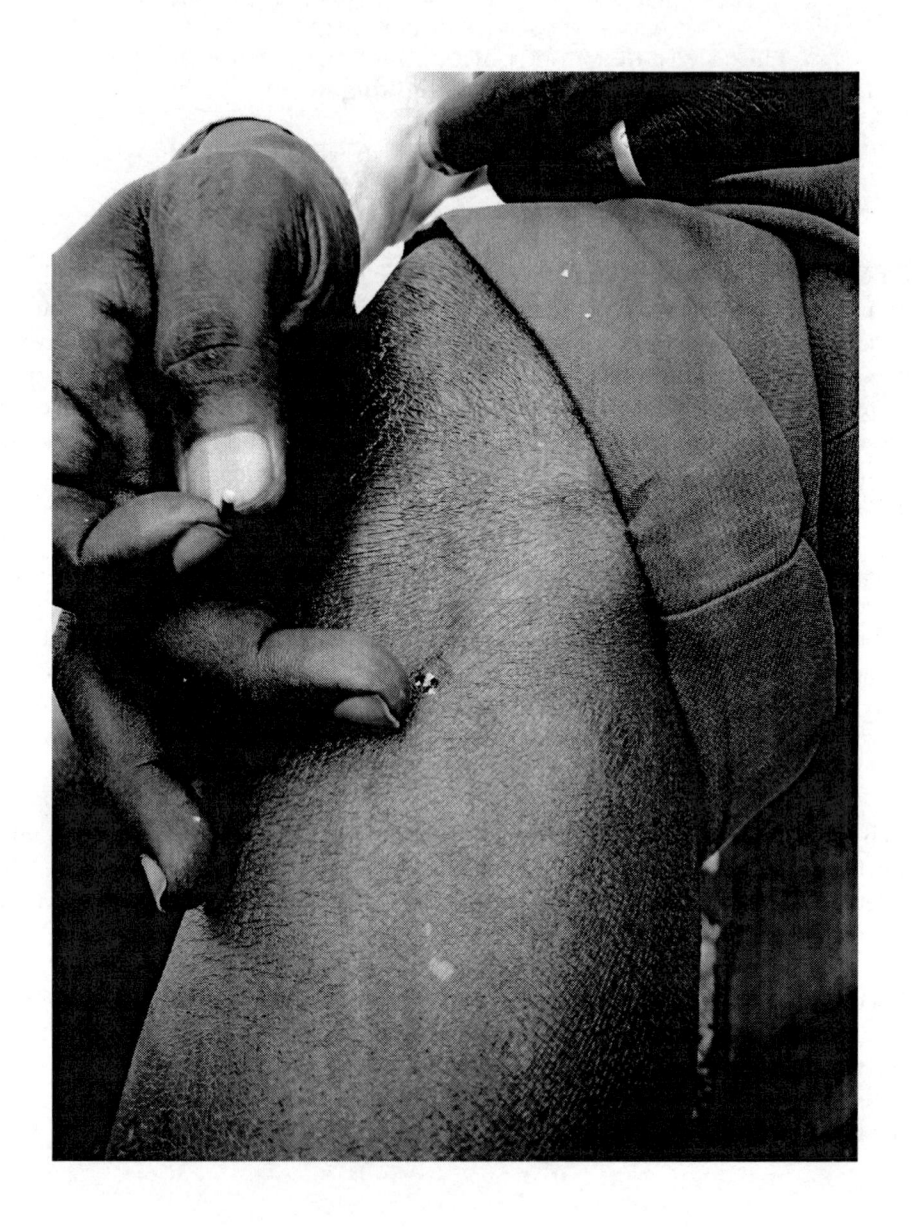

Appendix 1

Preparing and applying small moxa cones

The first, and perhaps the most important, step is to obtain appropriate high quality moxa specifically refined for direct moxibustion, meaning that burning temperatures can be minimised, that smaller cones can be more consistently prepared, and that there will be no spitting from pieces of leaf matter in the nap.

Equipment needed:

>Bowl of water
>Incense sticks/tapers
>Lighter/matches
>Pen for marking the points
>Moxa

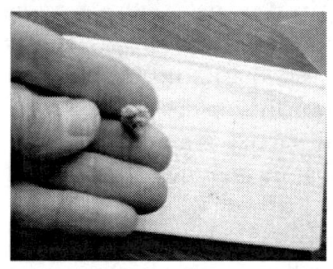

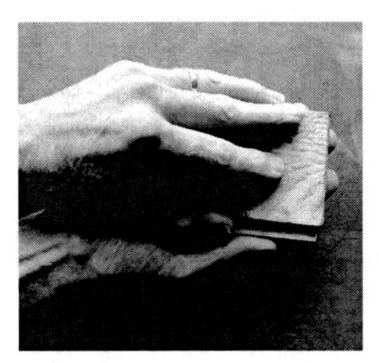

It is important to prepare cones of reproducible size and density. The easiest way to do this is to first roll some moxa into a thin thread.

Place a small amount of moxa between two flat pieces of wood or board, and rub the boards gently together from side to side until the moxa is formed into a long thin shape about 2mm wide.

It is important not to press too hard or the moxa will be too dense and will burn too hot.

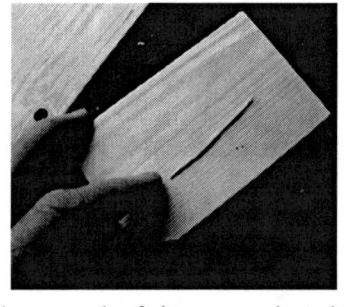

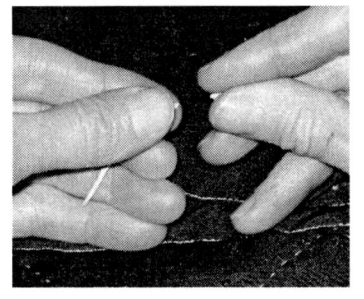

Making sure that your hands are dry and not greasy, hold one end of the moxa thread in your left hand (for right handed people) between thumb and first finger, and then tear off the smallest possible length of moxa with the thumb and first finger of your other hand. To maintain the shape of the cone you may need to roll it a little between your fingers.

The Moon over Matsushima

You should always aim for the smallest 1mg size, or even smaller (the size of half a grain of dry rice). Patients taught at the clinic how to do this technique on themselves at home may find this difficult at first but with practice they should soon be able to make cones of equal size and shape.

The cone should be placed upright so that only one end is touching the skin and it is not bent over. Although the term most commonly used it "cone", the general idea is that the base of small-cone moxa cones should be no wider than the rest of the cone – and if anything a little narrower, like a rice grain.

Moisten the skin very slightly using a lightly moistened fingertip (the "pinkey" little finger is best) that is not holding moxa. Stand the moxa upright on the point, so that only a small tip of the moxa is in contact with the skin. (Don't use too much water or the cone will not burn)

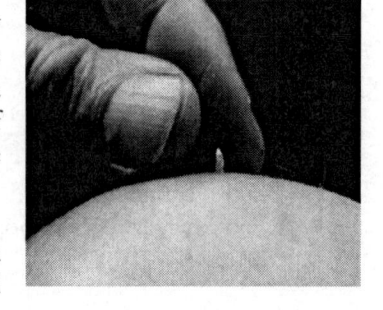

Light the taper and hold it as you would a cigarette between your right first and second fingers of your right hand.

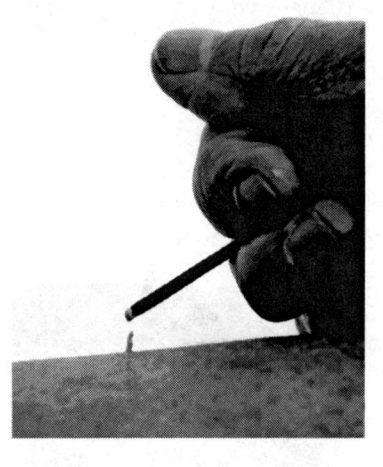

Light the top of the moxa by gently touching it with the incense stick and twisting it slightly. Rest your right hand on the skin to keep it steady.

Allow the moxa to burn down to the skin.

The beauty of holding the taper this way is that the moxa thread can still be held in the other hand and can be torn off by the thumb and forefinger of the taper-holding hand: nothing need be put down or picked up, and a swift and rhythmic technique can be developed.

If you are doing repeated cones, leave the ash on the skin and put the next cone on top. Repeat with 3, 5, or 7 cones.

When you have finished, wipe off the ash.

The same points should generally be treated again every day.

A brown stain and probably a blister will form but this will soon heal and form a hard layer. This reduces the sensation from the moxa as treatment is continued meaning that slightly bigger cones can be considered if appropriate or the cones made a little denser.

Appendix 1 – Clinical Treatments

Moxa treatment is very simple and quite safe if used properly. The only side effect (from direct moxa) might be a small scar.

If the treatment is too strong, however, the patient might possibly show signs of over-treatment such as dizziness, hot flushes, or nausea but these can all be avoided. Unusual reactions like this are almost always due to overdosage, which is why building up the dosage is so important. Restarting and continuing treatment at a lower dosage should be both safe and potentially effective.

Occasionally symptoms such as joint pains can temporarily worsen but may then be seen to resolve. If these effects occur they should only last a day ot two or less, but reduce treatment if there is any concern. If they last longer than a couple of days the treatment should be discontinued.

Patients should always be started on a low dosage and this can be increased gradually as long as the patient is not showing any adverse reactions.

Check for signs of any sort of infection at the moxa points whenever the patient is seen, and warn the patient accordingly as well. Immune compromised patients need particularly careful monitoring, but the potential benefit for them is great if care is taken.

It is very important for patients to understand that bigger cones are <u>not</u> more effective. Sometimes patients believe that this will be the case. As long as the cones are kept small, any blisters that develop will be tiny, and should not cause any risk to the patient. Small scabs will form over any tiny blisters, and this is actually a good sign. They should not be scratched or removed and should be allowed to heal and to drop off naturally – suggesting that the moxa treatment is helping the body's powers of healing. This may not happen so rapidly in the earlier stages of treatment, however, and if there is any concern that the skin is not healing or there is any sign of infection, treatment should be stopped and the blistering should be allowed to heal.

Once a scab has formed and fallen off a couple of times at any point, some positive effects will probably have already been noticed by the patient, and treatment should be continued. When the scab comes off by itself it is a sign that the tissue beneath has recovered. On darker or black skin, it is more likely that some tiny scarring will remain.

Never use moxa on broken skin or oedema.

Due to the possibility of blisters becoming infected it is advised against treating diabetic patients with this particular technique, rather using larger cones and a "snatch moxa" technique.

Extra special care should be taken not to over-treat pregnant women.

Treatment with moxa should be built up carefully and gradually, particularly in weaker patients and also those with more advanced illness. Every patient should be evaluated individually to assess the dosage they will need – the more advanced the illness, the lower the starting dosage and the slower the increase. Always start with a low dosage (one or 3 cones per point), and increase this gradually as long as the patient is not showing any adverse reactions.

The patient should quickly realise that the treatment only takes a few minutes if done once there is familiar with the technique, and that the benefits are well worth the small effort required.

The heat of the moxa and therefore the dosage can be adjusted in several ways:

1. Varying the number of cones repeated on each point.
2. Varying the density of the moxa (more tightly rolled cones burn hotter).
3. Adjusting the size of the cones.
4. Cowling.
5. Leaving the ash on the skin and burning repeated cones on top of this or removing each cone.
6. Removing the cone or snuffing it out before it burns down to the skin.

IN ALL CASES, WHERE MEDICATION IS PRESCRIBED IT MUST BE CONTINUED. Daily moxa treatment may well make medication more effective as the patient's own recovery instincts rally, and it should also help reduce side-effects from the drugs.

Traditionally, moxa is burnt in quantities of odd numbers, so always start with one or three cones on each points (equal numbers on both sides unless there is good reason) carefully locating the most reactive point. If no ill-effects are observed, and the patient has become accustomed to the treatment and accepts it, only then should the dosage be increased.

This will be an unfamiliar treatment. People are not used to moxa and may well be frightened of being burnt. Reassure them by demonstrating first on your own skin. Try to assess how sensitive a person is and start with a very low heat. This should feel quite pleasant and she/he will then be relieved and reassured. Later you may be able to increase the dose. If individual patients appear to be extremely sensitive to heat, the cone can be stubbed out immediately heat is felt – but it MUST still be felt by the patient to count.

The points will get a scab on them after a few times, and this will reduce the sensitivity. If there is any sign of blistering or a scab and the sensitivity increases stop moxa treatment immediately at this point.

Clinical treatments

Constitutional "whole body" treatments

These are indicated as being useful when nothing else has helped, when diagnosis is too complex, when the patient clearly needs constitutional fortification, or when the patient's condition is severe and chronic.

Sawada's "*Taiji*" or "*Taikokyu*" moxa treatment

Takeshi (Ken) Sawada (1877 – 1938) was a famous Japanese moxibustionist. He came from a family famous for its *kendo* traditions. He lived for twenty years working as a bodyguard in Korea, before studying the Chinese classics, learning and practising bone-setting and developing his famous skills in moxibustion. His work was initially brought to the attention of the public by a journalist investigating Japanese traditional medical practice. Sawada was known as a master of visual and palpatory inspection, relying primarily on observation and palpation to diagnose abnormalities of the internal organs which he treated with moxa, mainly on the back. He saw moxa as being particularly effective in the treatment of chronic disease by improving blood circulation. As such, many of the points he identified for treatment arose from years of systematic palpation and experience, and he "relocated" several classic acupoints as a result. His methods have held great influence over many followers, including Bunshi Shirota (1900-1974) who recorded his treatments and attempted to systematise them.

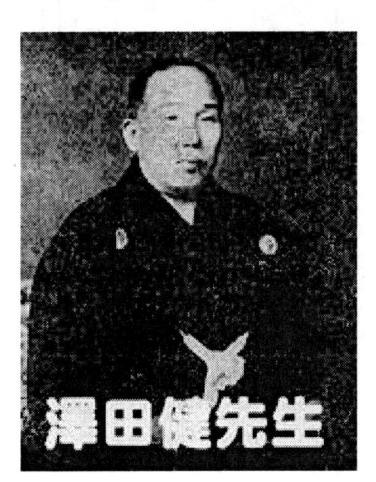

He used moxa for both symptomatic and constitutional treatment, considering that it could relax muscle tension, relieve inflammation and pain, improve circulation and strengthen the immune system. Points are generally selected by palpation and reactivity.

Sawada's original points for general constitutional treatment are listed below in the classic order of their application:

Ren 12, (left)TB4 (patient lying on back)
Bl23, Bl32 (patient lying face down)
Du12, Bl20 (patient sitting up)
LI11, Ki3 (patient sitting up or lying on back)

Shirota, who was also interested in the scientific explanations for these treatments, made some minor revisions based on his own experiences. He tended to omit TB4 and Ki3, and added **St36**, Du20 (often) and **Bl15, Bl17** and **Bl18**.

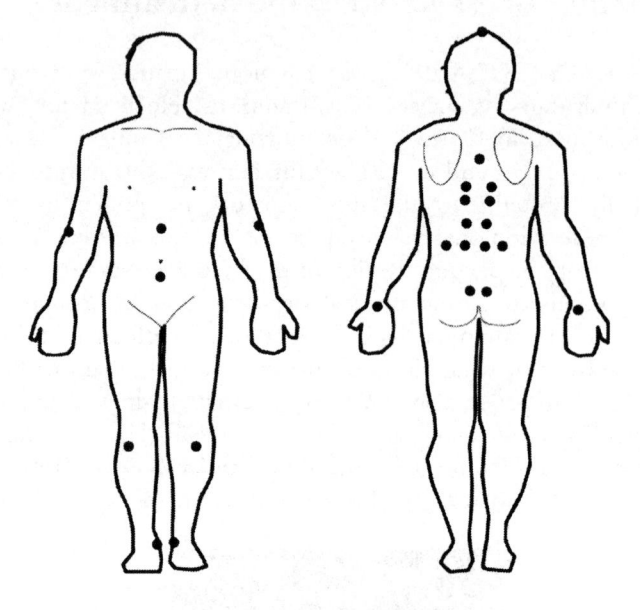

Sawada's Taiji Points

Shirota's adapted method is still widely used and taught as the classic Sawada *taiji* treatment. It can be developed into a flexible and fluid model for treatment, adding or removing points depending on the diagnosed disease and the palpatory findings either from initial diagnosis or as the treatment proceeds.

Shirota, it should be added, was inclined to use both acupuncture and moxibustion, whilst Sawada's approach was defined primarily by the use of moxa only (in fact it is not entirely certain that he was actually ever officially licensed as an acupuncturist at all, only as a moxibustionist).

Manaka's "Taikokyu" constitutional treatment

Dr Yoshio Manaka was both fascinated by moxibustion and impressed by the clinical results he saw in his patients from its application. He was a trained surgeon, but was renowned for successfully treating patients with very difficult conditions using his own creative take on acumoxa.

He was also heavily influenced himself by Sawada's approaches.

He was particularly guided in his adaptations by his own ideas on the topological influence of the meridian system. He focused large parts of his treatment approach on selected midline points and on special meeting points all of which he established based on the results of his own research, thus developing his own whole body treatment protocol.

Again, points are finally selected for treatment (and located) by pressure pain reactivity.

Ren 12, St25, Ren4 or 7,
Bl32, Bl52, Bl23
Bl18, Bl20
Du12
Du20
TH 8
GB31, GB40, GB34, Ki7, Liv3, Liv4 and 2 *cun* above Sp10

Manaka also developed his own specific points for different conditions which he would incorporate within his *Taikokyu* treatment. Many of these are listed later within this appendix.

Fukaya's approaches

Isaburo Fukaya (1901-1974) contracted tuberculosis whilst a student and recovered with moxibustion. Two particular aspects in his approach distinguish him from others: his use of the bamboo tube (which we have examined in Part 3 – the Branches), and his focus on the intrascapular area.

He considered abnormalities in the positions of the scapulae to be indicative of specific types of disorder – abnormalities which could be treated by searching and treating palpable points in the intrascapular areas themselves.

His method he proposed for locating such points was systematic:

1. First he would run his middle and ring fingers down the spine, the inner Bladder line and the outer Bladder line looking for points or areas which were sticky.
2. Next he would review these by palpating, looking for stiffness or rigidity in the musculature.
3. Then he would refine his point selection further by testing each point to see which would elicit the most pressure pain response.
4. Finally he would check by applying pressure with the bamboo tube for around 5 seconds, and then removing it to see whether there was any abnormal discolouration left behind, indicative of stagnant blood.

He categorized the abnormalities of the scapulae as follows:

Aspects of the scapulae	Disorder
Normal	General good health
Bottoms of both scapulae rotated towards spine	Digestive disorders
Bottoms of both scapulae rotated away from spine	Respiratory disorders
Bottom of right scapula rotated away from spine	Joint pain
Bottom of left scapula rotated away from spine	Cardiac/hypertension
Bottom of right scapula rotated towards spine	Reproductive disorders
Bottom of left scapula rotated towards spine	Intestinal disorders

As a general rule he advocated only selecting the four most reactive points, but would then recommend keeping repetitively applying cone-on-ash until the pain or the stiffness had cleared. His approach was to treat the uppermost points first and work downwards.

We can consider this as a root treatment approach, but he often treated additional points, many of which were extra-meridial for added effect.

He applied a few general rules to his treatment:

- The same points do not necessarily work at each treatment
- Live points often move
- The most famous points are not always the most effective
- The number of cones and their size should be adjusted to suit the patient, so that they feel a comfortable heat.

Fukaya also had a few unusual point location methods which he adapted from traditional lay sources. In these instances he would loop a string around the problem area, and then use the same loop around the neck as a measuring device, hanging the loop down the back and stretching it to a point on the spine which would then be the indicated point for moxa. The system evolved as follows:

- For problems of the head, loop the string around the widest part of the head
- For problems of the feet, loop the string around the perimeter of both feet when placed together on the floor
- For problems of the arm, form a loop from a length of string stretched down the length of the arm from LI15 to the tip of the middle finger
- For problems of the chest, loop the string around the chest at the level of the nipples.

Some of his special points also occur in the lists of indicated treatment points which follow later in this appendix.

Nam su Kim's Korean Formula – "Mu-guk-bo-yang-tm"

Otherwise known as "Gudang", Dr Kim is a nonagenarian living and working legend in Korea, albeit shrouded with some controversy. He has been accused of having illegally trained 4,000 unqualified Koreans in the practice of moxibustion, but a Korean court upheld his right of practice.

His simple constitutional treatment is intended more as a lay health maintenance regime to be done regularly. It is very popular in South Korea.

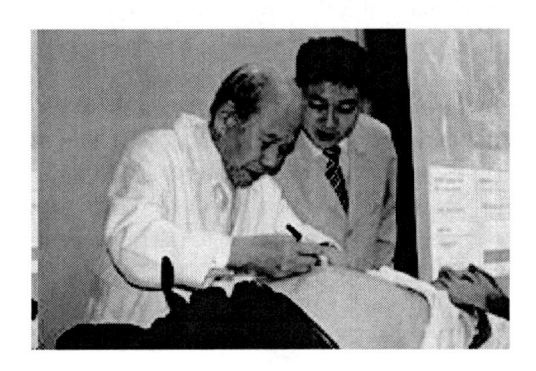

Points used:

Ren12, St36 & LI11 - to invigorate Spleen and Stomach
andeither **Ren6 & Ren4 (male)**
or: **Ren 3 & St28 (female)** - to strengthen Kidney function
Bl13 - to tonify respiration
Bl43 - for cardiac function and chronic disease
Du20 - for the mind

Doctor Hara's Treatment of (almost) all Types of Diseases

Doctor Shimetaro Hara (1883-1991) started his medical career in 1901 and began doing medical research in 1924. By 1927 he was so fascinated by the actions of moxibustion that he began a series of experiments on five groups of guinea pigs, deliberately infecting them all with the TB bacillus. (Guinea pigs are subjects of choice for such research, because (unfortunately for them) they have no natural resistance at all to the TB bacillus).

The first group was treated with moxa for a month before their infection and treatment continued afterwards. The second group had their moxa started three weeks after their infection. The third group had moxa started ten weeks after infection. And the fourth group received moxa for a month before their infection but then had their moxa treatment discontinued. A fifth group was the control, with no moxa at all. All the moxa treatments consisted of three 1mg cones on nine points "under the waist", with the frequency and dosage reducing as the experiment progressed if there were any observable signs of overdosage.

The first group did the best; the second group did nearly as well; the third group did not do so well but still compared favourably to the control group; and the fourth group survived an average two months longer than the control group.

His results amazed him. "Disease is not cured by someone else outside but through regenerative powers within," he wrote, and he specifically advocated the use of moxa for the treatment of TB which was a common killer disease in 1930s Japan.

For general health maintenance he simply advocated daily moxa on St36, 7 cones on each leg, although he also approved of the "eight day method" (see below) particularly when starting out. "This is all you have to do and something great will happen" he said, and he went on to form the "Great Japan National Health Alliance". On joining, members had to swear to carry on doing moxa at St 36 for the remainder of their life.

For "all types of disease" he advocated St36 together with his eight "loin points".

It is unclear exactly how he originally chose their exact locations but he described them as being both logical and convenient, hidden from sight, and more pleasant in terms of heat perception than any other points on the body. He was far from dismissive of meridian points, but was not dogmatic in their use. He was sure that part of moxa's effects could be obtained from applying moxa anywhere on the body, but considered that this was only a part of the story. He poetically compared those who believed that the effects of moxa were simply down to the effects of random micro-burns to be like people who claim to appreciate the sight of flowering fruit trees in springtime but ignore the colour of the cherry blossom or the fragrance of the plum blossom – they deprive themselves of an appreciation of the whole experience of the phenomenon.

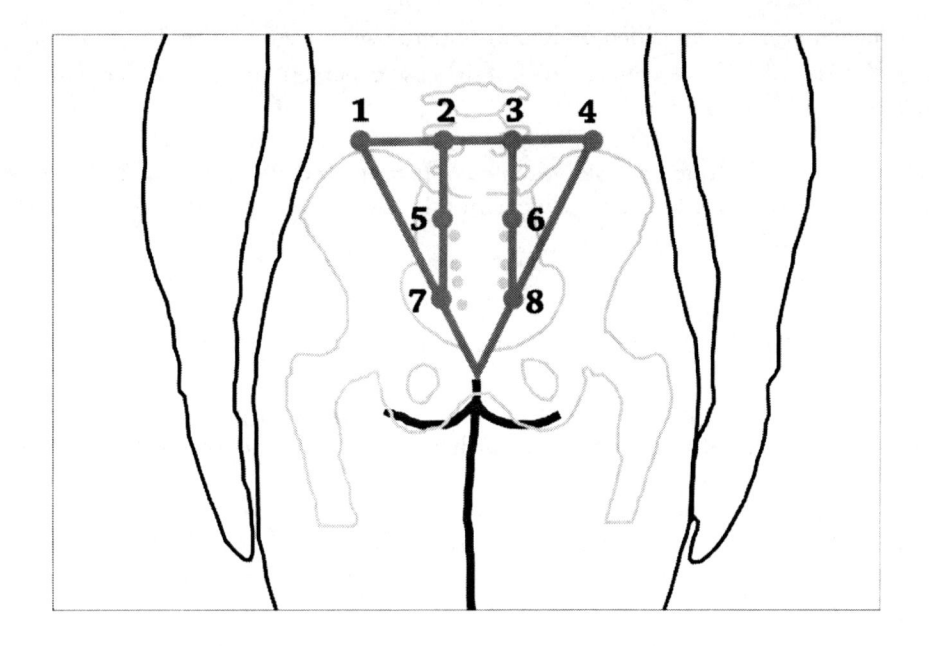

The location of Hara's "eight loin points":

First a triangle is formed by locating the highest points of the PSIS and the tip of the coccyx.
Points 1 & 4 are at the two highest points on the PSIS
Points 2 & 3 are located equally between 1 & 4.
Lines are then drawn parallel to the spine from Point 2 & 3.
Points 7 & 8 are located where these two line intersect the triangle
Points 5 & 6 are equidistant between 2& 7 and 3&8.

For Doctor Hara "all types of disease" included stiff shoulder, asthma, anaemia, eye disease, wrist pain, sinusitis, epilepsy, hypertension, hysteria, depression, headaches, tuberculosis, diabetes, heart disease, gynaecological disease, arthritis, venereal disease, and even typhoid.

Cancer was about the only disease he was prepared to consider might not be helped.

New Moon Moxa for Nourishing Life – the Eight Day Method

The new moon was considered the best time to use moxa on ST 36 for nourishing life 養生. This was a Chinese idea, enabling a person to grow older without deteriorating or losing function.

The principles are quite simple. Moxibustion is applied to *Zu San Li* (St36) daily for the first eight days of every lunar month, each treatment using three or five cones on each leg.

Nourishing Life – Spring and Autumn Treatments

Usually, nourishing life treatments are not begun before a person is 30 years of age. The intensity of the treatment is furthermore often recommended to increase with the person's age.

Wilcox describes how, from the age of forty, moxa should be applied in the spring to Ren6, and in the autumn to Ren4. She also suggests using ten separate applications on a daily basis from around January 30th to February 8th and August 2nd to 12th, either with small cones or with moxa on ginger, as many as 30 cones a day on each point. Liu Jie-Sheng, a contemporary Chinese acupuncturist, endorses Dou Cai's opinion that moxa can help to restore original *yang* and similarly encourages Nourishing Life treatment. In his case he recommends applying date-sized moxa cones on ginger at Ren6 for just five days at the beginning of spring and at Du4 for five days at the beginning of autumn each year.

A similar tradition exists in Japan for older people just in the spring but in this case the second day of the second lunar month after the New Year was identified as the most favourable time (known as *futsuka kyu* or *futsuka yaito*). This would place the treatment most often in March or April.

Treatments for specific conditions

The remainder of this particular appendix focuses on points indicated for specific medically diagnosed conditions. The conditions are listed under various categories, with various sources for the indicated points listed alongside in brackets*. As a general guideline, points should only be selected on the basis of palpable reactivity.

It should be understood that it is the responsibility of the practitioner to assess each patient on an individual basis, and to refer on whenever appropriate. Some of the treatments listed are for extremely serious conditions, and come from a time before there was widespread access to orthodox medical care. Generally, all treatments are for small cone direct moxa unless otherwise identified. Those attributed to Sawada should always be considered in combination with his general constitutional treatment (at least with Ren12, Du12, LI11 & St36) to create a larger single homogenous flowing moxa treatment primarily led by palpatory findings. Likewise, Manaka's should be best considered in combination with his own "*taikokyu*" treatment.

The numbers of cones to be applied are not often identified. Dr Manaka suspected that feeling heat from three cones at each point was enough. Sawada suggested three, five or seven cones were appropriate depending upon the constitutional condition of the patient. More acute conditions often require more cones. Since most patients seen in an acupuncture clinic in the West are deficient, the total number of points used should always be decided upon with discretion, particularly early on in treatment.

"PPP's" are pressure pain points. **"Key" points** are shown in **bold**. "EP" denotes an extra-meridial or non-standard point. The locations for some of these extra-meridial points may not be so familiar to some acumoxa practitioners, or they may entail specific Japanese variations to the normally accepted locations. Most of these are listed later in this appendix, but more familiar extra points do not have their locations described. The term "through moxa" refers to the use of points on opposite sides of limbs at the same or similar levels. These are often very useful for musculo-skeletal disorders. Ideally, the moxa should be ignited at both points at the same time so that the "hits" from the moxa occur simultaneously. This can be tricky, but, if longer twists of moxa are used on one point, and shorter ones on the other, there is no need for both cones to be lit exactly simultaneously. (The technique is said to mimic "through needling".)

*Note that those protocols denoted as "Newman Turner & Low – Japanese" were in turn derived from three separate sources originally published by the *Ido No Nippon* publishing company between 1973 and 1976:

   (a) "Neuropathy" by H Kinoshita
   (b) "Diseases of the Locomotor Apparatus" by H Mori and
   (c) "Circulatory, Renal and Skin Diseases" by H Kurushima

Respiratory:

Asthma	Ren12, Ren14, **Ki27**, Du12, Bl12, Bl11, Du10, Bl17, Bl20, **Lu5**, Ki3 (Shirota/Sawada) Bl18, Lu7, Ren12, Liv4 (Manaka) Asthma *yu* point by Bl17 (Ida) Scarring moxa: Bl12, Bl13, Bl43, Ren17 (Auteroche et al) Fukaya's respiratory point (Fukaya)
Bronchitis	**Lu1, Lu5**, Du12, Bl12, Bl11, Du10, Bl17, Ki3, Ren12, Ren14 (Shirota/Sawada) Lu6, Ren12 (Manaka) Moxa x3-5: Du14, Bl12, Bl13, Ren17 (Newman Turner & Low)
Closed nose	Du23, GB12, Bl40 (Manaka) Du22-23 to puffy PPPs (Ida) from Du22, Bl10, LI10, Ht3, St36, LI4 (Shirota) Medial Sp1 (Fukaya)
Colds	**Bl12**, Du12, Lu5 - moxa x21 at beginning stages (Shirota/Sawada) Sore points between scapulae, Du14, GB20, Bl12, LI4 (Manaka) With headache - okyu Du14 or 15, 3/5/x7 (Ida) Bl12, Du12 (x12) (Shirota) Du14 (moxa multiple cones (Shudo)
Cough	"Stop coughing" point (Birch) Du14 - x15 (Shudo)
Emphysema	GB23 - palpate, may be nearer GB22: if it feels hot x7 cones, if not, x15-30 (Mizutani) Fuakya's respiratory (Fukaya)
Flu	SI3, *Huatuo* Bl11, Du12, Sawada's GB33 (Shirota) Du14, Bl11, LI4 (protects against *Gan Mao* - flu etc (Auteroche et al)
Haemoptysis	Pc4, TB8, Ki3 (Shirota)
Nasal problem	Du23 (moxa (Shudo) (severe) Check LI7 (or LI6) for tenderness

Appendix 1 – Clinical Treatments

Pleuritis	**Pc4**, Bl12, Du9, Bl17, Bl18, GB21, GB36, above Liv14, Ren12 (Shirota/Sawada)
Pneumonia	**SI3**, Bl12, Du12, Bl11, Lu5, Du14 (Shirota/Sawada) SI3, *Huatuo* Bl11, Du12, Sawada's GB33 (Shirota)
Rhinitis	LI20, Du12, Bl12, GB20, LI11, LI10, LI4 (Shirota/Sawada) Hypertrophic: Du12, Bl12, Bl11, **Bl10, Du22, LI10, St36**, LI20 (Shirota/Sawada)
Running nose	LI7 (Fukushima)
Shortness of breath	Pc6, Pc7, GB40, Liv4 (Manaka) Fukaya's respiratory (Fukaya)
Sinusitis	Du12, Bl12, Bl11, **Bl10, Du22, LI10, St36**, LI20, occasionally add Bl15, Du16, Ht3, Ren12, Ren13 (Shirota/Sawada) Du23, LI11, LI4, St36 (Manaka) Chronic - Du22-3 (all nasal problems) (Birch) *Yintang* & LI20 - *chinetsukyu*; around nose, lower back, SI16, Du12, Bl12, Bl19, Bl20 - *chinetsukyu* followed by scattered needling (Fukushima) Middle Liv1 (Fukaya)
Whooping cough	Du12, Du14, Bl12 (Shirota/Sawada)

Special Senses:

Astigmatism	GB20, Sawada's LI4 (Shirota/Sawada)
Blepharitis	LI11, TB22 (Shirota)
Blocked ears	GB20
Conjunctivitis	**LI11, TB22**, Bl15, Bl18, GB34, St36 (Shirota/Sawada) TB21, St41, Du12 (Manaka)
Dizziness	GB43, GB12 (Shirota) Medial Liv1 (Fukaya)

Earache	From: TB17, GB2, Ki3, Ht3, TB9, LI10 (Shirota)
Ear disorders	Du20, GB20, TB8, GB34, St36 (Manaka) Palpate on line directly above affected eartip. Check movement of neck (forward/back etc) and look which elicits most reaction. Sotai movements from difficult to easy on Px's exhalation - at end of motion, apply resistance & moxa sore point. x3 overall (Ida)
Eye diseases	EP sore point on pupil line behind hairline, GB2, Bl18, LI1, LI4, St36 (Manaka) EP's on ipsilateral finger joints (dorsal) - DIP 5th & index, PIP middle finger (Birch)
Eye pain	From TB22, LI11, Huatuo Bl23, Sawada's LI4 (Shirota)
Headache	Du12, LI11, Lu7, St36, GB34 (Manaka) From Du20, Du16, Bl10 (or above Bl10), Du12, LI10 (Shirota) Du12, LI11, Lu7, St36, GB34 or Du20, Du16, Du12, Bl10, above Bl10, LI10 - okyu (Birch) *Kyutoshin* Bl10, GB20 affected side (Birch) Okyu: Bl10, SI14, Bl18, Bl21, St36 (Birch) Chronic – Bl10 – regularly for 6 months (Newman Turner & Low - Japanese) Medial Liver 1 (Fukaya
Headache-occipital	Du10, Bl9, Bl10, GB21, SI14, Bl28 (Birch)
Haemorrhaging at back of eye -	EP above Bl10, LI4 (Shirota/Sawada)
Inflammation of canthi -	**LI11**, Du12, Bl12, Bl20 (Shirota/Sawada)
Iritis	As scleritis plus GB5 and GB3 (Shirota/Sawada)
Keratitis	As trachoma plus Bl13, Bl25, Du16 (Shirota/Sawada)
Loss of smell	Bl12, Du22, needle LI20 (Shirota/Sawada)
Migraine	**GB17**, Du20, Bl10, Du12, LI10, TB9 (Shirota/Sawada)

Appendix 1 – Clinical Treatments

from Bl10, TB15, GB17, Bl7, Du20 (Shirota)
GB17, Du20, Bl10, Du12, LI10, TB9 (Birch)
GB20, GB21 x7 (Fukaya)

Otitis media	SI19, TB17, GB12, Ht3, **Ki3**, Bl23, Bl11, Bl12 (Shirota/Sawada) Ki2 *chinetsukyu* (Fukushima)
Pharyngitis	(see also "sore throat") Ren12, Bl12, Bl11, TB17, Lu5, Ki27, needle St9 (Shirota/Sawada)
Retinitis	EP one *cun* above Bl10, LI4 - this also helps haemorrhaging in the capillaries at the back of the eye (Manaka)
Scleritis	TB22, Bl12, Du12, Bl42, **LI11**, Bl18, St36, Sawada's LI4 (Shirota/Sawada)
Sore throat	From infection: **Lu5**, Ki27, Bl12, Bl11, TB17 (Shirota/Sawada) from Ki3, Lu5, Du12, *Huatuo* Bl11, Lu7, TB17 (Shirota) Medial Sp1 (Fukaya)
Styes	SI19 (Manaka) Sawada LI2 x5 (Mizutani)
Swollen glands	Parotitis: TB17, LI10, Lu5 (Shirota/Sawada)
Tired eyes	*Chinetsukyu* with eyelids closed, not letting cones get hot. (Inoue) *Yintang - chinetsukyu*, check Bl43 for reactivity (Fukushima)
Tinnitus	**Ht3**, TB17, GB2, SI19, St24 (Shirota/Sawada) Ht3, Pc4, St36, Sp6, LI11 – if younger loosen neck and shoulder and treat points on TB channel (Mizutani)
Tonsillitis	**Lu5, Bl11, Du14**, Bl12, Lu6, Lu7, Ki3 (Shirota/Sawada) St9, LI4, LI1, Ki7 (Manaka) LI4, *Bo-shi-ri-ou-mon* (Mizutani)

"Cold moxa" poultice of crushed purple skinned garlic on LI4 (Auteroche et al)

Trachoma **TB22**, Bl20, Bl21, LI11, St36 (Shirota/Sawada)

Ulceration of tongue or mouth –
Ren12, Bl20, Bl21, Bl12, LI15, LI15, St36, and needling around mouth (Shirota/Sawada)
from Bl14, LI11, LI15 (Shirota)

Cardiovascular:

Angina **Ht7**, SI11, **Pc4**, Ren14, **Ren17**, Du12, Bl15, Du10 (Shirota/Sawada)

Arrhythmia Ren12, Ki23, Du12, Bl14, Bl23, Bl20, Bl18, Du12, Bl15, Du20, Pc4, Ht7 (Shirota/Sawada)

Chest pain SI11, Bl43, for vertical chest pain add Ki3, for horizontal chest pain add Japanese Liv14, for whole chest Pc4 (Shirota)

Cold from poor circulation –
Reactive points alongside spine (T1-L5), Bl32, Ki7, Ren4, Sp10 (Manaka)

Cold hands and feet Bl11 (hands), St37 and St39 (feet), Bl32 moxa x21 rice size (Newman Turner & Low)
Ki2, GB33, St36, GB34, GB41, GB43 rice size (Newman Turner & Low - Japanese)

Cold in lower limbs Ki1 (Fukaya)

Hardening arteries Bl43, Bl18, Bl23, Ht7 (Manaka)

Heart pain from Pc4, SI11, Ht7, Du10, Ren17, Ren14 (Shirota)
Chungchuan - heat for 5 minutes moxa stick (Newman Turner & Low)

Heart valve disease **Pc4, Ren14**, Ren12, Bl17, Bl15, Du10, Du12, Bl12, SI11, Ht7 (Shirota/Sawada)

Appendix 1 – Clinical Treatments

Hypertension	**Du20, Du12, TB15, Du10, Sawada's SI10**, Sawada's LI4, Ren12, Ren9, Bl18, Bl15, Bl32, LI11, GB34 (Shirota/Sawada) Ren17, Ren12, Ren4, St36, Ki3, Du20, Bl10, GB21 (Manaka) GB20, GB21, Bl43, LI11, LI10, St36 x3 for one week, then break for a week and repeat (or treat every other day for as long as possible). Add *Bo-shi-ri-ou-mon* (Fukaya) *Shitsumin* (Fukaya) *Kyutoshin* technique: palpate and treat from Bl10, GB20, GB21, ashi points on upper back and lumbar region with px sitting, & St36 (Akabane/Birch/Ida) GB20, GB21, Bl43, LI11, LI10, St36, *Bo-shi-ri-ou-mon* – x3, but if no sensation felt continue till heat is felt (Mizutani) Du4, Ren9, Sp8, Du20, Du12, TB15, Bl32 – with insomnia add GB20, Ht7 (Newman Turner & Low - Japanese) St36 & St40 (Auteroche et al)
Hypotension	Ren12, St21, LI11, St36, Du12, TB15, Bl10, Bl17, Bl20, Bl23 (Newman Turner & Low - Japanese)
Irregular Pulse	Ren12, Ki23, Du12, Bl14, Bl23, Bl20, Bl18, Du12, Bl15, Du20, **Pc4**, Ht7 (Shirota/Sawada)
Palpitations	**Pc4**, Ren12, left Ki25, Ren14, Bl11, Du12, Bl14, Bl17, Bl10, Ht7, GB17 (Shirota/Sawada) Pc6, Pc7, GB40, Liv4 (Manaka) Pc4, Ht7 (Shirota)
Peripheral circulatory disturbances -	Sp6 & GB34 to increase circulation (Shudo)
Tachycardia	Ren17, Ht3, Ht7, GB34, Du9, Du12, TB15, SI11, Sp8, Pc4 x5; with hyperthyroidism add Ki27, Ki6 (Newman Turner & Low - Japanese)
White blood cell def.	St36

The Moon over Matsushima

Central Nervous System:

Bell's Palsy
: **Bl18**, Du8, Bl10, Du12, Bl18, LI10, TB9, St7, St5, LI20, SI18 (Shirota/Sawada)
TB17 (*kyutoshin*), with local needling (Birch/Ida)

Epilepsy
: Bl18, Du8, Du12, **left GB17**, GB34, Du16 Shirota/Sawada)
Du20, Du12, Bl18, GB41, TB5, Ren14, Liv14, GB29 (Manaka)

Facial paralysis
: **LI10**, GB34, Bl18, Du8, St4 (very small cones) (Sawada)
TB5, LI4, St36, GB41, plus touch and scratch needle technique around the face (Manaka)
Moxa on garlic St3, St4, St6, St7, SI18, TB22, EP *Taiyang*; or rice grain TB22, GB20, TB17, Du11, LI11, Bl13, Bl21- bilateral (Newman Turner & Low - Japanese)

Hemiplegia
: Point on posterior aspect of lateral malleolus, between its tip and Bl60; point on ulnar styloid, 0.5 *cun* above SI5 - moxa x50, with greenstick pecking, add 3-5 moxas on Bl60 or SI6 as required - take care with heat reaction. (Newman Turner & Low)
Bl62 (3 cones) & SI3 (5 cones) on affected side (Fukushima)

Inflammation of spinal cord -
: Du12, Bl11, Bl18, Du8, Bl23, Du3, Bl32, Ren3 (Shirota/Sawada)

Intercostal Neuralgia
: Ren17, Ren14, Ren12, Liv14, Liv13, Bl18, Bl19, Du9, Bl17, Bl15, Du12, Ht3, Pc4, GB34, GB41 (Shirota/Sawada)
Sore points in intercostal spaces along border of sternum and spine (Manaka)

Neuralgia of arm associated with median nerve –
: Pc4 & Pc7 or Pc6 (Shirota/Sawada)

Neuralgia of arm along the ulnar nerve –
: Ht3, Ht7, Ht4 (Shirota/Sawada)

Appendix 1 – Clinical Treatments

Neuralgia of inguinal joint	Liv8, Sp10, slightly lateral to St34, Bl20, Bl22, Bl23, GB30 (Shirota/Sawada)
Neuralgia of lumbar area	**Bl18**, Bl20, Bl23, Bl25, above Bl53, Bl27, Bl32, GB31, lateral to Bl37, Bl17, St36, GB34, Ki3 (Shirota/Sawada)
Neuralgia of upper arm	Du12, TB15, SI10, LI15, SI11, Bl15, LI11, Lu6, Pc4, TB4, Ht7, Ren14, Lu1, Bl27 (Shirota/Sawada)
Numbness	Of arm: Sore points just behind top of shoulder (Manaka)
Occipital pain	Du12, Bl12, **Bl10**, Du16, Du20, LI10 (Shirota/Sawada)
Paralytic diseases	*Chinetsukyu* on deficient areas (Fukushima)
Sciatic neuralgia	Bl32, GB30, Bl37, GB34, St36, EP 3 *cun* above Bl37 atlateral edge of muscle, Bl59, Bl60, Ki3, slightly lateral to St34, Bl23, Bl25, Bl20, Bl18, Ht3, Ren3 (Shirota/Sawada) Bl23, Bl25, Bl37, Bl58, Ren17, Ren4, GB31, St36, Sp6, sore points along or below PSIS (Manaka) In pregnancy - *Kyutoshin* GB31 (Ida) Palpate and select points on and around L2-5, both on and just to the sides of the spine, and on PSIS, lateral to lumbar eye points. Also on affected limb, treat pressure pain point on buttock. If pain is on back of leg only, Bl37, if wider, GB31, GB33, or Bl40 *kyutoshin*. Don't do more than three times on each point. (Akabane)
Speech disturbance	Du15 (Shirota)
Trigeminal Neuralgia	TB22, GB12, Bl10, Bl11, Du12, Bl18, LI10, TB9, St7, St5, LI20, SI18 (Shirota/Sawada) Sore spots on face, GB20, GB12, TB4, GB34 (Manaka) Triangle points: Du14 & Bl12, Du13 & Bl13 (Mizutani)

Gastrointestinal:

Appendicitis	**Ren6** (30-50 cones if in extreme acute pain**),** **St34**, Bl23, Sawada Ki3, Bl25, Ren12, Bl18, Liv8 (Shirota/Sawada) Ren12, TB4, R-St25, R-St27, Ren6 (x15-30), R LI10, LI11(x20-30), Bl25, Bl25, Bl23, St36 (x5-7) (Mizutani) Special point level with spine of 3rd vertebrae, 3 *cun* from midline on right – moxa x40, then needle Bl18 (Newman Turner & Low)
Appetite disorders	Medial St45, St 36 (Fukaya)
Beri-beri	St36, GB34, GB41, Sp6, slightly lateral to St34, GB31, Ki3, Ki9, *Xiyan*, Pc4, plus *taiji* treatment (Shirota/Sawada)
Cirrhosis	Bl18 (Newman Turner & Low)
Constipation	**SawadaHt7, left SP14**, Bl25 (Shirota/Sawada) Du20, Bl25, Ht7, Sp4 (Manaka) Sawada's Ht7 (between Ht & SI channel), left Sp14 (Shirota) St28 (12) Special point 0.5 *cun* inside St25, and Ki16 x7 each (Newman Turner & Low) Ren12, St25, Ren6 - *chinetsukyu* (Fukushima)
Crohn's disease	St37, Ren6 moxa on ginger, St25, St39
Diabetes	**TB4, Ren12**, left St21, Ki16, Ren6**, Bl20, Bl22**, Bl23, Du12, Du20, St36 (Shirota/Sawada) Any type, Magnificent Six (*Ino-mutsu-kyu*) – Bl17, Bl18 & Bl20; Du6 & Du7) (Ida) Du6, Du7 – find sore spots which may be bilateral *Huatuo* points, max x5 (Mizutani) Bl27 (heavy), tips of little fingers and toes (moxa stick), cervical vertebrae from atlas to C7, point 0.5 *cun* right of Ren9 (moxa according to age) (Newman Turner & Low) – moxa with extreme care Du6 okyu; *chinetskyu* Sp4 (2 cone), Pc6 (1 cone)- (Fukushima)
Diarrhoea	**St34, Bl60**, Bl33 (Shirota/Sawada)

Appendix 1 – Clinical Treatments

With intestinal gurgling: **Bl60** (Shirota/Sawada) watery: St34, Bl33; explosive: Bl60 (Shirota)
Ren 8 or Ren9, Ren7, Ki16 *chinetsukyu* (acute hotter, chronic cooler) (Fukushima)

Digestive disorders	Chronic - Magnificent Six (*Ino-mutsu-kyu*) – Bl17, Bl18 & Bl20 (Ida) Medial St36 (Fukaya)
Diverticulitis	Special points between St25 & 26, and St26 & 27: needle St25, moxa x5 and needle first special point, needle St26, and needle second special point, moxa x5 and needle St27 (can be used in many bowel complaints) (Newman Turner & Low)
Dyspepsia	Ren6 moxa on ginger (Auteroche et al)
Enteritis	Chronic: sore points alongside spine (T10-L5), Ren8 (Manaka) Acute: St25, EP *Uraneitei* (Manaka)
Food allergy	EP *Uraneitei* (many times) (Fukushima)
Food poisoning	St44, EP *uraneitei* (if one foot doesn't feel it, moxa this foot and only count after patient starts to feel it, 15-20 times) (Shirota) If heat is felt after 5 cones on *uraneitei* it is not food poisoning. Keep applying until heat is felt (Mizutani)
Gallbladder stone	**Above Liv14**, St21, Ren12, **Bl19**, Bl20, **right Bl50**, GB34, slightly lateral to St34, GB41, Du9, Bl17, right SI11 (Shirota/Sawada) from Ren12, right St21, above right Japanese Liv14, above right St19, right *Huatuo* Bl19, Bl50, GB36 or GB40 (Shirota) GB41 (3 cones)-TB5 (2 cones) repeated till pain subsides (Fukushima)
Gastric spasms	**St34**, Ren12, Ren14, St21, Bl20, **Bl50**, **Liv13**, Bl17, Bl12, St36 **uraneitei** (Shirota/Sawada) Bl20, St34, St36, *uraneitei* (Manaka)
Gastritis	LI10, St36 (Manaka)

Gastroenteritis	Acute: **uraneitei**, Ren12, Ren9, Ren6, St21, **St34**, St27, Bl21, Bl20, **Bl50**, Bl33, St37, St36; Chronic: **Ren12**, St21, Ren9, Ren6, St27, Bl20, **Bl21**, **Bl50**, Bl17, Bl32 (Shirota/Sawada) Mild: *Kyutoshin* St36 & PPPs on back (Birch/Ida)
Gastroptosis	Ren12, Ren13, Bl15, Du9, Bl21, Bl20, Bl10, Du20, Ren9, St24, Ren6, Ki16, Bl23 (Shirota/Sawada) Ren12, St25, St34 (Manaka)
Haemorrhoids	**Lu6**, Du20, Bl32, Bl33, Du3, Du2 (Shirota/Sawada) Bl32, Du20, Lu6, Sp7 (Manaka) EP *yaoqi*, Du2, special point caudal to Du2 in notch of coccyx, Du1, special point anterior to Du1 on rim of anus, x20, pecking technique with greenstick, 3 treatments at weekly intervals (Newman Turner & Low)
Haemorrhoid pain	Japanese Lu6, Bl33, Du2 (Shirota)
Haemorrhoidal haemorrhage	Lu6, Bl32, Bl33, Bl27, EP *josen*, Bl23, Du3 (Shirota)
Heartburn	Medial St45 (Fukaya)
Hepatitis (chronic)	Liv8, Liv3 (Manaka)
Hernia	As gastric spasms, plus St27, Ren6, Ren7, Bl25, Bl32 (Shirota/Sawada) Points between Ren14 & 15 and Ren 15 & 16, and 1 *cun* lateral to Ren15 (Newman Turner & Low)
Hyperacidity	Bl17, **Bl43**, *jiaji* Bl17 (**avoid St36**) (Sawada) **Bl17**, **Du9**, Ren12, Ren14, above St19, Bl50, GB34, Liv4 (***not*** St36) (Shirota/Sawada) Bl14, Bl15 (Mizutani)
Indigestion	(acute) moxa tips of fingers and thumb – left for male, right for female (Newman Turner & Low)

Intussusception	**Du4**, *Huatuo* of Bl23, Ren12, St27, TB4, Ren6 (Shirota/Sawada)
Liver diseases	**Liv14**, above St19, Ren12, **Bl18**, SI11, Liv4 (Shirota/Sawada)
Loss of appetite	Stimulate alongside spine (T8-L2) and around navel (c. 3 *cun* circumference) (Manaka) Palpate & treat reactive points to sides of navel, Ren12, on right subcostal region, around Bl20 & Du9 (Akabane)
Oesophageal spasms	Ren12, Ren14, Bl17, Du9, Bl15, Du12, Bl12, Ren17 (Shirota/Sawada)
Parotitis	TB17, LI10, Lu5 (Shirota/Sawada)
Peritonitis	**Liv13**, Ren9, Liv8 (Shirota)
Periodontitis	LI11, LI10, Bl14 (Shirota)
Prolapse of anus	Bl32, Bl33, Du20 (Shirota)
Stomach-ache	When hungry: Du9, Bl17, Ren16, Ren14 (Shirota) Medial St45 (Fukaya)
Stomach atony	Ren12, Ren13, Bl15, Du9, Bl21, Bl20, Bl10, Du20 (Shirota/Sawada)
Stomach cramps	St34, Bl50, Liv13 (Shirota)
Stomatitis	Ren12, Bl20, Bl21, Bl12, LI15, LI11, St36 (Shirota/Sawada)
Ulcers	**LI10, LI4,** SI6 (Shirota/Sawada) Bl21-22 (Ida) Haemorrhaging: GB34 (Shirota) Peptic – Ren8, Bl17, Sp8, GB34 (Newman Turner & Low) Stomach – **GB34**, St34, Bl20, Bl18, Bl21, Bl50, Bl17, above Bl53, above St19 (Shirota/Sawada) Duodenal – as Stomach but add right Bl50, Bl51, Bl53 (Shirota/Sawada) Gastric or duodenal: scarring moxa to Ren9, Ren4, Ren6, St36 (Auteroche et al)

Skin:

Allergic skin problems	Bl12, Du12, **LI15**, LI11, LI10 (Shirota/Sawada) EP *Uraneitei*, & bleed vascular spiders St36-7 (Ida)
Acne	LI11 & LI4 daily (Fukushima)
Carbuncle/boils	LI11, LI10, LI4, SI6 (Shirota) LI4, LI10, LI11, SI6 (add SI10, SI11 for upper body; add Bl25, Onodera point for lower body) (Newman Turner & Low – Japanese) Moxa on garlic slice on boil (Auteroche et al)
Eczema	As allergic skin problems (Shirota/Sawada) Bl43, Bl18, Bl20, Bl23, Pc6, Liv3, Ren17, Ren14, Ren12, St25 (Manaka) LI15, LI11, Du12, Bl12 (Shirota)
Erysipelas	*Datsumei* (on induration) 20-50 cones (Sawada)
Furuncles	LI10, SI6 (20-50 cones 2-3 times a day) (Sawada) EP *Zhoujian* (moxa opposite side) LI4, LI11 (Manaka)
Herpes Zoster	Burn cone on top of blister – will become dark and peel off – with early attention will go away in a fortnight (Mizutani)
Itchy skin	Allow cone to get more than a little warm (Inoue)
Open ulcers	LI10, LI4, SI6 (Shirota/Sawada)
Ringworm	LI11, LI15 5x sesame seed size daily for a month; on fingers Pc4, Pc7, TB4, Du12 x5 daily; on toes GB40, Ki6, Sp4; on larger areas enclose area with points around it (Newman Turner & Low – Japanese)
Scrofula	EP *Zhoujian* (opposite side) **LI10**, LI11, Ht3, Bl12, Du12, Bl15, GB21, St36, Lu7, Lu6 (Shirota/Sawada)
Sweat rash	As allergic skin problem (Shirota/Sawada)

Appendix 1 – Clinical Treatments

Ulcers (chronic)	EP *Zhoujian* (deep-rooted); Bl59 (leg)
Urticaria	EP *Uraneitei* (Ida) LI15, Bl12, LI11 (Shirota) LI10, LI11, LI15, TB15, Du9, Du12 x5 (Newman Turner & Low – Japanese)
Verrucae	x20-30 daily for three days; if unsuccessful, repeat 2-3 times (Newman Turner & Low – Japanese)
Verrucae plana juveniles	locate parent (largest wart) x20-30 daily (Newman Turner & Low – Japanese)

Musculo-skeletal:

Ankle pain	Through moxa Sp6-GB39 (Birch)
Arthritis	As rheumatoid arthritis (Shirota/Sawada) Palpate points above and below, and moxa sensitive ones (Shirota)
Arthritis of ankle	Periodic heated needle St41, St42 (Newman Turner & Low)
Arthritis of elbow	Thread moxa (up to 20) around area of inflammation (Birch) Periodic heated needle: LI11 (Newman Turner & Low)
Arthritis of foot	Simultaneous moxa: Sp6 & GB39, Ki6 & Bl62 5-7x (Ida)
Arthritis of knee	Periodic heated needle: Bl39, EP *Hsihsia* (Newman Turner & Low) EP *xiyan*, St36, Sp10, Bl27, Bl40 (okyu is "indispensable") (Shudo)
Arthritis of lower jaw	Periodic heated needle: St7 (Newman Turner & Low)
Arthritis of shoulder	Periodic heated needle: LI15, EP *Chupi* (Newman Turner & Low)

Arthritis of thumb	Periodic heated needle: LI5 or occasionally Lu9 (Newman Turner & Low)
Arthritis of wrist	Periodic heated needle: TB4 or occasionally SI4 (Newman Turner & Low)
Back pain	Acute: *Kyutoshin* Bl58 (Ida)
Elbow pain	Through moxa x5-7: LI10 & Lu6, LI12 & Lu4 (Ida)
Finger pain	Through moxa x5-7 SI4 & SI5 (Ida)
Frozen shoulder	LI15, SI11 (Manaka) *Kyutoshin* LI15 (Ono)
Herniated lumbar disc	Bl23, Bl52, Bl25, GB30 (good with *sotai*) (Manaka)
Knee inflammation	St25 (moxa on needle, when caused by dampness and cold) (Maciocia) Points around knee, Liv8, Sp9, Bl40, GB34 (Manaka) GB30 with Bl23 *Kyutoshin* as step 2 tx (Ida) x5-7 simultaneously: St34, Sp10; GB34, Sp9; Liv9, GB32; Liv6, GB35 (Ida) Bachmann knee points - acute: anticlockwise, cold/chronic moxa clockwise; best not if knee is swollen
Lumbago	*Kyutoshin* PPP in lower left quadrant of abdomen, plus Bl23, Bl25, Bl52, Bl18, Du3 – x3-5 (Birch/Ida) GB31, Bl56, Bl60; add Bl23, Bl47 upper lumbar; add Bl23, Bl24, Bl25 middle lumbar; add Bl25 (medial), Bl31 lumbo-sacral (Newman Turner & Low – Japanese)
Lumbar pain	Bl22, Bl23, Bl25, Bl52, St27, Bl58 (Manaka) Acute – *kyutoshin* Bl57, Bl58 or GB34 (Birch) From prolonged standing: point lateral to 1.5 *cun* lateral to Bl47 – 3 large moxa cones blown on to hasten combustion (Newman Turner & Low)

Appendix 1 – Clinical Treatments

Rheumatoid arthritis	**Bl27, Bl32**, Bl33, Ren14, Ren12, Ren6, Bl15, TB15, SI10, Bl20, Bl25, TB4, Ht7, **Pc4**, St36, GB34, Ki3, Liv8; also treat points around swollen joints and gently needle St9 until needle vibrates against carotid artery (Shirota/Sawada) Upper limbs (x10) Bl13, Bl14, Bl15, Bl17; lower limbs Bl25, Bl27, Bl28 (Ida) As upper or lower limbs above and add through moxa to affected joints – St34-Sp10, Sp9-GB34, Liv9, GB32, Liv6-GB35, GB39-Sp6, Pc6-TB5 (Mizutani) Knee: points around knee and okyu *taiji* treatment (Manaka) Bl14 & Bl15 (look for indurations, and moxa till they go) (Shirota)
Rheumatism	GB21, Du12, Bl43, Bl18, Bl20, Bl23, Ren12, St25, Ht7, Ki3, "ring moxa" around affected joint, 6-8 points, 3 cones each (Manaka)
RSI	Bl17 (Birch)
Shoulder pain	with difficulty moving: Du12, **TB15, SI10, LI15**, SI11, Bl15, LI11, Lu6, Pc4, TB4, Ht7, Ren14, Lu1, Bl27 (Shirota/Sawada) GB21, SI11, GB34 (Manaka) SI11 *kyutoshin* (Manaka) Through moxa x5-7 SI9, Pc2 (Ida) *Kyutoshin* LI15 or GB21 (Birch) *Chientungtien*: heat 10-20 mins (Newman Turner & Low) Difficulty raising: point on acromion between LI15 & 16, x7 and add drainage needle to LI15 & LI16; painful point on tip of acromial process –3 large blown moxas (Newman Turner & Low) Spontaneous dislocation: SI11, SI9, TB13 moxa x7 (Newman Turner & Low) Moxa x6 indurations Bl13-17, SI11, LI11 (Shudo)
Shoulder stiffness	With stomach problems – GB21, Bl43, Bl17; from occupational strains – Bl10, GB20, SI15, SI14 (Mizutani)

Spinal deformity	Points below edge of 11th rib close to spine, level with Du6 (Newman Turner & Low)
Sprained ankle	Liv3, Liv4, sore points around medial malleoli (Manaka) Tip of medial malleolus x3; point at centre of posterior aspect of heel at edge of plantar skin moxa x7 (Newman Turner & Low)
Tempero-mandibular syndrome –	St7, Bl13 (Shudo)
Tennis elbow	Bl17 (any arm/tendon problem) (Ida) Up to 20 thread moxas over area of tenderness (Birch) Okyu lateral epicondyle of humerus (Shudo)
Thumb pain	LI11 –moxa x5 (Mizutani)
Trigger finger	Ashi's on palmar side of metacarpo-phalangeal joints (Shudo)
Whiplash	Sore points on back of neck, Du20, Bl18, Liv4 (Manaka) PPPs beside cervical vertebrae, Du20, Bl18, Liv4 (Birch)
Wrist pain	Through moxa x5-7 TB5, Pc6 (Ida) PPP LI10; through moxa Pc6-TB5 (Birch)

Endocrine:

Hyperthyroidism	Du12, Bl12, Bl11, Ki27, Ren22, LI10, Bl23, Bl18 (Shirota/Sawada) Lu3 (x50) (Newman Turner & Low) – it should be noted that this point has been frequently contraindicated for moxa across many centuries.

Appendix 1 – Clinical Treatments

Male and female reproduction:

Abnormal foetal position – Bl67 (5 cones for ten days in eighth month) (Maciocia)
Sp6 *Kyutoshin* x4-5; compare sensitivity left/right Bl67 & moxa least sensitive x3-7 (35th week) (Ida)
Sp6, Bl67 (Shudo)

Abnormal menstruation – As endometritis plus Bl27 (Shirota/Sawada)

Amenorrhoea — As endometritis without Bl31 but particularly with Bl25 (Shirota/Sawada)

Breast pain — **SI11**, Ren17(Shirota/Sawada)

Breast inflammation — Ren17 (Manaka)

Difficult childbirth — **Bl67** (Shirota/Sawada)
Bl67, tip of little toe (Shirota)

Dysmenorrhoea — Du20, Bl18, Bl32, Sp10, Liv4 (Manaka)
Point between Ki3 & Ki4, slightly posterior, Ki3, Ki5, heat around tip of medial malleolus, Ren4, Ren2, EP *Tzukung*, EP*Bafeng*. Moxa pole 10-20 mins. (Newman Turner & Low)

Endometritis — Ren12, Ren6, St27, Ren3, Bl23, Bl20, Bl18, Bl31, Bl32, Sp6, GB34 (Shirota/Sawada)

Frigidity — See "impotence" (Newman Turner & Low)

Gonorrhea — Ren6, St27, Ren3, **Ren2, Liv8**, Bl23, Bl52, Bl32, Bl33, GB34, Sp6 (Shirota/Sawada)

Impotence — Ren12, Ren6, St27, Ren3, Ki12, Bl23, GB25, Bl32, Bl18, Liv4 (Shirota/Sawada)
Points 0.5 *cun* from midline and 0.75 *cun* below umbilicus – Moxa x5 and needle Ren7, and can add moxa x5 to point 6 *cun* below navel and 1 *cun* from midline (Newman Turner & Low)
Ren6, St36 scarring moxa (Auteroche et al)

Infertility (men) — Bl32, Ren12, Ren4, Sp6, EP *sanjiaojiu* (Manaka)

315

Infertility (women)	Ren12, Ren6, St27, Ren3, Bl23, Bl20, Bl18, Bl31, Bl32, Sp6, GB34, Bl27 (Shirota/Sawada) As infertility for men (Manaka)
Insufficient lactation	As breast pain, add Bl20, Bl21, Ren12, TB4 (Shirota/Sawada) GB21, SI11, Bl43, LI10, Ren17, St36 (Manaka) Ren17, St18 moxa pole for 10-20 mins (Newman Turner & Low) Ren17 *chinetsukyu*; also GB21, Bl14, Bl15, Bl43 orBl44 (Fukushima)
Irregular menses	as endometriosis, add Bl27 (Shirota/Sawada)
Loss of libido	Ki7, Liv3, Liv4, Sp10 (Manaka)
Menopausal disorders	Du20, Bl10, GB21, Bl43, Bl18, Bl23, Pc7, St36, Liv3, Ren14, Liv14 (Manaka) Du12, Du11, Du10, Du9, Du8, Sp6, Sp10 x7 (Mizutani)
Menorrhagia	GB34 (Shirota)
Morning sickness	**Ren12, TB4**, Bl17(Shirota/Sawada) TB4, Ren12, Ren14 (Shirota)
Orchitis	**TB4**, Bl52 or just beneath (Sawada)
Pregnancy maintenance	Sp6 (x5 daily in 5th month, x7 in 6th, x9 in 7th, x11 in 8th, x13 in 9th for easier delivery) (Shirota) Bl14 & 17 4-6 months, Bl15 & 14, 10 months-birth – *chinetuskyu* (Fukushima)
Premature ejaculation	From empty cold, moxa on ginger lower *jiao* points (Auteroche et al)
Spermatorrhea	Point between Bl23 & Bl47 moxa7, Bl23 moxa10, Bl43 x10 (Newman Turner & Low)
Syphilis	Bl41, Bl43, *Kichikuba*, Bl46 (Sawada)
Tilted uterus	(either anterior or posterior) **TB4, Ren12**, Ren6, Bl23, Bl20, Bl31, Bl32 (Shirota/Sawada);

Appendix 1 – Clinical Treatments

	(left or right) **TB4** (left for tight incline, right for left incline) (Sawada)
Uterine bleeding	**Bl27**, GB34 (Shirota/Sawada) GB34, Bl27 (Shirota)
Uterine haemorrhage	Liv1 moxa x7 (x3 if after abortion) (Newman Turner & Low)
Uterine retrovertion	Tip of spinous process of T5 – heat for 5 mins and needle Ren3 (Newman Turner & Low)
Vaginal discharges	Bl23, Bl52, Bl32, St27, Ren4, Ren3, Sp6 (Manaka)

Renal:

Bladder problems	Moxa x3-9 tip of spinous process of L3 and Bl28 (Newman Turner & Low)
Bladder/urethral pain	bladder – Ren3, Ren4, St28, Ren6, Liv8, Bl32 urethra – Liv8, Ren2, Ren3, Ki12 (Shirota)
Cystitis	Ren9, **Ren3**, Ki12, **Liv8**, Bl23, Bl32, Bl33, Bl59 (Shirota/Sawada) Ki12, St29 (Mizutani)
Enuresis	Ren9, Ren6, **Ren3**, Bl32, Du3, Bl23, Liv4 (Shirota/Sawada) Du12, Bl32, Ren4, Ki7, (also lightly tap along Ren, St21-29, Bl13-24, Lu& LI channels from elbow to wrist, Sp4-Sp9, & GB34-41) (Manaka) Du20, Du4, Ren4, Ren12-moxa 2-3 points daily (Newman Turner & Low)
Kidney problems	*Shitsumin* – has diuretic effect – if no sensation is felt continue until hot (Mizutani) Ki16, Bl23, Bl52, Bl58, EP *shitsumin* okyu (Shudo) *Shitsumin* (Fukaya)
Nephritis	**Du9, Ren7, Ki16**, Ren12, Ren3, Bl23, Du4, Bl22, GB25, Bl20, Ren9, Sp6, Ki3, Ki1, **Du20**, Bl32, Ren3, Ren9, Bl31, St36 (Shirota/Sawada)

317

	Shitsumin (Fukaya) Special point anterior to Sp10 on outer border of sartorius muscle x7 (Newman Turner & Low)
Pyelonephritis	Bl23, **Bl22**, St24, slightly lateral to St34, Ki16. (Shirota/Sawada)
Renal atrophy	As nephritis (Shirota/Sawada)
Renal calculus	Ren7 (Newman Turner & Low)
Renal Tuberculosis	As nephritis. If accompanied by bladder tuberculosis, treat Ren3, Bl32, Bl33, Liv8 as well (Shirota/Sawada)
Urethritis	Ren6, St27, Ren3, **Ren2, Liv8**, Bl23, Bl52, Bl32, Bl33, GB34, Sp6 (Shirota/Sawada)
Urinary tract disorders	(Flow difficulties) point between Bl62 and Bl64 moxa x5 (Newman Turner & Low)
Urine retention	Bl22, Bl27, Ren3, Bl67, or Du28, Liv4, Liv3 (alternate formulae) (Newman Turner & Low)
Urinary incontinence	Special point below Ren2 immediately below the pubic bone – moxa x7 with care (Newman Turner & Low)

Mental Health:

Anxiety	Du10 (Shudo)
Depression	Bl15 & 44, Ren6 (Maciocia)
Insomnia	Du20, Du22, Bl10, Du12, Bl18, Ht7, St36, Ki2 (before going to bed) (Shirota) Du20, Bl18, Liv4, insomnia point *shitsumin* (Manaka) *Shitsumin*, Bl17; T3-9 check for tender points (Ida) Reactions at Bl17 & Du9 x20; or Du12, Du11, Du10, Du9, Du8 x5, with GB20 or Bl10, GB21, Bl43, Bl15, Bl17, Lu4, LI11, LI10, St36 (Fukaya)

Appendix 1 – Clinical Treatments

GB2, GB17, Bl14, Bl18, GB34, Ren12, Ren4, 5-7x daily (Newman Turner & Low – Japanese)

Neurosis — **Du20**, left GB17, **Bl10**, Du12, Bl15, **Bl18**, Bl23, LI10, **Ht7**, St36, GB34, Ren12, Ren14, **Bl17** (Shirota/Sawada)
Tender points on intravertebral sopaced between T3 & T9 (Fukaya)
GB20, Du11, Bl14, Bl18, Bl23, Ren12, GB34, Sp6 x3-5 daily long-term (Newman Turner & Low – Japanese)

Psychosis — As neurosis (Shirota/Sawada)

Shen disturbance — *Chintesukyu* Du12 (Fukushima)

Staring into space — *Gui lin* (ghost eyes) – Sp1 & LI11 moxa x3 alternately

Stress — Du20 (Birch)

Special points — Du11, St36 (Mizutani)

Childhood illnesses

Allergic skin problems – thread moxa from Bl12, Du12, LI15, LI11, LI10 (Birch)

Asthma — Ren14, Lu1, Liv14, Du12, Bl13 (Manaka)
Du 12, asthma *yu* point (& Lu1 if reactive). Also thread moxa Du12 (Birch)
Thread moxa Ren14, Lu1, Liv14, Du12, Bl13 (Birch)

Baby night crying — Du12 (Manaka)

Cerebral palsy — Whole body shonishin. *Okyu* to Du14 & 13 for upper limb, and Du4 for lower. (Birch)
Thread moxa Du12, Du8 (x3-5), & shonishin around Du12 (Birch)

Diarrhoea in nursing child –
Du12, Ren7 (Shirota/Sawada)

The Moon over Matsushima

Eneuresis	Thread moxa: Ren3, Du12, "moving Liv1" between Liv1&2 (x1-5) (Birch) Thread moxa Du12, Bl32, Ren4, Ki7 plus "shonishin" pediatric acupuncture whole body tx (Birch)
Epilepsy	Thread moxa Du8, Du12, GB8 (x3) (Birch) Bl10, Du11, Bl13, Du21, GB34 (5 cones daily for 20 days, then rest 14 days and repeat (Newman Turner & Low – Japanese)
Fretful child	Thread moxa **Du12**, Du4 (Birch)
Indigestion	Thread moxa: Du12, Du4, Bl21 (x3-5) (Birch)
Otitis media	Add whole body shonishin, especially tapping around affected ear. For chronic, add Ki2 & Ki3 (Birch) Thread moxa from SI19, TB17, GB12, Ht3, Ki3, Bl23, Bl11, Bl12 (Birch)
Tonsillitis	Don't treat if temperature over 100deg. Thread moxa from Lu5, Bl11, Du14, Bl12, Lu6, Lu7, Ki3 (Birch)
Vomiting milk	**Du12** (Shirota/Sawada) Du12, Bl17 (Manaka) Thread moxa to Du12, Du4, Ren16 (x1-3) (Birch)
Weak constitution	Thread moxa: Du12, Du4, (boy) left Bl18, right Bl20 (girl reverse) (x1-3) (Birch)
Whooping cough	Thread moxa **Du12**, Du14, Bl12 (Birch)

Miscellaneous/ First Aid/ Emergency:

Balance general body functions –	Du12, St36; 5 cones (Newman Turner & Low – Japanese) St 36; *Shinsenko* (Fukaya)
Bites (insects)	Local*chinetsukyu* on bite, burning hot (Inoue)

Appendix 1 – Clinical Treatments

Bleeding incl. internal   Sp1
    GB34 (Mizutani)

Broken treatment/needle shock –
    Du14, Ren6(5-10 cones until improvement) (Inoue)

Bruises   *Chinetsukyu* (1 cone) quite hot at acute stage; as the bruise ages – surround whole area and burn one thread moxa at each point; and when yellow use mild *chinetsukyu* around edges (Nakada)

Cerebral Haemorrhage – from Du20, Bl20, LI10, St36, LI4 (Shirota)

Cerebral Anaemia   Japanese Pc4, LI10, St36, Ht7, SI1, Du22 (Shirota)

Collapse of *yang* inc. trembling, sweating & dizziness –
    Ren6 or 4 (Auteroche et al)

Detoxification   Ki9 (Shirota)

Drunkenness   Ki9 (Shirota)

Fever   SI2, SI3(intermittent) (Shirota)
    Du14(let cones burn hot repeatedly. Fever may break into sweat and drop after as many as 10 cones) (Inoue)

Flushing (counterflow *qi*) –
    Ki1 (Fukaya)

Hiccoughs   Liv4 with sotai stretch (rotating foot outwards and relaxing at point of heat as little toe touches couch surface (Manaka)

Jetlag   Shitsumin (Mizutani)

Nosebleed   Sore points on back of neck, TB8, GB34 (Manaka)
    from Du16, Du23, Du14 (Shirota)

Paronychia (infection on side of nail) –
    Sawada's Lu11 (Sawada)

Preventing postoperative infection –
LI11 (Sawada)

Stroke
Du20, Bl10, **Du16**, Bl12, Du12, Bl15, TB15, SI10, Bl18, Bl23, Bl32, Ren12, TB4, LI10, St36, GB34 (Shirota/Sawada)
Bl18, GB20, LI15, LI11, GB31, Bl51, St36, Bl56, GB39, lateral gluteal point – best if started within 10 days of onset; results poor if after 6 months (Newman Turner & Low – Japanese)
Tip of toes of affected limb x1 after 3 weeks (Mizutani)

Tonify upright *qi*
St36, ten minutes moxa every 5-7 days (over thirties) (Maciocia)

Tonify original *yang*
Ren4 and Bl23 moxa (Auteroche et al)

Tonify *qi* and blood:
Bl17 & 19, moxa (Four Flowers), Bl17, Bl18 & Bl20 (Magnificent Six) (Maciocia)

Toothache
LI7, Bl14, TB17 (Shirota/Sawada)
Sore point on side of head above ear, LI11, LI4, St36, GB34 (Manaka)
Point between Pc5 and Pc6 (Newman Turner & Low – Chinese)

Toothache – lower
Sawada's LI7, Bl13, LI4 (Shirota)

Toothache – upper
Bl14, St 44, TB10, LI10 (Shirota)
Point on ulnar styloid process, just proximal to SI5, opposite side to pain (Newman Turner & Low)
Du20, left GB17, Bl10, Du12, Bl15, Bl18, Bl23, LI10, Ht7, St36, GB34, Ren12, Ren14, Bl17 (Shirota/Sawada)

Locations for the extra points listed above:

Asthma *yu* point – Around Bl17, usually superior and lateral – a clear knot.

Bachmann knee points – 5 points on lower limb clustered on the patella: one in its centre, one on top edge, one on the bottom edge, and one on the edge at each side.

Bafeng – On leg. In web between each of the toes: four on each foot. (Six of the eight are Liv2, St44 & GB43).

Bo-shi-ri-ou-mon – On bottom of big toe in middle of crease where it connects to foot.

Chientungtien – On back, at middle of lateral border of scapula.

Chungchuan – Between TB4 and LI5.

Chupi (Jubi) – 3.5 *cun* below and anterior to acromion

Datsumei – On the line between LI11 & LI15 slightly distal to the midpoint.

Fukaya's medial Liv1 – on centre line of top of big toe between Liv1 and Sp1.

Fukaya's medial Sp1 – at end of the fold of the base of the big toe when it is bent.

Fukaya's medial St45 – on centre line of top of second toe, level with St45.

Fukaya's respiratory – on underside of middle toe in centre of crease at the base of the toe itself where it meets the foot.

Hsihsia (Xia xia) – Just below patella, on patellar ligament, midway between the 2 *Xiyan* points.

Japanese Liv14 – In subcostal region, at tip of 9th costal cartilage, slightly medial to mammary line, level with Ren13.

Japanese Lu6 – On forearm, $\frac{1}{3}$ to $\frac{1}{2}$ distance between wrist and elbow.

Japanese Pc4 – On forearm, $\frac{3}{10}$ distance between wrist and elbow creases

Josen – On back, below spinous process of 5th lumbar vertebrae.

***Kichuba* points** – Bilateral on back, one *cun* above the level of Bl18 and one *cun* lateral to the midline of the spine.

Onodera point – More a reactive area than a point – becoming reactive in the presence of peptic ulcers, diseases of upper gastrointestinal tract and pain in leg and hip joint: a reactive point appears about 5cm below iliac crest on back.

Sawada's Bl27 – 0.5 *cun* above Bl31, at the margin of the sacrum.

Sawada's Du4 – Bilateral points on the *huatuo jiaji* line for Bl23 (mainly for emergency teratment)

Sawada's Ht7 – On wrist crease between Heart and Small Intestine channels.

Sawada's Ki3 – Nearer to the standard Ki6.

Sawada's LI2 – at radial aspect of crease in first finger between distal and middle phalanx.

Sawada's LI4 – On dorsum of hand at junction of first and second metatarsal but proximal to LI4, where one can feel a small pulse.

Sawada's LI7 – With index fingers and thumbs of both hands interlaced with index finger over styloid process of other hand, the point lies in a depression between the muscles under the tip of the index finger.

Sawada's Lu11 – On centre line of nailbed, $\frac{1}{3}$ from tip.

Sawada'a SI10 – Midway between the top of the posterior axillary crease and the tip of the acromion.

Shinsenko – "Heart of the Foot" a little nearer to the heel than Ki1.

Shitsumin – In centre of plantar surface of heel.

"Stop coughing" – 0.5 *cun* distal to Lu5, sometimes proximal.

Tzukung – On abdomen, 3 *cun* beside Ren3.

Uraneitei – On plantar surface of foot, at base of second toe, where a dot placed in the centre of the underside of the second toe touches the foot when the toe is bent over.

Xiyan(Eyes of knee) – On leg, below patella in hollow on either side of tendon (one is St35).

Yaoqi – On the *Du* channel line, level with the S2-S3 space, between left & right BL28/BL32.

Zhoujian – On the tip of olecranon process – right side for left side symptoms and vice versa.

Sennenkyu's easy guide to stick-on moxa treatment

The following is adapted directly from a commercial company's "easy guide to moxa points", and can be easily further adapted to suit many patients. The list was drawn up specifically for the use of stick-on moxas, such as Sennenkyu or Neo, but could equally be adapted for small cone direct moxa.

The categories of complaints are divided into four sections:

Relieving fatigue

Tiring easily	St36, Bl23, Du12, Ren12
Blurry eyes and poor vision when tired	LI11, St36, Bl15, Bl10, Du12
Body always feeling weary	St36, LI11, Ren12, Du12
So tired that sleep is difficult	Ki3, Ht7, Bl18, St36, Liv4, Du12
Bloated face when tired	Sp6, Ki6, Bl23, Ren8, Du12
Difficulty concentrating when tired	Liv4, TB15, Bl10, Du12
Catching colds easily when tired	Bl12, Du12, Du11
Irritable when tired	Ren17, Bl18, Pc6, Ki6, Ren22, Du12
Heavy or dull lower back when tired	Bl23, St36, Bl53

Circulation

Constant chills	Ki6, St36, GB33, Ren5, Ren12
Cold feet even when head or face is flushed	Ki6, GB34, Du12, Bl10, TB15
Dizzy upon standing	St36, Pc6, Du12, Bl15, Bl10
Frequent urination when cold	St36, Bl23, Bl33, Ren4
Lethargy when in air conditioning	LI11, St36, Bl23, Du12
Headaches if body is cold	Ki6, LI11, St36, Bl23, Du12
Painful or swollen feet after walking	St36, Sp6, Ki7, Bl23, Du12
Menstrual pain when cold	Sp6, Bl33, Ren5, Ren4
Lower abdominal pain during menstruation	Sp6, Sp10, Ren2, Ren5, Bl33

Gastrointestinal

Tendency to constipation	Ht7, Sp14, TB6, GB34, Ki6, St25
Tendency to diarrhoea	Bl60, Ki3, St34&25, Bl32, Ren8& Ren4
Stomach pain	Pc6, St36, St25, Ren12
Stomach hurts when hungry	Sp6, GB34, Ren12
Poor digestion and distended stomach	St36, Pc6, Ren12, Bl17, Liv13, Ren8
Lack of appetite	St36, Ren12, Ren5
Frequent burping	Pc6, Bl40, Bl17, Ren12, Ren22
Urge to move bowels (but uncomfortable bowel movements)	Bl25, St27, Ren12, Bl33
Unpleasant taste in mouth	GB34, Pc6, Bl20, Bl21, Ren12

Neuralgia and muscle pain

Stiff shoulders	GB21, LI11, Du12
Shoulder stiffness with headaches	TB15, LI11, GB20, TBB Du12
Stiffness/pain (extending from shoulders into back)	LI11, Bl12, Du12, Ren12
Shoulder stiffness (with loose teeth or swollen gums)	LI7, Bl14, LI4, LI10
Tired arms after shopping	LI11, LI10, LI15, TB15, Ht3
Tired legs after returning home	St36, Bl58, Bl23
Tight calves after sporting activity	St36, GB34, Bl58, Bl40
Lower back won't straighten after crouching	GB34, Bl52, Bl25, Bl53

Appendix 2

A selective list of research papers particularly relating to immune response.

1. **Histological study of skin treated with moxa.** Shimetaro Hara. Fukuoka University Medical Journal. 1929; 22:2. Old Japanese.

2. **Recovery tendencies of tuberculous animals treated with moxa.** Shimetaro Hara. Fukuoka University Medical Journal. 1929; 22: 5. Old Japanese.

3. **Tuberculosis and moxibustion.**Shimetaro Hara. Jiechi Ika to Rinsho. 1929: 6: 9. Old Japanese.

4. **Effects of moxa on subcutaneous histocyte cells. (1 & 2).** Shinji Ota 1930. Nihon Biseibu-tsugaku Zasshi; 24: 4.Old Japanese.

5. **Effects of moxibustion on splenic function of leucocytes and in gamma-irradiated mice under general and local anasthaesia.**Chinese Publication of uncertain provenance – 1980 Taiwanese.

6. **Effects of Electronic Moxibustion on Immune Response 1**. Watanabe S, Hakata H, Matsuo K, Hara H, Hara Shimetaro. Journal of Japan Society of Acupuncture and Moxibustion 1981;31(1): 42-50. Japanese.

7. **Accuvaccination.** Singh, B.K. Paper delivered to World Acupuncture Conference, Colombo 1982.
http://www.bhupendratechniques.com/Research/Theories/Acuvaccination

8. **Effects of Electronic Moxibustion on Immune Response 2**. Watanabe S, Matsuo K, Hara H, Hirose K, Hara Shimetaro. Journal of Japan Society of Acupuncture and Moxibustion 1982;32(1): 20-26. Japanese.

9. **Effect of moxibustion on the phagocytic activity in mice.** Okozaki M, Furuya E, Kasahara T, Sakamoto K. American Journal of Chinese Medicine 1983. Vol XI; No. 1-4: 112-122.

10. **Effect of moxibustion on the cellular immunocompetence of gamma-irradiated mice.** Hau D M, Wu J C, Chang Y H, Hwang J T. American Journal of Chinese Medicine. 1988; 3: 157-163.

11. **An electron microscopic study of the acupuncture or moxibustion stimulated regional skin and lymph node in experimental animals.** Kimura M, Mastrogiovanni F, Toda S, Kuroiwa K, Tohya K, Sugata R, Ohnishi M. American Journal of Chinese Medicine. 1988: 16(3-4): 159-167.

11. **Changes of content of blood serum through moxibustion on acupoint equivalents.** Sakamoto K, Kasahara T, Sakurai Y. Journal of Japanese Society of Acupuncture and Moxibustion. 1988; 320-325. Japanese

12. **Suppression of the DTH reaction in mice by means of moxibustion at electro-permeable points.** Tohya et al. American Journal of Chinese Medicine 1989; 17(3-4):139-144.

13. **A study on Radical Scavenging Effects of Moxa.** Ohnishi M, Toda S, Sugata R, Tohya K, Kuroiwa K, Kimura M. Journal of Japanese Society of Acupuncture and Moxibustion. 1990; 40(4): 377-379. Japanese

14. **Protective effect of moxibustion for mountain sickness** Homma Y, Murai M. Journal of Japanese Society of Acupuncture and Moxibustion.1991; 41(6): 346-352.

15. **Effect of moxibustion on the growth of primary tumor, pulmonary metastases and immune responses in mice bearing Lewis lung carcinoma.**(LLC). Utsunomiya Y. Bulletin of Meiji University Oriental Medicine.1995; 16: 27-38.Japanese.

16. **The immune system and acupuncture moxibustion.** Amagai T, Itoi M. J Japan Society of Acupuncture and Moxibustion. 1996; 46(4): 315-25. Japanese.

17. **Studies on anti-inflammatory and immune effects of moxibustion.** Tang Z, Song X, Li J, Hou Z, Xu S. Chen Tzu Yen Chiu 1996;21(2):67-70. Chinese.

18. **Immunohistochemical expressions of HSP and CGRP induced by moxibustion stimulation in the peripheral neurons of CH3/HENCrJ mice.** Nakanishi H.; Chiba A, Chichibu S. Neuoroscience Research. 1997; 21(1): 79-79.

19. **Influence of direct moxibustion with moxa cones the size of a rice grain on cell count and proportion of leucocytes in rabbit and human peripheral blood.** Yamashita H, Tanno Y, Ichiman Y, Nishijo K, Takahashi M. Japanese Journal of Oriental Medicine. 1998; 48: 599-608. Japanese.

20. **Effects of Moxibustion on the Enhancement of Serum Antibody in Rabbit against *Staphylococcus aureus*.** Yamashita H, Ichiman Y, Takahashi M, Nishijo K. American Journal of Chinese Medicine 1998:26.1;29-37. (also Japanese Journal of Oriental Medicine. 1996; 47: 457-64. Japanese)

21. **Appearance of peculiar vessels with immunohistological features of high endothelial venules in the dermis of moxibustion-stimulated rat skin.** Tohya K, Urabe S, Igarashi J, Tomura T, Take A, Kimura M. American Journal of Chinese Medicine 2000; 28: 425-33.

22. **Changes in peripheral lymphocyte subpopulations after direct moxibustion.** Yamashita H, Ichiman Y, Tanno Y. American Journal of Chinese Medicine. 2001; 29 (2): 611-621.

24. **Effects of moxa-cone moxibustion at Guanyuan on erythrocytic immunity and its regulative function in tumor-bearing mice.** Wu P, Cao Y, Wu J. Journal of Traditional Chinese Medicine 2001 Mar; 21(1): 68-71.

25. **Diverse biological activities of moxa extract and smoke.** Hitosugi N, Ohno R, Hatsukari S et al. In Vivo. 2001 May-Jun; 15(6) 249-54. Japanese.

26. **Present Research on Moxibustion.** Aizawa S, Menjo Y, Tohya K, Nakanishi H, Toda S. Journal of Japanese Society of Acupuncture and Moxibustion. 2003; 53(5): 601-613. Japanese.

27. **Acute lymphangitis treated by moxibustion with garlic in 118 cases.** Zhou W. Journal of Traditional Chinese Medicine. 2003; 23(3):198.

28. **Effects of moxibustion at shenque (CV 8) on serum IL-12 level and NK cell activities in mice with transplanted tumor.** Qiu X; Chen K; Tong L; Shu X; Lu X; Wen H; Deng C. Journal of Traditional Chinese Medicine. 2004 Mar; 24(1): 56-8. .

29. **Effects of moxibustion at Zusanli (St36) on alteration of Natural Killer Cell activity in rats.** Choi G S, Han J B, Park J H, Oh S D, Lee G S, Bae H S, Jung S K, Cho Y W, Ahn H J, Min B I. American Journal of Chinese Medicine. 2004 Mar; 32(1): 303-312.

30. **The study of Standardisation Plan and Usefulness of Moxa Combustion.** Geon-mok L, Kil-soong L, Seung-hun L, Jong-duk C, Eun-mi S, Jung-sun C, Yang-jung K. Journal of Korean Acupuncture and Moxibustion Society 2003; 20(6):63-79. (reprinted in Journal of JSAM 2004; 54(4): 604-619.

31. **Assesment of the Function of Peritoneal Macrophages in Rats treated with long term direct moxibustion.** Matsuo T, Kasahar Y, Kubayashi K Journal of the Society of Acupuncture and Moxibustion 2005; 1:36-42.

32. **Effect of moxibustion on the hemodynamics of cutaneous and sub- cutaneous tissue.- comparison between five-cone and seven-cone moxibustion.** Tawa M, Kitakoji H, Sakai T, Yano T. Japan Journal of Acupuncture and Moxibustion 2005; 55 (4): 538-548. Japanese.

33. **Literature Documentation of Basic Research on Immunological Effect by Acupuncture and/or Moxibustion Treatment Immunological Research Committee for Acupuncture and Moxibustion.** Tohya K, Fukazawa Y, Kasahara Y, Okuda M, Tahara S, Kuribayashi K. Japan Journal of Acupuncture and Moxibustion 2006; 56 (5): 767-778. Japanese.

34. **Do Japanese Style AcupunctureandMoxibustion Reduce Symptoms of theCommon Cold?** Kawakita, Shichidou et al - EBM working group, Research Department, the Japan Society of Acupuncture and Moxibustion (JSAM), 2007.http://ecam.oxfordjournals.org/cgi/content/full/nem055v1

35. **Study on Moxibustion: Elucidation of Characteristics of Moxa.** Ozaki A, Aizawa S, Toda S, Kumamoto K, Ebara S, Koike T. Journal of the Japan Society of Acupuncture and Moxibustion, 2008. 58 (1): 32-50. Japanese .

Appendix 3 - **Resources**

In the UK good supplies of Japanese moxa can be obtained from:

>**Oxford Medical Supplies**
>http://www.oxfordmedical.co.uk/index.asp?cat=25&scat=71&t=Japanese+Moxa+Supplies

>**Scarborough's** http://www.scarboroughs.co.uk/acupuncture/acupuncture-moxa.html

>**Dulwich Acupuncture**
http://www.dulwichacupuncture.com/index.php?cPath=202

In Germany they can be obtained from:

>**Docsave**
http://www.docsave.eu/start/index.php?page=shop&k1=moxa&k2=moxa_uebersicht&kat=moxa_uebersicht

In the US they can be obtained from:

>**Kenshin Trading**
http://kenshin.com/acupuncture.php

In Australiasia they can be obtained from:

>**Helios**
www.heliosupply.com.au

Direct from Japan:

>**Sankei** (a good range)
http://oq83.jp/index_e.html

>**Khobayashi**
http://www.kobayashi-rouho.com/item/index-e.html

>**Yamasho**
www.moxa.net

Further Reading –

Moxibustion

Lorraine Wilcox 2008 "**Moxibustion, the Power of Mugwort Fire**" (Blue Poppy Press)

Lorraine Wilcox 2009 "**Moxibustion: a Modern Clinical Handbook**" (Blue Poppy Press)

Subhuti Dharmananda 1998 "**Relationships of Borneol, Artemisia and Moxa**" Institute for Traditional Medicine, Portland, Oregon. (Online article) http://www.itmonline.org/arts/borneol.htm

Subhuti Dharmananda 2004 "**Moxibustion: Practical Considerations for Modern Use of an Ancient Technique**" Institute for Traditional Medicine, Portland Oregon. (online article)
http://www.itmonline.org/arts/moxibustion.htm

Japanese Acumoxa

Stephen Birch and Junko Ida 1998 "**Japanese Acupuncture, a Clinical Guide**". (Paradigm Publications)

The Society of Traditional Medicine 2003 "**Traditional Japanese Acupuncture, Fundamentals of Meridian Therapy**" (Complementary Medicine Press)

Masakazu Ikeda 2005 "**The Practice of Japanese Acupuncture and Moxibustion – Classic Principles in Action**" (Eastland Press)

Shudo Denmei 1990 "**Japanese Classical Acupuncture. An Introduction to Meridian Therapy**" (Eastland Press)

Shudo Denmei 2002 "**Finding Effective Acupuncture Points**" (Eastland Press)

Yoshio Manaka, Kazuko Itaya and Stephen Birch 1995 "**Chasing the Dragon's Tail**" (Paradigm Publications)

Acupuncture (general)

Stephen Birch & Robert Felt 1999 "**Understanding Acupuncture**" (Churchill Livingstone)

Koryo Sooji Chim Korean Hand Therapy (KHT

Tae-Woo Yoo "**KHT Korean Hand Therapy Vol 1**" (Eum Yang Mek Jin Publishing Company)

Sotai

Keizo Hashimoto MD "***Sotai* Balance and Health through Natural Movement**" (Japan Publications Inc.)

The Mawangdui texts

Donald Harper 1998 "**Early Chinese Medical Literature – The Mawangdui Medical Manuscripts**" (Keegan Paul)

Early Chinese Medicine

Keiji Yamada 1998 "**The Origins of Acupuncture, Moxibustion, and Decoction**" – (Kyoto: Nichibunken, International Research Centre for Japanese Studies)

Nathan Sivin 1995 "**Text and Experience in Classical Chinese Medicine**" in "Knowledge and the Scholarly Medical Tradition"(Cambridge University Press)

Vivienne Lo 2005 "**Imaging Practice: Sense and Sensuality in Early Chinese Medical Thought**" (Metailie and Dorofeeva)

Paul Unschuld 2003 "**Huang Di Nei Jing Su Wen – Nature, Knowledge, Imagery in an Ancient Chinese Medical Text**"(University of California Press)

David J Keegan 1988 (doctoral dissertation) "**Huang-ti Nei-Ching: the Structure and Compilation; the Significance and the Structure**" (University of California, Berkeley)

The History of Japanese Medicine

Wolfgang Michel "**Far Eastern Medicine in seventeenth and early eighteenth century Germany**"
http://www.flc.kyushu-u.ac.jp/~michel/publ/aufs/73/73.htm

U.A.Casal "**Acupuncture Moxibustion and Massage in Japan**".http://nirc.nanzan-u.ac.jp/publications/afs/pdf/a136.pdf

The Moon over Matsushima

Haiku and Bashō

Matzuo Bashō 1694; translated by Nobuyuki Surwasa and published in 1965 "**The Narrow Road to the Deep North and Other Travel Sketches**" (Penguin Classics)

The Tarim Mummies

J.P.Mallory & Victor Mair 2008 "**The Tarim Mummies: Ancient China and the Mystery of the Earliest Peoples from the West**" (Thames and Hudson)

Elizabeth Barber 2000 "**The Mummies of Urumchi**" (W.W.Norton & Co)

The Silk Road

Colin Thubron 2006 "**Shadow of the Silk Road**" (Chatto & Windus)

David Christian 2000 "**Silk Roads or Steppe Roads? The Silk Roads in World History**" (Journal of Word History, Vol 11)

Kos, Hippocrates and the Vegetable Cauterisation

Elizabeth Craik "**Knife and Fire – Medical Practice of East and West**" http://www.hmn.bun.kyoto-u.ac.jp/report/2-pdf/4_bungaku1/4_11.pdf

The Kushan Empire

I have yet to find a good book on the Kushans. My starting point, however, was Michael Wood's stimulating 2007 "**Story of India**" (BBC Books)

Or http://kushan.org/

The VOC

Two books are worth reading for quite different reasons, but both offering real flavours of the VOC enterprise.

One is Simon Winchester's 2003 "**Krakatoa – the Day the World exploded**" which describes the early history of Batavia in colourful detail.

The other is David Mitchell's wonderful 2010 novel "**The Thousand Autumns of Jacob de Zoet**" (Hodder and Stoughton) which offers a frighteningly authentic insight into life in the tiny Dutch outpost at Deshima.

Index

Abo, Toru, 206
Achamaenid Empire, 38
acidosis, 181
aconite, 125, 153, 236, 237
actions of moxa, 180
acupoint, 8, 75, 237
Africa, 52, 214, 248, 249
ageing of mugwort, 19, 65, 91, 92, 93, 103
agricultural theory, 7
Ainu, 96
Akabane, Kobei, 82
Alay Valley, 42
alkanes, 227
Allen, Katherine, 268
alpha thujone, 227
Anglo-Saxons, 93
animal experimentation, 211
Artemis, 96
Artemisia, iii, 22
   argyii, 86
   chinensis, 86
   douglasiana, 97
   gnaphalodes, 96
   indica, 86
   montana, 86, 103
   princeps, 86, 101, 103
   vulgaris latiflora, iii, 22, 86
artemisia acetate, 101, 102, 227
Artemisia the First, 39
Artemisia the Second, 39
Asia Minor, 37, 38, 61
Australia, 25, 273
auto-immune disease, 199
autonomic nervous system, 181, 206, 207, 213
Bactria, 49, 50, 51
Bai Shi
   Mister White, 18, 55, 56, 57
Banckes' Herbal, 98
Barber, Elizabeth, 44
Bashō, Matsuo, 1, 6, 22, 34, 141, 281, 334

Batavia, 22, 24, 25, 26, 27, 28, 31, 57, 58
Beauty of Xiahe, 55
beifuss, 94
Beijing Declaration, 279
Beijing Olympic Games, 49
bian, 1, 67, 72
Bian Que, 18, 55, 56, 73, 77
Bianque Xinshu, 137, 149
Birch, Stephen, vii, 18, 66, 81, 216, 226, 332
borneol, 101, 102, 227, 230, 332
Brand, Eric, 93, 232
Breech presentation, 257
British Acupuncture Council, 233
Budd, Sarah, 260
Buddha
   the, 179
Buddhism, xiv, xv, xvi, 49, 51, 53, 77
Burning of the Books, 2, 10, 56, 64
Busschof, Hermann, 22, 23, 24, 25, 28, 30, 32, 33, 34, 57, 58, 59, 78
button cautery, 33, 59
CAM. *See* Complementary and Alternative Medicine
Cancer, 150, 212
Cardini, F, 258
Caria, 37, 38, 39, 40
Carians, 39
Casals, U.A., 77, 333
Causes of disease
   Endogenous, 191
   exogenous, 192
cell count, 208
Central Asia, vii, 37, 41, 45, 48, 49, 54, 57
Central Nervous System, 264
Chace, Charles, 66, 72, 75, 157
Chang'an, 56
Changbai Mountain Range, 86
channel frequencies, 251
channel sinews, 158
chemistry of mugwort, 91, 101, 271

Chernobyl, 95, 204
chinetsukyu heat perception moxa, 82, 227, 241, 242
Chiron, 96
Chunyu Yi, 11, 13, 66
cineole, 101, 102, 103, 227, 230
Cingulum Sancti Johannis, 97
Cleyer, Joseph, 23, 32, 78
Clonal Ignorance Theory, 200
Cochrane Library, 257, 267, 268, 269, 276, 277
Coen
    Jan Pieterzoon, 25, 28
Complementary and Alternative Medicine, 266, 268, 276, 283
Confucianism, 1, 14, 15
Confucius, 14, 15, 64, 65, 263, 283
cowling cones, 111, 122
cowrie shells, 37, 48
Craig, Jenny, vii, 92, 183
Craik, Elizabeth, 9, 36, 45, 46, 58
Ctesias, 37
Cui Zhidi, 76
Culpepper, Thomas, 86, 93
Cyrus the Great, 40
danokyu, 110, 244
Daoism, 1, 14
De Vegetabilus, 94
Deadman, Peter, 134, 144
denatured proteins, 226
Denmei, Shudo, 254, 332
Deshima, 28, 32
Divergent Channels, 154, 157
divination, 20
dosage, 211
Dou Cai, xv, 137, 149, 150, 153
double-blinding, 272
Dragon Boat Festival, 98, 99, 100
Duanwu. See Dragon Boat Festival
Dutch East India Company. See *VOC*
"Easy Delivery Moxa", 261
Eckman, Peter, 78, 81
Egyptian mummy, 45
Ehrenreich, Barbara, 193
Eight Extraordinary Vessels, 3, 82, 261
Elbow Tip, 132
electronic moxibustion, 202, 203

Eleven Vessel Foot-Arm Moxa Classic, 62
Eleven Vessel Yin-Yang Moxa Classic, 62
eschar, 250
Essay upon the Cure of the Gout, 30
etymology of ideograms, 8, 18, 20, 21, 65, 89, 100
Evidence Based Medicine, (EBM) 264, 266, 272, 280
Exeter Cathedral, 97
Extra Cephalic Version, 267
fan zhen, 158
Far Infra-Red, 237
Felt, Robert, vii, 18, 66, 81, 332
Festival of St. John, 98, 99
filiform needle, 17
FIR. See Far Infra Red
five pole moxibustion method, 78, 172
Four Flowers, 20, 196, 198, 212
Four Treasures, 87
Frois, Luis, 33, 46
Fu Hao, 48, 49
Fukaya, Isaburo, 76, 81, 82, 251, 252, 253
Fukushima, Kodo, 119, 139
Galen, 245
Gaohuang Shu Xue Jiu Fa "Moxibustion on *Gaohuang shu* Bl43", 76
garlic, 31, 76, 124, 126, 153, 236, 237, 239
Ge Hong, 75
ginger, 124, 125, 126, 138, 171, 231, 236, 237, 239, 296
golden age of Confucianism, v, 14, 15
Gonzan, Goto, 78
gout, 22, 28, 30, 32, 58
Grabowska, Christine, 268, 269
granulocytes, 201, 207, 208, 213
Great Compendium of Acupuncture and Moxibustion, 80, 185, 244
Great Japan Health Alliance, 141
Greek medicine, 9, 38
Guangdong, 86
Gudang, 293
Guo Yu
    Discourse on the States, 6, 7, 8

Halicarnassus, 38
Han, 1, 2, 5, 8, 10, 11, 12, 13, 14, 15, 16, 17, 18, 19, 20, 41, 42, 48, 55, 56, 57, 60, 72
hao zhen, 18, See also filiform needles
Hara, Dr Shimetaro, ix, 82, 136, 139, 140, 141, 144, 187, 188, 202, 205, 211, 212, 216, 218, 222, 226, 246, 247, 248, 249, 251, 272, 294, 295, 327
Harper, Donald, 8, 61, 67, 69
Hashimoto, Kaizo, 159, 160
He Xian Gu, 96
health promotion moxa of Sayama, 120
Heat Shock Proteins, 226
heat-sensitivity meridian-balancing, 164
heptatriacontane, 102, 103, 228
herbal fire buttons, 33, 34
Herodotus, 39
Het Podagra, 22, 58
hexagram 63 "Already Completed", 148
Hippocrates, 30, 35, 36, 37, 38, 45, 57
Hippocratic medicine, 9, 35, 58
Hiroshima, 141, 142, 204
histotoxin, 182
HIV/AIDS, 212, 214, 248, 249, 283
Hội An, 26, 27, 28, 34
hormesis, 247
horoku kyu, 126
Huang Di, 14, 15, 16, 18, 55, 67, 73, 76, 333
Huangfu Mi, 12, 14, 56, 75
Hubei, 62, 86
hypertension, 252
Ibuki, Mount, 86, 87, 88, 89, 100, 103
Ikeda, Masazaku, 110, 113, 119, 120
immune cells
    B cells, 202
    CD4, 202, 205, 212, 250
    CD8, 205
    granulocytes, 207
    Lymphocytes, 207
immune system, 194
immunological effects of moxibustion, 104, 265
India, xiv, 21, 24, 25, 28, 35, 49, 50, 51, 53, 60

Indirect Moxa, 123
Infra-red, 236
Inoue, Keiri, 118, 119, 154, 166, 242
intermediary materials, 9, 123, 239, 241, 242
Investigational Medicinal Product (IMP), 270
Iron working in China, 70, 71
Itaya, Kazuo, 183
jade, 41, 44, 48, 49, 55
Japan, iii, ix, 22, 26, 27, 32, 33, 34, 63, 76, 77, 79, 81, 82, 333
Japanese moxa growing prefectures, 86
Jesuit missionaries, 33
Ji Xianlin, 54
Jia Yi Jing, 19, 75
Jin Ping Mei, 79
jingluo, meridian, 3, 4, 13, 62, 67, 70, 188
jiu moxibustion, 19, 21, 46, 59, 60, 65
Jiu Jia Yi Jing
    The Systematic Classic of Acupuncture and Moxibustion, 12
Jumna River, 51
Kabul valley, 51
Kaempfer, Engelbert, 78
Kalama Sutra, 179
Kamp, Doortje van der, 131
Kanishka, 49, 51, 52, 53
Kashgar, 42, 43, 50
Kashmir, 51
Keats, John, 283
Keegan, David, 14, 18, 73, 333
Khotan, 48, 49
Kim, Nam su. *See* Gudang
Kobo Daishi, 77
Korea, iii, 26, 53, 87, 203, 209
Koryo Sooji Chim, 167, 169
Kos, 12, xii, 36, 37, 38, 39, 40, 45, 57, 61
Kosinko, 96
Kunlun Mountains, 7, 41, 43, 49
Kushan Empire, 41, 49
kyu kon shin, 175
kyutohinaishin, 171
kyutoshin moxa-with-needle, 82, 92

337

Lacnunga, the, 85
lapis lazuli, 44
laudable pus, 245
Lavier, Jacques, 120
Leamington-Acupuncture (LA), 174
Legalism, 1, 14, 15
leukaemia, 255
Li Shizhen, 80, 86, 89, 100, 253
Li Tang, 146
Lingshu, 11, 13, 14, 17, 19, 56, 62, 66, 67, 68, 69, 71, 72, 73, 74, 75
Liu Bang, 15
Liu Jie-Sheng, 138, 296
Lo, Vivienne, 5, 8, 79, 333
longevity, 37, 75, 76, 77, 96, 134, 135, 136, 137, 140, 150, 152, 186, 212
long-snake technique, 124
Low, Roger, iv
luo channels, 122, 191
Luoyang, 53, 56
Lyantonde, Uganda, 248
lymphocytes, 200, 201, 207, 209, 213, 226, 229
macrophages, 193, 201, 204, 207, 208, 213
Mai Fa, 61
Mai Jing
   Pulse Classic, 3
mai vessel, 3, 5, 6, 8, 9, 10, 62, 68, 70
Mair, Professor Victor, 44, 54
malaria, 98, 243
Maldive Islands, 38
Manaka, Dr Yoshio, 6, 81, 82, 122, 131, 133, 146, 147, 158, 159, 160, 161, 162, 167, 172, 175, 182, 183, 244, 247, 250, 251, 253, 291, 297, 298, 299, 300, 301, 302, 303, 304, 305, 306, 307, 308, 309, 310, 312, 313, 314, 315, 316, 317, 318, 319, 320, 321, 322, 332
Mandell, Richard, 249
manga comic books, 51
Manpei, 136
Manson, Sir Patrick, 98
Matsushima Islands, i, vii, 141, 281, 282
Mausollus, 39

Mawangdui, 2, 3, 4, 5, 6, 7, 9, 10, 18, 19, 46, 60, 61, 62, 65, 66, 67, 68, 69, 70, 71, 73, 79
Medical Practitioner's Law, 81
Meng Zi
   Mencius, 14, 57, 64, 65, 66
Meridian Therapy, 119, 174, 332
metallurgy, 1, 70, 72
metronome, 251
mibyo-chi self-healing, 131
Middletown, Pennsylvania, 143
Ming Dynasty, v, 14, 26, 75, 76, 79, 82, 100, 199, 212, 253
Mister White (see *Baishi*)
Mitchell, Mary, 268
Mizutani, Junji, 182, 253, 255
mochse, 59
mogusa, 21, 22, 33, 34, 46, 58, 60
Mongolia, iii, 51, 105
Moxa and temperature, 214
moxa harvest, 99, 100
moxa on ceramic, 126
moxa on loquat leaf, 126, 236
moxa on miso, 126
moxa on tangerine peel, 126, 236
moxa pole, 123, 128, 235, 262
moxa processing, 86, 87, 89, 90, 93, 101
moxa smoke, 233
moxa temperature, 20, 91, 92
Moxafrica, vii, viii, ix, 183, 212, 218, 248, 283
moxa-with-intradermal, 171
moxa-with-needle, 82, 127
Moxibustion Method for Consumptive Disease, 76
mugwort, iii, iv, v, vi, 1, 12, 19, 20, 21, 22, 32, 33, 34, 39, 45, 57, 59, 61, 62, 63, 64, 65, 66, 73, 75, 79, 80, 75, 85, 86, 88, 90, 91, 93, 95, 96, 97, 100, 101, 244, 232, 264, 270, 271, 272
mugwort pillows, 95, 97
mummies, 44, 54
mycgwyrt, 59, 93
myxa (μυξα), 58
Nan Jing, 56, 67, 69, 72, 73, 79

338

Narrow Passages in the Back Country, 141
NASA, 237, 276, 278
Native American tribes of the Great Plains, 96
Natural Killer Cells, 193, 205
needle-shock, 256
Nepal, iii, 89
neutropenia, 208, 256
Newman Turner, Roger, iv
nine healing herbs, 93
Nobuyaso, Dr Ishino, 261
Nogier, Dr Paul, 59
nomads, 37, 39, 41, 45, 50, 56
Nourishing Life, 137
Nursing and Midwifery Council, 268
Obaidey, Edward, 112, 113, 115, 116
Oda, Ryuzo, 87
Of Internal Affections, 46
Of the Places of Man, 45
Ohmura, Yoshiaki, 142, 212
o-kyu, 22
Ono, Bunkei, 195
Oracle Bone Inscriptions, 20
Ötzi, the Ice Man, 47
Pamirs, 41, 42, 43, 44, 45, 49
Pamphile, 36
Pan African Acupuncture Project, 248
Papal Donation, 24
parasympathetic nerves, 209
Persia, xii, 37, 41
Persian Empire, 37, 38, 39, 40, 44
peyote, 97
photonic release, 242
Pigen, 149
Pliny the Elder, 36, 37, 42
poison, 85, 126
Polybius, 52
Pope Alexander VI, 24
Post-Viral Syndromes, 283
PRC, People's Republic of China, 54, 101, 181, 182, 255
prime growing areas for moxa, 86
progenitor cells, 201, 202
qi
   wei, 188
   xie, 68, 190, 191, 195

ying, 188
zheng, 68, 190, 195, 196
qi manipulation, 67, 68, 72
Qibo, 15, 53
Qin Dynasty, 2, 11, 12, 14, 15, 16, 18, 53, 70, 73
Qizhou, 86
radiation sickness, 142, 144
RCT's (randomised control trials), 260, 266
realgar, 233
Ride the Bamboo Horse, 132, 133
Roman soldiers, 94
Ross, Ronald, 98
Rubinstein, Aaron, 171, 172
rusalsky, 143
sagging pulse, 109
Salamis, 39
salt, 44, 76, 86, 118, 126, 236
Sawada, Ken (Takeshi), 78, 81, 82, 145, 198, 289, 290, 291, 297, 298, 299, 300, 301, 302, 303, 304, 305, 306, 307, 308, 309, 310, 311, 313, 314, 315, 316, 317, 318, 319, 320, 321, 322, 324
Seres, the, 37, 54
Shan Hai Jing (the "Classic of the Mountains and Seas"), 53
Shang Dynasty, 20, 37, 41, 48, 56
Shi Jing "Book of Odes", 64
Shiji
   Classic of History, 11, 13, 19, 66, 71
Shima, Miki, 157
Shinto, 96
Shirota, Bunshi, 289, 290, 298, 299, 300, 301, 302, 303, 304, 305, 306, 307, 308, 309, 310, 311, 313, 314, 315, 316, 317, 318, 319, 320, 321, 322
Shuangbaoshan figurine, 4, 63
Shudo, Denmai, 145, 174, 254, 298, 303, 311, 313, 314, 315, 317, 318, 332
silk, 2, 26, 36, 37, 42, 45, 62, 71
silk roads, 42
Silk, Jonas, 280
Sima Qian, 11, 13, 19, 48, 49

Sivin, Nathan, 11, 13, 333
Slavonic names for mugwort, 95
smokeless moxa, 232
snail shell moxa, 128
snatch moxa, 81, 213, 254
sō, 131, 198
soft heat, 154
sotai, 158, 159, 160
Soulie de Mourant, George, 3
South Africa, vii, ix, 25
Spanish Civil War, 245
St John the Baptist, 63
St Thomas Aquinas, 263
St. John the Baptist, 97
St. John's Plant, 97
St. John's Wort, 97
Stone Tower, 42
Strabo, 50
subduction zone, 7
Suffering Gate, 10, 140, 148
Sugiyama, Waichi, 77
Sun Simiao, 76, 263
Sunda Straits, 25
Sushruta Samhita, 98
Suwen, 11, 13, 15, 16, 18, 19, 45, 56, 60, 66, 67, 68, 69, 71, 74, 75
Sydenham, Thomas, 34, 35
sympathetic nerves, 208, 209
syphilis, 124
Systematic Classic, xiv, 12, 56, 66, 74, 75, 245
Taklamakan Desert, 41, 43, 49
Tamura, Shoichi, 187
Tang dynasty, 14, 20, 65, 75, 76, 100
tannins, 102, 103, 227
Tarim Basin, 12, 37, 41, 43, 48, 54
Taulakääpä, 47
techne, 35
technology, 8, 17, 18, 38, 45, 57, 70, 72
Temple, Sir William, 30, 32
Thambarijah, Radha, 80
thermocouples, 216
Three Mile Island, 143
Tian Shan
    Tian Mountains, 7, 43
Tin Yao So, James, 80
tinder fungus, 46, 47, 48

Tohya, K, 228
tomb findings, xii, xiii, 2, 4, 5, 10, 12, 13, 16, 17, 18, 45, 48, 71
tomb of Prince Liu Sheng, 17, 71
toonetsukyu penetrating moxa, 82
Toyohari, 119, 220, 242
Transient Receptor Potential
    TVRP1, 226, 227, 230
    TRPV2, 226
    TRPV3, 226, 227, 230
Transient Receptor Potential (TRP) channels, 226
triangle Moxibustion, 132
tuberculosis, viii, 76, 82, 196, 197, 207, 214, 248
    drug resistant, 283
tubes, 9, 115, 116, 117, 170, 251
Uganda, vii, ix, 248
Unschuld, Paul, 14, 16, 63, 68, 74, 333
Veith, Ilsa, 142
Verwaal, Ruben, 30
Vietnam, iii, 22, 23, 26, 27, 34, 81
VOC
    Vereenigde Ooost-Indische Compagnie, 24, 25, 26, 27, 28, 32
Walloon, 59
walnut shell spectacles, 128
Wang Chao, 135
Wang Dao, 76
Wang Kenliang, 244
Wang Xuetai, 60
Wang Zhizhong, vi
warming moxibustion, 46, 60, 107, 109, 114, 123, 124, 146, 152, 153, 154, 164, 166, 175, 237, 254
Warring States, 1, 2, 6, 14, 17, 35, 64, 70
warts, 256
wei qi, 188
white blood cells, 181, 202, 256
Wilcox, Lorraine, v, 19, 47, 75, 79, 80, 100, 180, 244, 332
Wild Sage, 96
Wiseman, Nigel, 9
Woolmer, Bob, 126
Wu Shi Er Bing Fang, 60
Xinjiang, 48, 54, 71

Xiongnu, 49, 50, 56, 57
Yamada, Keiji, 6, 19, 62, 65, 333
Yamashita, Hitoshi, 205, 206, 213, 220
Yanagishita, Toshio, 220
Yanagiya, Sorei, 82, 113
Yang Jizhou, 80, 185, 212
Yellow River, 7, 8, 56
Yi Jing, 74, 108, 109, 148
Yin Yang Mai Sihou
    Death Signs of the Yin Yang Vessels, 10
Yin Yang Shuyi Mai Jiu Jing, 7, 62
Yingpan Man, 54
Yoo, Tae-Woo, 167, 168, 172
Yuan dynasty, 79, 255

Yueren. *See* Bian Que
Yuezhi, the, 41, 48, 49, 50, 55, 57
Yurungkash (White Jade) river, 49
Zhang Gao, 140
Zhang Jiebin, 80, 131, 134, 139, 145, 147, 153, 199
Zhang Qian, 37, 42, 44, 50
Zhang Zhuo, 144
Zhangjiashan, 3, 4
Zhen Jing, 75, 108
Zhou dynasty, 15
zhuang, 75, 131, 148, 150, 198
Zhuang Zi (Chuang Tzu), 57, 65, 66
Zu Pi Shuyi Mai Jiu Jing, 62

A few things about the author...

Merlin Young is a happily married acupuncturist living and working in the Black Country which was, until recently, the industrial heartland of the UK.

Before discovering acupuncture he was in turn: a failed English Literature undergraduate (as a result of reading and enjoying the works of Kurt Vonnegut Jr more than those of William Shapespeare); a youth worker in inner-city Birmingham; a bench joiner; a building estimator; and a stressed-out construction project co-ordinator.

After studying acupuncture he developed specific interests in Japanese acumoxa techniques particularly on account of their finesse and delicacy: he is a registered academic member of the Toyohari Medical Association of Tokyo.

After coming across the extraordinary work of Dr Paul Farmer in Haiti and Peru, he became increasingly interested in fundamental issues of global healthcare inequalities, especially in relation to the growing threat from drug-resistant TB, and he began to ponder what traditional East Asian medicine might truly have to offer the bottom billion (or two) of humankind in the twenty-first century.

In 2008 he co-founded the Moxafrica charity with Jenny Craig PhD. The charity was set up specifically to investigate whether small-cone direct moxa might have a part to play today in the desperate battle against drug-resistant TB in the developing world, particularly in Africa with its terrifying rates of co-infection with HIV-AIDS. Most of his energies over the last four years have been focused on this quest which is ongoing. At the time of publication, this has developed into a collaboration with a team of pharmacologists at the famous Makerere University in Kampala, Uganda resulting in a Phase II RCT looking at the serological, immunological and radiological responses to adjunctive moxa treatment for TB patients in Uganda – the first time that this has been attempted.

He now wishes so very much that he'd paid more attention in his science classes when he was at school.

He considers the Moon over Matsushima to be as much a foundation stone for the Moxafrica project as much as it is a general book on moxibustion.

In his spare time he pretends to garden, has fun in the kitchen with variable success, tries to stay healthy and does his best to keep a sense of humour.

He also considers himself to be one of the worst meditators on the planet.

For more information on Moxafrica, please go to www.moxafrica.org

The Moon over Matsushima